£51.30

Cariology Today

Dedicated to Professor Dr. *Hans-R. Mühlemann*
on the occasion of his retirement as chairman of the
Department of Cariology, Periodontology and Preventive Dentistry
of the University of Zürich

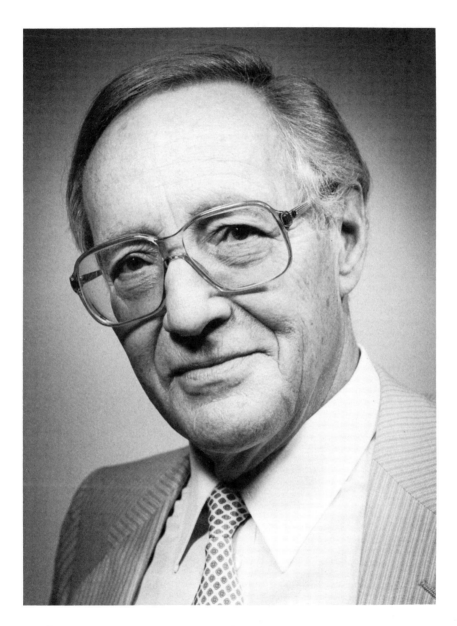

International Congress in Honour of Professor Dr. Hans-R. Mühlemann,
Zürich, September 2–4, 1983

Cariology Today

Editor: *B. Guggenheim*, Zürich

34 figures and 36 tables, 1984

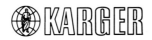 **KARGER**

S. Karger · Basel · München · Paris · London · New York · Tokyo · Sydney

National Library of Medicine, Cataloging in Publication
Cariology today: international congress in honour of Professor Dr. Hans-R. Mühlemann,
Zürich, September 2–4, 1983
Editor, B. Guggenheim. – Basel; New York: Karger, 1984.
1. Dental Caries – congresses I. Guggenheim, B., II. Mühlemann, Hans Rudolf, 1917–
WU 270 C2765 1983
ISBN 3–8055–3761–1

Drug Dosage
The authors and publisher have exerted every effort to ensure that drug selection and dosage set forth in this text are in accord with current recommendations and practice at the time of publication. However, in view of ongoing research, changes in government regulations, and the constant flow of information relating to drug therapy and drug reactions, the reader is urged to check the package insert for each drug for any change in indications and dosage and for added warnings and precautions. This is particularly important when the recommended agent is a new and/or infrequently employed drug.

© Copyright 1984 by S. Karger AG, P.O. Box, CH-4009 Basel (Switzerland)
Printed in Switzerland by Schüler AG, Biel
ISBN 3–8055–3761–1

Contents

Diet

Plaque

Fluoride and Enamel

Contents

Prevention and Therapy – Where from Here?

Summaries of Panel Discussions

Preface

This volume contains the papers presented at the 'Cariology 1983' congress, held in Zurich from September 2 to 4, 1983. This conference, addressed by world authorities in their fields, was held in honour of Prof. *Hans-Rudolf Mühlemann,* who retired as chairman of the Department of Cariology, Periodontology and Preventive Dentistry of the University of Zurich. When he stepped into office in 1953 the Department of Operative Dentistry still taught and practised restorative dentistry not far moved from the principles established by *G. V. Black* more than 40 years previously. Besides including Periodontology into the official designation of the department, which at the time was a novelty in Central Europe, *Hans Mühlemann* challenged the established principles of a dormant discipline. His present high reputation and recognition is not based on a single major invention but on his credo that dentistry is a science and not an art. It would be beyond the scope of this preface to rate and assess the fruits of his 30-year professional career, which was restless yet full of sparkling imagination. I shall, however, try to detail some highlights based on a rather personal and contemporary view.

The high prevalence of dental caries in the early fifties within the Swiss population led *Hans Mühlemann* to the conclusion that this problem could not be managed by major improvements in therapy, but rather by well-founded prophylactic measures. He realized early on that solid foundations for caries prophylaxis demanded an interdisciplinary approach. A team was gradually recruited, able to tackle relevant questions in caries research employing epidemiological, biochemical, microbiological, immunological, and pharmacological methods.

Hans Mühlemann fed and sometimes overfed his collaborators with ideas, born in his ever-combining mind often inspired by scientific literature in unrelated fields. On the other hand, these budding scientists were left sufficient freedom to be creative themselves. This unique environment enabled several of these people, influenced by *Hans Mühlemann's* perceptions of dentistry, to develop and attain faculty positions in and outside Switzerland. Other assistants who preferred to enter private practice were perceptive to a well-balanced and scientifically based form of preventive dentistry.

This Mühlemann-spirit, solidly based on a pole position in international caries research and on success at the level of community dentistry, slowly but definitely changed the political stage on many levels.

Research began to flourish not only in other departments of the Zurich Dental School but also in the other Swiss Dental Institutes. *Hans Mühlemann's* efforts produced considerable changes within the curriculum and also brought about the establishment of several departments devoted to basic research. This required changes in the then-existing Swiss Federal Education Laws. He was further able to convince the Swiss Dental Association to acknowledge and implement the advantages of prophylaxis-orientated dentistry. This was a laborious task and many others having encountered such adversity, might have succumbed. Only with the support of the Swiss Dental Association could the education of dental hygienists begin and be recognised as a profession. He has in addition prepared the scene for the establishment of other types of auxiliary dental personnel.

Another feather in the cap for *Hans Mühlemann* was the way in which he actively propagated knowledge and awareness of dental health to the Swiss population at large. In this field, of course, he required considerable assistance from industry. He was able to furnish the relevant industries with ideas to produce better and more efficient products for dental home care. He also encouraged the food industry to produce hypoacidogenic sweets, chewing gums, chocolates, snacks, and pharmaceutical products. When these products complied with the standards set by in vivo intraoral pH testing, they were labeled as 'safe for the teeth'. It was a masterpiece that *Hans Mühlemann* could convince the Swiss Health Authorities to register the label 'safe for the teeth' for items which were shown to be non- or hypoacidogenic by the pH telemetry test.

On a personal level, the essence of *Hans Mühlemann's* pacemaking contributions to the science of dentistry was the dynamic manner in which these highlights have been brought to fruition. In consequence of these, Switzerland is distinguished from its neighbouring and other countries by its high level of dental education, its achievements in preventive dentistry, and its standards in dental research. The high reputation of this man, the esteem within which he is held by his colleagues, and the many distinctions which he has received during his active career are well-deserved.

The chapters of this book, reflecting the state of the art in cariology today, document once more that *Hans Mühlemann's* contributions during the past three decades were exceptional and substantial. On behalf of the international research community in cariology I would like to express our sincerest respect and gratitude.

B. Guggenheim

Epidemiology

Moderator: P.J. Holloway, Manchester, England

Cariology Today. Int. Congr., Zürich 1983, pp. 1–12 (Karger, Basel 1984)

Changing Patterns of Disease in the Western World

M.C. Downer

Scottish Home and Health Department, Edinburgh, UK

Introduction

Evidence is accumulating from many parts of the Western World which indicates that dental caries experience among children and young adults has declined since at least the early 1970s. A recent collection of studies, in which available data from several countries were examined, recorded a fall in caries prevalence among younger age groups in areas as far apart as Northern Europe [1–7], North America [8, 9], and Australasia [10].

A decrease in caries prevalence will have important implications for the planning of dental services in terms of the number and type of dental personnel required, the content of their professional training, the provision of facilities, and the way in which dental care is provided. From the point of view of the scientific community, a detailed consideration of changes in the pattern of caries may provide further insight into the nature of the disease and its prevention.

The object of the present investigation is to document changes in caries experience in a number of developed countries of Western European culture and to examine in particular the role of fluoridation, and its benefit when viewed against the background of the general decline in disease prevalence. The overview presented does not provide a comprehensive review of all the information available. Data were included rather, for their usefulness in affording comparison, their probable reliability, and because they were expressed in a form which facilitated uniformity of presentation.

Downer 2

Table I. Changes in caries experience of 3- to 6-year-old children in four European countries

	Reference	Age years	n	Mean dmft/deft	Mean dmfs	Caries reduction %	Compound annual reduction rate, %
England							
Hertfordshire (south)	11						
1973		3	263	1.37		62	11.4
1981		3	252	0.52			
Scotland							
Edinburgh (east)	2						
1970		5	403	5.08		36	4.3
1980		5	200	3.26			
Lewis (Western Isles)	12						
1971		5–6	230	7.29		37	4.6
1981		5–6	235	4.75			
Finland							
National (16 towns)	22						
1975		3		1.5		67	16.7
1981		3		0.5			
1975		5		5.0		64	15.7
1981		5		1.8			
The Netherlands							
The Hague	13						
1972		5	175		13.15[1]	48	10.4
1978		5	170		6.79[1]		

[1] Includes radiological data.

Materials and Methods

The data were derived from the following sources: (1) local prevalence studies conducted at two points in time in which the clinical examinations were undertaken on each occasion by the same standardized examiner, or group of examiners, in the same locations using the same methods [1, 2, 4, 9, 11–16]; (2) national surveys employing random samples drawn at different points in time, but using similar methods of data collection on each occasion [3, 8, 17–19], and (3) routine epidemiological data collected in a standardized way for the purposes of providing statistics on service provision at national or local level [20–22].

Although some sources of information included data for a wide spectrum of ages, those selected referred to the three broad age groups most commonly encountered in studies of the epidemiology of caries, namely, children of 5 or 6 years of age or under, 11- to 12-year-old children, and young adults in the 16- to 25-year age range. In the majority of epidemiological studies of caries, data are expressed in terms of dmft/deft or DMFT, and these were the indices preferred. However, most of the US, Danish, and Dutch data were available only as dmfs/DMFS and have, therefore, been presented in this form. The minimum period between studies was 5 years. The use of data from the period before 1970 was generally avoided because in many early surveys the criteria of examination were either not well documented, or there was a possibility that diagnostic standards were different from those employed more recently.

In some studies in the first category, the data were collected for different purposes on the two occasions. For example, the first set of data represented baseline examination findings in a clinical trial, while the follow-up data were collected for the purpose of comparison with them [1, 2, 9, 12, 14, 15]. In other instances, follow-up data collected locally were compared with data from broadly the same area obtained in previous national surveys [3]. Where such studies have been cited, the original reports confirmed that the examinations were conducted to similar standards. With regard to fluoridated communities, only longitudinal studies have been included in which comparable data for adjacent non-fluoridated areas were also available [1, 3]. Unless stated otherwise, radiological findings were not included. The annual decrease in caries experience in the locations specified was calculated as a percentage compound rate [23].

Results

Table I presents the changes in caries experience for the youngest age group in four European countries. There is evidence of a general decline in mean dmf levels since 1970 with Scottish children having apparently experienced the lesser reductions. The data from The Hague, unlike those from the other locations, were expressed as dmfs and included radiological findings, so that reservations must be expressed about their comparability.

Table II presents the data for 11- to 12-year-old children and

Table II. Changes in caries experience of 11- to 12-year-old children in five European countries and in the United States

Location	Reference	Age years	n	Mean DMFT	Mean DMFS	Caries reduction %	Compound annual reduction rate, %
England							
Bristol (south-west)	14						
1970		11–12	397	4.58		37	5.0
1979		11–12	520	2.89			
Devonshire (south-west)	1						
1971		12	460	5.32		49	6.6
1981		12	537	2.70			
Oldham (north-west)	2						
1970		11–12	249	4.99		33	4.0
1980		11–12	207	3.32			
Shropshire (West Midlands)	1						
1970		12	966	4.53		32	3.8
1980		12	1,196	3.08			
Scotland							
Lewis (Western Isles)	12						
1971		11–12	139	5.69		41	5.2
1981		11–12	307	3.35			
Denmark							
National	20, 21						
1976		11	56,450		7.3	22	4.8
1981		11			5.7		

Finland								
National (16 towns)	22							
		1975	11		5.5		49	10.6
		1981	11		2.8		42	8.7
		1975	12		6.9			
		1981	12		4.0			
The Netherlands								
The Hague	13							
		1972	11	188		10.30[1]	21	3.8
		1978	11	162		8.18[1]		
USA								
National	8							
		1972	11	4,088		4.58	35	5.2
		1980	11	3,479		3.00		
		1972	12	4,116		6.36	34	5.1
		1980	12	3,601		4.18		
Norwood (Mass.)	9							
		1972	12	455	5.45		16	2.8
		1978	12	421	4.60			

[1] Includes radiological data.

Table III. Changes in caries experience of 16- to 25-year-old adults in three European countries

Location	Reference	Age years	n	Mean DT	Mean MT	Mean FT	Mean DMFT
England and Wales							
National	18						
1968		16–24	371	2.1	5.2	8.2	15.5
1978		16–24	576	2.0	4.7	7.7	14.4
Scotland							
National	17						
1972		16–24	382	2.7	6.7	6.8	16.2
1978		16–24	211	2.2	6.4	8.4	17.0
Denmark							
Military recruits	4, 16						
1972		17–25	1,476	2.5	2.0	12.1	16.6
1982		17–25	1,007	0.6	0.3	10.9	11.8

includes five European countries and also the United States. Apart from Finland, which again showed evidence of an exceptionally marked decline in caries experience, the annual reduction rates in DMF were generally consistent and in the range of 3–7%. It is noteworthy that DMFS levels recorded in the US national surveys were very little higher than DMFT levels for comparable years reported in local prevalence studies in England.

The changes in caries experience of young adults in the United Kingdom and Denmark are presented in table III. Whereas a small decline in overall caries experience was recorded in England and Wales between 1968 and 1978, in Scotland between 1972 and 1978, a slight increase occurred. The difference lay mainly in the filled component of the index which fell from 8.2 to 7.7 in England and Wales, but rose from 6.8 to 8.4 in Scotland. The mean DMFT of Danish military recruits showed a decrease amounting to nearly 30% during a similar period, with particular improvements in numbers of decayed and missing teeth.

Table IV considers the reductions in caries experience of life-long child residents of fluoridated areas of England and Ireland and relates these to decreases in comparable non-fluoridated localities. For the fluoridated Irish communities, the pre-fluoridation baseline indices are shown. The additional benefit conferred by fluoridation over and above the general decline in caries experience is readily apparent.

Unlike the data presented in tables I–III, those for Ireland in table IV covered a period from the beginning of the 1960s, and it is evident that the annual reduction rates in non-fluoridated areas of Ireland over this much longer time period were considerably lower than those recorded since 1970 in other non-fluoridated parts of Europe. This would be compatible with a view that most of the general decline in caries has occurred during the last decade.

Discussion

The recorded changes in caries experience over time documented in this study are likely to be real within the range of error introduced by possible changes in population structure or shifts in diagnostic standards. In each location, the clinical assessments were made according to the same criteria, often by the same standardized examiners, on both occasions. Although any shifts that may have occurred cannot be measured, it is reasonable to suppose that they were minimal. However, where national data are concerned, whether collected for routine statistical purposes or in the course of surveys, large numbers of examiners were involved, and the possibility of examiner variability was, therefore, greater.

It would be inadvisable to place too much reliance on any direct comparisons of caries levels at particular points in time between the various locations specified, except for the direct comparisons between fluoridated and neighbouring non-fluoridated localities. Mostly, different examiners were involved, and the examination environment, equipment, and the methods and criteria of examination may also have been different.

A decrease in caries experience is apparent in each of the three widely separated age groups considered. However, the data available for young adults were sparse, and it is only in Denmark that any appreciable decline in caries in that age group is yet discernible. In the youngest age band, a particularly marked decline was observed in Finnish children. In this respect, it is interesting to note that fluoride preventive programmes, and the provision of dental health advice to parents of young children, form an integral part of children's dental

Table IV. Changes in caries experience of children in fluoridated (F) and non-fluoridated (NF) areas of the British Isles

	Reference	F/NF	Age years	n	Mean dmft	Mean DMFT	Caries reduction %	Compound annual reduction rate, %
England	1							
Dudley (West Midlands)								
1970		NF	5	366	5.07			
1980		NF	5	301	3.45		32	3.8
Northfield (Birmingham)								
1970		F	5	364	2.63			
1980		F	5	188	1.22		54	7.4
Sutton Coldfield (West Midlands)								
1970		F	5	304	2.65			
1980		F	5	215	1.13		57	8.2
Ireland	3							
County Limerick (Limerick City)								
1961		NF	5	306	7.1			
1980		F	5	169	2.5		65	5.4
County Galway (Loughrea and Tuam)								
1962		NF	5	428	5.5			
1980		NF	5	98	3.8		31	2.0

County Waterford (Waterford City)							
1961	NF	5	431	6.4		59	4.4
1981	F	5	186	2.6			
County Waterford (Dungarvan and Dunmore)							
1961	NF	5	431	6.4		42	2.7
1981	NF	5	142	3.7			
County Limerick (Limerick City)							
1961	NF	11	310		4.0	48	3.3
1980	F	11	182		2.1		
County Galway (Loughrea and Tuam)							
1962	NF	11	376		4.0	10	0.6
1980	NF	11	126		3.6		
County Waterford (Waterford City)							
1961	NF	11	334		4.4	52	3.6
1981	F	11	227		2.1		
County Waterford (Dungarvan and Dunmore)							
1961	NF	11	334		4.4	23	1.3
1981	NF	11	209		3.4		

services in Finland [24]. Apart from the development of a systematic preventive programme, there is also well-documented evidence from Finland of particularly large changes in a number of other parameters of importance in dental health. Thus, there was a noticeable fall in sucrose consumption between 1970 and 1979 and at the same time, large increases in fluoride tablet consumption and sales of toothbrushes and fluoride-containing dentifrices [24].

Despite possible differences in diagnostic standards, age-specific caries levels among children in the United States nationally, are generally lower than those in Europe, and in this connection it is important to record that the number of persons in the United States using fluoridated water supplies doubled during the 1960s from approximately 40 to 80 million. Many of the 11- to 12-year-old children in the 1980 survey could thus have had lifelong exposure to water fluoridation. There is evidence of a fluoridation influence among American children from the finding that DMF levels in 1980 in urban areas of the United States were in general lower than those in rural areas. Urban areas have the higher proportion of the population with access to fluoridated water supplies [8]. It is interesting to note that in Norwood, Mass., USA, where water supplies were not fluoridated [9], the caries levels were similar to those in non-fluoridated English localities [1, 2, 15]. As well as water fluoridation, there was a considerable increase in the use of topically applied fluoride agents in the United States during the 1970s. The results of a detailed analysis of the pattern of caries reduction in individual tooth surface types in the national survey were indicative of a fluoride effect [8], and the same finding has been reported elsewhere [14].

Many epidemiological studies, including some of those cited, show that data used in summarizing levels of caries experience often conceal large local [25, 26], regional [2, 17–19], and subcontinental [8] variations. Some of this variability is probably accounted for by fluoride-based preventive programmes. However, another major determinant of DMF experience is the level of provision of dental treatment services. For example, where service provision is generous, it is found that a high proportion of DMF is attributable to the filled component of the index [27]. From the epidemiological viewpoint, the F component represents the outcome of diagnostic decisions by a large number of clinicians and is beyond the control of the investigator.

In conclusion, this overview has demonstrated that caries experience among children and some young adult groups has fallen in many countries of the Western World. Many of the studies cited also showed a corresponding decrease in prevalence, in terms of noticeably improved proportions of caries-free children, although for the purposes of the present study this index of the changing pattern of disease was not examined. There is strong evidence that fluoridation of the water supplies, where implemented, has produced marked additional benefits over and above the general decline that has occurred. Although many factors have probably contributed to the decrease in caries, it is the effects of fluoridation and the provision of preventive and restorative dental care that epidemiological research has so far succeeded in isolating and elucidating the most extensively.

Acknowledgements

The author is indebted to the late Dr. *Erik Randers Hansen* of the Danish National board of Health and Dr. *Heikki Tala* of the Finnish National Board of Health for supplying national statistics on child dental health for their respective countries.

References

1   Anderson, R.J.; Bradnock, G.; Beal, J.F.; James, P.M.C.: The reduction of dental caries prevalence in English schoolchildren. J. dent. Res. *61:* 1311–1316 (1982).

2   Downer, M.C.: Secular changes in caries experience in Scotland. J. dent. Res. *61:* 1336–1339 (1982).

3   O'Mullane, D.M.: The changing patterns of dental caries in Irish schoolchildren between 1961 and 1981. J. dent. Res. *61:* 1317–1320 (1982).

4   Fejerskov, O.; Antoft, P.; Gadegaard, E.: Decrease in caries experience in Danish children and young adults in the 1970's. J. dent. Res. *61:* 1305–1310 (1982).

5   Von der Fehr, F.R.: Evidence of decreasing caries prevalence in Norway. J. dent. Res. *61:* 1331–1335 (1982).

6   Koch, G.: Evidence for declining caries prevalence in Sweden. J. dent. Res. *61:* 1340–1345 (1982).

7   Kalsbeek, H.: Evidence of decrease in prevalence of dental caries in The Netherlands: an evaluation of epidemiological caries surveys on 4–6- and 11–15-year-old children, performed between 1965 and 1980. J. dent. Res. *61:* 1321–1326 (1982).

8   Brunelle, J.A.; Carlos, J.P.: Changes in the prevalence of dental caries in US schoolchildren, 1961–1980. J. dent. Res. *61:* 1346–1351 (1982).

9   Glass, R.L.: Secular changes in caries prevalence in two Massachusetts towns. J. dent. Res. *61:* 1352–1355 (1982).

10   Brown, R.H.: Evidence of decrease in the prevalence of dental caries in New Zealand. J. dent. Res. *61:* 1327–1330 (1982).

11   Silver, D.H.: Improvements in the dental health of 3-year-old Hertfordshire children after 8 years. Br. dent. J. *152:* 179–183 (1982).

12   Hargreaves, J.A.; Thompson, G.W.; Wagg, B.J.: Changes in caries prevalence of Isle of Lewis Children between 1971 and 1981. Caries Res. *17:* 554–559 (1983).

13   Truin, G.J.; Plasschaert, A.J.M.; König, K.G.; Vogels, A.L.M.: Dental caries in 5-, 7-, 9- and 11-year-old schoolchildren during a 9-year dental health campaign in The Hague. Community Dent. oral Epidemiol. *9:* 55–60 (1981).

14   Clerehugh, V.; Blinkhorn, A.S.; Downer, M.C.; Hodge, H.C.; Rugg-Gunn, A.J.; Mitropoulos, C.M.; Worthington, H.V.: Changes in the caries prevalence of 11–12-year-old schoolchildren in the north-west of England from 1968 to 1981. Community Dent. oral Epidemiol. (in press).

15   Andlaw, R.J.; Burchell, C.K.; Tucker, G.J.: Comparison of dental health of 11-year-old children in 1970 and 1979, and of 14-year-old children in 1973 and 1979: studies in Bristol, England. Caries Res. *16:* 257–264 (1982).

16   Antoft, P.; Gadegaard, E.; Lind, O.P.: Social inequality and caries studies in 1,719 Danish military recruits. Community Dent. oral Epidemiol. *2:* 305–315 (1974).

17   Todd, J.E.; Whitworth, A.: Adult dental health in Scotland 1972 (Her Majesty's Stationery Office, London 1974).

18   Todd, J.E.; Walker, A.M.: Adult dental health, vol. 1: England and Wales 1968–1978 (Her Majesty's Stationery Office, London 1980).

19   Todd, J.E.; Walker, A.M.; Dodd, P.: Adult dental health, vol. 2: United Kingdom 1978 (Her Majesty's Stationery Office, London 1982).

20   Hansen, E.R.: Evaluation of preventive dental programmes for schoolchildren; in Frandsen, Dental health care in Scandinavia, pp. 83–98 (Quintessence, Chicago 1982).

21   National Board of Health, Denmark: National Statistics (National Board of Health, Copenhagen 1982).

22   National Board of Health, Finland: National Statistics (National Board of Health, Helsinki 1982).

23   Alman, J.E.: Declining caries prevalence – statistical considerations. J. dent. Res. *61:* 1361–1363 (1982).

24   Tala, H.; Ainamo, J.: Changes in general behaviour and environmental factors; in Frandsen, Dental health care in Scandinavia, pp. 137–156 (Quintessence, Chicago 1982).

25   Downer, M.C.; Teagle, F.A.; Whittle, J.G.: Field testing of an information system for planning and evaluating dental services. Community Dent. oral Epidemiol. *7:* 11–16 (1979).

26   Blinkhorn, A.S.; Downer, M.C.; Wight, C.: Dental caries experience among Scottish secondary schoolchildren in relation to dental care. Br. dent. J. *154:* 327–330 (1983).

27   Holloway, P.J.; Davies, G.N.; Downer, M.C.: The Danish Oral Health Care Service for Children; a comparison with alternative systems. Int. dent. J. (in press).

Dr. M.C. Downer, Department of Health and Social Security,
Alexander Fleming House, Elephant and Castle, London SE1 GBY (UK)

Cariology Today. Int. Congr., Zürich 1983, pp. 13–23 (Karger, Basel 1984)

Explanations for Changing Patterns of Disease in the Western World

T.M. Marthaler

Division of Applied Prevention, Department of Cariology, Periodontology and Preventive Dentistry, Dental Institute, University of Zurich, Switzerland

Introduction

For the last three decades, the majority of dental scientists have regarded fluoridation of drinking water as the most effective means of preventing dental caries in large groups.

With the exception of intensive programs with small groups, there are no reports demonstrating that any other single method of caries prevention is as effective as water fluoridation. Part of a resolution of the 28th World Assembly [WHA 28.64, May 29, 1975] summarizes this situation: 'Noting that, while optimization of the fluoride content of water systems remains the most effective known means of preventing dental caries, other systems of securing some of the benefits of fluoride protection . . .'.

In view of these circumstances, it must be concluded that the well-documented, rapidly declining caries prevalence in large populations cannot be attributed to one single method of caries prevention. It is therefore necessary to estimate the total cariostatic effect when several measures of caries prevention are combined.

Cariostatic Effect of Combined Use of Several Caries-Preventive Methods

In a dentifrice study of 740 children observed over a period of 3 years, *Andlaw and Tucker* [1975] found an average DFS increment of 7.68 in the control group as compared to 6.07 in the fluoride group. Usually, the difference of 1.61 is expressed as a reduction of caries increment of 21%. In a 7-year study, *Driscoll* et al. [1978] found an average of 5.22 new DMF surfaces in children who chewed, rinsed with and swallowed an acidulated phosphate-fluoride tablet containing 1 mg fluoride. The control group, using tablets without fluoride, developed 7.25 new DFS. The resulting reduction is equivalent to 28%.

How large is the total effect when both methods are used in a group of children? Let us imagine a group of children who, in the absence of other preventive fluorides, develop 100 DFS in the course of 4 years. Presuming that these children used the mentioned fluoride dentifrice, they would develop 79 new DFS instead of 100 (assuming ideal conditions, devoid of random variations). If, in addition, they also used the chewable fluoride tablets as tested by *Driscoll* et al. [1978], the DFS increment of 79 would be reduced by an additional 28%, leaving 57 new DFS instead of the original 100. Assuming that a third method of caries prevention, with a known effectiveness of 30% DFS reduction, was also applied, the increment would be further reduced from 57 to 40 new DFS.

The corresponding general formula for the total effect of combined measures, R_T, is straightforward. Let R_A, R_B, R_C ... be the percentage reduction of measures A, B, C ... Then the total percent reduction of the combined use of these measures would amount to

$$R_T = 100 - 100[(1 - R_A/100)(1 - R_B/100)(1 - R_C/100) ...].$$

It is obviously difficult to obtain high caries reductions, say above 60%, by combining several methods with low or moderate effectiveness. If, for example, $R_A = 15\%$, $R_B = 20\%$, and $R_C = 25\%$,

$$R_T = 100 - 100(0.85)(0.8)(0.75) = 49\%.$$

In this formula it is assumed that the percentage effect obtained by a given method is constant regardless of whether it is used alone or in combination. If this assumption does not hold, R_T overestimates the total effect.

Haugejorden and Helöe [1981], for example, cite eight papers supporting the hypothesis of an additional (not 'additive') cariostatic effect when different systemic and topical methods of fluoridation are combined. In contrast, four papers reported a limited or no effect of the combined use of fluorides. A full appraisal of the extensive literature on this topic is beyond the scope of this paper. Nevertheless, in view of several papers reporting statistically significant additional effects, the null hypothesis of no additional effect is rejected. It is only a question of its magnitude under given conditions which needs to be further studied.

There are three reasons why it must be assumed that R_T overestimates the effect, particularly when effective caries-preventive measures have already been introduced previously:

(1) In populations with low caries activity there are subjects who will not develop lesions. An additional method cannot reduce caries in this subpopulation. An example is given by *Glass* et al. [1983].

(2) Certain types of lesions (e.g. smooth surface lesions) or caries in certain segments (e.g. incisors) are more easily prevented than fissure and pit lesions. The latter type contributes the main share of DF experience once caries has substantially declined [*Hugoson and Koch,* 1982; *Marthaler,* 1981].

(3) When two measures act identically or by similar mechanisms, it is unlikely that the combined effect is proportionally stronger than one or the other measure alone. *Okazaki* et al. [1981] found that the decrease in relative solubility of fluoridated hydroxyapatites was proportional to the logarithm of the fluoride content. Similarly it may be argued that in a white spot lesion, remineralization may be favored once the necessary fluoride concentration is attained, and that additional fluoride is not useful. (Recent work suggests that other ions are indispensable for thorough remineralization – *Featherstone* et al. [1982] and *Silverstone* et al. [1981].)

Suggested Reasons of the Decline

Real and assumed reasons for the decline may be grouped under four headings, namely: (1) increased use of fluorides; (2) improvements of oral hygiene; (3) dietary changes, and (4) other, e.g. microbial, host, salivary factors.

Water fluoridation will not be discussed in this connection. There is no doubt that where it has been in operation for at least a decade, it is an important factor. Conversely, changes in levels or principles of restorative treatment are not considered as having feigned the decline of DMF experience.

Table I. Reasons of reduced caries prevelance as suggested by authors from 14 countries from which a decline of caries prevalence has been reported

Country or region author and year	Fluorides	Diet	Additional reasons, remarks
Denmark [*Fejerskov* et al., 1982][1]	dentifrices rinsing programs		better knowledge, health education
England [*Anderson* et al., 1982][1]	dentifrices		other factors are thought to have had an effect
Ireland [*O'Mullane*, 1982]	dentifrice	decrease in sugar consumption	increases in dentifrice sales are mentioned
Netherlands [*Kalsbeek*, 1982][1]	dentifrices tablets topical	no change in national sugar consumption	'no beneficial effect of dental health education could be demonstrated' other factors played a role
New Zealand [*Brown*, 1982][1]	dentifrices tablets		other factors
Norway [*von der Fehr*, 1982][1]	rinse/brush dentifrice		preventive programs (with F rinsing or brushing) reach 90% of the schoolchildren
Scotland [*Downer*, 1982][1]	dentifrices	slightly lower sugar consumption	dental health education
Sweden [*Koch*, 1982][1]	rinses dentifrices	less frequent sugar intake	basic and supplementary preventive programs for most children and adolescents; oral hygiene? F and diet

USA [Brunelle et al., 1982][1]	rinses		supervised programs at school
Two towns Mass., USA [Glass, 1982b]	dentifrices tablets		absence of organized preventive programs
Mass., USA [DePaola et al., 1982][1]	dentifrices topical	changes in intake patterns	systemic F effect negligible? changes in oral flora? antibiotics?
Australia [Carr, 1982]	dentifrice supplements		dental health promotion by school dental services and dental profession
Finland [Hausen et al., 1983]	programs dentifrices	sucrose consumption constant	preventive measures, mainly utilization of fluorides
Switzerland [Marthaler, 1983]	dentifrices brush-ins salt	sucrose consumption constant, less frequent intake assumed	the control effect of fluoride cannot explain the total reduction from 1963/64 to 1979/80

[1] These papers are all contained in *Glass* [1982a].

A great many authors have expressed their opinion on the present problem. The examples compiled in table I show that the use of fluoride dentifrices is the most commonly accepted factor. In several countries, fluoride-free dentifrices were substituted by fluoride-containing dentifrices within periods of a few years. Some authors go so far as to consider the use of fluoride dentifrices as the only certain reason. *DePaola* et al. [1982] surmised that life-long use of a dentifrice, providing fluoride during the critical eruption period with its enhanced responsiveness of the enamel, may be of greater benefit than that observed in 2- or 3-year clinical trials.

Fluoride supplements (tablets, fluoride vitamin drops) and topical fluoride are mentioned by several authors as a factor in caries reductions. In Scandinavian countries, Switzerland and New Zealand, rinsing and brushing with fluoride preparations forming part of school-based programs were related to dental (and often gingival) health.

In 7 of the 14 papers, dietary changes are not mentioned at all, while constant sugar consumption is suggested in three papers. Changes in sugar intake patterns, or less frequent consumption, are alluded to by three authors, but no scientific data is available supporting this assumption.

Improved oral hygiene has been discussed only by *Koch* [1982]. Pertinent work summarized by *Andlaw* [1978] suggested that it could be justified to regard this factor as minor or even negligible. With respect to free smooth surfaces, however, better oral hygiene, coupled with regular fluoride contact through dentifrices, should not be completely disregarded. Increasing sales of dentifrices have been reported by *O'Mullane* [1982].

Changes of the plaque microflora are considered by *Kalsbeek* [1982] and *DePaola* et al. [1982]. The latter authors consider intraoral fluoride as interfering with transmission and implantation of organisms as well as with the intraoral spread of infection from open caries lesions. They also refer to the widespread use of antibiotics.

Dental health education per se does not inhibit caries. It operates through promoting the use of fluorides, changes in dietary patterns and improvements of oral hygiene. About half of the authors, especially those from the Scandinavian countries, regard such programs as important. *Glass* [1982b], on the other hand, pointed out that the improvements in children living in two Massachusetts towns without water fluoridation occurred despite the absence of any further organized preventive programs. The material presented by *Hugoson and Koch* [1982] provides strong support regarding the usefulness of educational measures in a broad sense. These authors presented data indicating a very rapid decline of caries prevalence: children at age 15 showed 27.1 DFS in 1973, but only 13.7 in 1978.

Analysis of the Situation in the Canton of Zurich

A decrease from 23.7 DFS to 6.9 DFS was reported in 14-year-old children from 7 communities in the Canton of Zurich between 1963 and 1979 [*Marthaler,* 1981]. In 1963, 0.86 first molars were missing on average compared to only 0.053 in 1979. Assuming 3 decayed sites on average per extracted first molar, the actual decrease would have been from 26.3 to 7.1. These two averages will be used for the following discussion which is based on a more detailed analysis [*Marthaler,* 1983].

With respect to fluorides, four points have to be considered: (1) fluoride containing domestic salt; (2) fluoride applied with supervised toothbrushing exercises at school; (3) fluoridated dentifrices, and (4) other fluorides.

Domestic salt containing 90 ppm fluoride was introduced in 1956. From 1962/66 until 1974, 85% of the domestic salt used in the Canton of Zurich was fluoridated. However, due to the insufficient fluoride content, only 0.45 mg fluoride was sold per person per day. In addition, only part of the salt used in the kitchen is actually ingested (in May 1983 the fluoride content of domestic salt has been elevated to 250 ppm). Based on all available information, minimal and maximal effect in the total population were estimated at 13 and 21%.

Similar considerations regarding the *supervised toothbrushing exercises with fluoride preparations* resulted in estimates of 15% as minimal and 30% as maximal effect.

According to *Balbi* [1978], 58–63% of the dentifrices sold in the period 1972–1975 contained 1,000–1,250 ppm fluoride, and *Dal Vesco* [1980] reported that 72–80% of children used *fluoride toothpastes.* Assuming that 80% of the children use fluoride dentifrices and that the true effect is in the range of a 25–35% reduction [*von der Fehr and Møller* 1978], the resulting limits for the total child population are between 20 and 28%.

Table II. Total reduction, R_T, to be expected in the population from (1) the use of fluoride salts; (2) toothbrushing exercises with fluoride preparations; (3) fluoride dentifrices, and (4) other fluorides (gels, tablets)

	Estimated caries reduction, %		
	minimal	maximal	average
F salt	13	21	–
F brush instructions	15	30	–
F dentifrices	20	28	–
Other F	5	15	–
R_T	44	66	55
DFS 1963	26.3	26.3	26.3
Reduced by R_T	14.7	8.9	11.8
DFS 1979	7.1	7.1	7.1
Percent reduction not explained by F	52	20	40

Other fluoride measures recommended are weekly use of a fluoride gel used with a toothbrush and the daily ingestion of fluoride tablets. Sales of fluoride-containing products and scientific data [summarized by *Marthaler,* 1983] suggest that these methods of using fluorides are applied to an extent which can have produced a minor effect only. This was estimated to have caused a 5–15% DFS reduction.

Minimal and maximal percent DFS reductions for the combined effect were computed with the aid of the formula for R_T, developed above (table II). Minimal and maximal estimates of R_T are 44 and 66%. It is improbable that for each of the four fluoridation measures the maximal estimate corresponds to the real situation. In addition, it was discussed above that R_T tends to overestimate the total effect of combined fluoride measures. Therefore it is justified to assume a total effect of fluoride in all forms in the range of 44–55% rather than the above average of 55%.

Factors Other Than Fluorides

Total fluoride effects as analyzed in the preceding section are likely to have resulted in a reduction not exceeding 55%, equal to the decline of the DFS average from 26.3 to 11.8. The residual change from 11.8 to 7.1 DFS corresponds to a reduction of 40%. Besides fluorides, changes in dietary habits and better oral hygiene are assumed to have had a beneficial influence.

Total sugar consumption has remained within the range of 39–46 kg/person/year for 30 years. There are no scientific reports indicating a tendency of children to consume less sugar. Any consideration of the effects of changes in sugar intake patterns and oral hygiene habits is fraught with uncertainties when their roles in the declining prevalence of caries are discussed. Due to this uncertainty, researchers may have been reluctant to discuss factors other than fluorides. The analysis of the situation in the Canton of Zurich as well as other data suggest, however, that the reduction clearly demonstrated in more than ten countries cannot be attributed to the effect of fluorides alone.

Concluding Remarks

This review shows that fluorides are regarded as the most important or even the only factor responsible for the decline in caries prevalence. Increases in the use of ingested and topical fluoride are relatively easy to assess in large populations, and the corresponding cariostatic effects can be predicted with some degree of certainty on the basis of extensive experimentation throughout the world. On the other hand, dietary changes, particularly sugar intake patterns, have not been followed over long periods. Averages of total sugar consumption were the only data cited. Since it is the frequency of sugar consumption or, more precisely, the time during which sugar is available to be fermented by plaque microorganisms, total sugar consumption figures are of very limited value. In addition, children up to age 16, in whom the decline was studied, constitute approximately one-fifth of the total population. Accordingly, a 25% reduction of sugar consumed in this age group would result in a decrease of only 5% of the nationwide average.

Data on oral hygiene habits are equally scant but the number of toothbrushes and the amounts of dentifrice sold could be useful indicators. Again, changes would reflect the situation in the entire population, but the reported changes are so large that they justify more detailed scrutiny.

References

Anderson, R.J.; Bradnock, G.; Beal, J.F.; James, P.M.C.: The reduction of dental caries prevalence in English schoolchildren. J. dent. Res. *61:* 1311–1316 (1982).

Andlaw, R.H.: Oral hygiene and dental caries – a review. Int. dent. J., Lond. *28:* 1–6 (1978).

Andlaw, R.H.; Tucker, G.J.: A dentifrice containing 0.8 per cent sodium monofluorophosphate in an aluminium oxide trihydrate base. A 3-year clinical trial. Br. dent. J. *138:* 426–432 (1975).

Balbi, A.: Entwicklung und Stand des Kaufs von Mundpflegemitteln auf Grund marktanalytischer Erhebungen. Med. Diss. Zürich (1978).

Brown, R.H.: Evidence of decrease in the prevalence of dental caries in New Zealand. J. dent. Res. *61:* 1327–1330 (1982).

Brunelle, J.A.; Carlos, J.P.: Changes in the prevalence of dental caries in US schoolchildren, 1961–1980. J. dent. Res. *61:* 1346–1351 (1982).

Carr, L.M.: Dental health of children in Australia 1977–1980. Aust. dent. J. *27:* 169–175 (1982).

Dal Vesco, V.: Der Einfluss von häuslichen Fluorgaben, Geschlecht, Schultypus und Einkommen auf den Kariesbefall von Schulkindern. Eine Erhebungsstudie. Med. Diss. Zürich (1980).

DePaola, P.F.; Soparkar, P.M.; Tavares, M.; Allukian, M., Jr.; Peterson, H.: A dental survey of Massachusetts schoolchildren. J. dent. Res. *61:* 1356–1360 (1982).

Downer, M.C.: Secular changes in caries experience in Scotland. J. dent. Res. *61:* 1336–1339 (1982).

Driscoll, W.S.; Heifetz, S.B.; Korts, D.C.: Effect of chewable fluoride tablets on dental caries in schoolchildren: results after six years. J. Am. dent. Ass. *97:* 820–824 (1978).

Featherstone, J.D.B.; Cutress, T.W.; Rodgers, B.E.; Dennison, P.J.: Remineralization of artificial caries-like lesions in vivo by a self-administered mouthrinse or paste. Caries Res. *16:* 235–242 (1982).

Fehr, F.R. von der: Evidence of decreasing caries prevalence in Norway. J. dent. Res. *61:* 1331–1335 (1982).

Fehr, F.R. von der; Møller, I.J.: Caries-preventive fluoride dentifrices. Caries Res. *12:* suppl. 1, pp. 31–37 (1978).

Fejerskov, O.; Antoft, P.; Gadegaard, E.: Decrease in caries experience in Danish children and young adults in the 1970s. J. dent. Res. *61:* 1305–1310 (1982).

Glass, R.L.: The first international conference on the declining prevalence of dental caries. The evidence and the impact on dental education, dental research, and dental practice. J. dent. Res. *61:* suppl., pp. 1301–1383 (1982a).

Glass, R.L.: Secular changes in caries prevalence in two Massachusetts towns. J. dent. Res. *61:* 1352–1355 (1982b).

Glass, R.L.; Peterson, J.K.: Bixler, D.: The effects of changing caries prevalence and diagnostic criteria on clinical caries trials. Caries Res. *17:* 145–151 (1983).

Haugejorden, O.; Helöe, L.A.: Fluorides for everyone: a review of school-based or community programs. Community Dent. oral Epidemiol. *9:* 159–169 (1981).

Hausen, H.; Milen, A.; Tala, H.; Nordling, H.; Paunio, I.; Heinonen, O.P.: Caries frequency among 6–17-year-old participants of the Finnish public dental care during 1975–79. Community Dent. oral Epidemiol. *11:* 74–80 (1983).

Hugoson, A.; Koch, G.: Community dentistry – the Swedish experience. Int. dent. J. *32:* 379–402 (1982).

Kalsbeek, H.: Evidence of decrease in prevalence of dental caries in the Netherlands: an evaluation of epidemiological caries surveys on 4–6- and 11–15-year-old children, performed between 1965 and 1980. J. dent. Res. *61:* 1321–1326 (1982).

Koch, G.: Evidence for declining caries prevalence in Sweden. J. dent. Res. *61:* 1340–1345 (1982).

Marthaler, T.M.: Interim report on DMF-reduction 16 years after the introduction of a preventive program. Community Dent. oral Epidemiol. *9:* 210–214 (1981).

Marthaler, T.M.: Resultate nach 16 Jahren prophylaxeorientierter Schulzahnpflege: welche Faktoren waren wirksam? (in press, 1983).

Okazaki, M.; Moriwaki, Y.; Aoba, T.; Doi, Y.; Takahashi, J.: Solubility behavior of CO_3 apatites in relation to crystallinity. Caries Res. *15:* 477–483 (1981).

O'Mullane, D.M.: The changing patterns of dental caries in Irish schoolchildren between 1961 and 1981. J. dent. Res. *61:* 1317–1320 (1982).

Silverstone, L.M.; Wefel, J.S.; Zimmermann, B.F.; Clarkson, B.H.; Featherstone, M.J.: Remineralization of natural and artificial lesions in human dental enamel in vitro. Caries Res. *15:* 138–157 (1981).

T.M. Marthaler, MD, Division of Applied Prevention, Department of Cariology, Periodontology and Preventive Dentistry, Dental Institute, University of Zurich, CH-8000 Zurich (Switzerland)

Cariology Today. Int. Congr., Zürich 1983, pp. 24–32 (Karger, Basel 1984)

Epidemiologic Trends in Caries: Impact on Adults and the Aged

James P. Carlos

National Caries Program, NIDR, Bethesda, Md., USA

We have been discussing recent reports of epidemiologic studies in several western countries, which have provided consistent and encouraging evidence for a major decline in the prevalence of dental caries among school-aged children. Although the reasons for these reductions cannot be established with scientific rigor, most investigators interpret the data as evidence of the effect of increased caries prevention efforts during the past two decades; in particular, to the large increase in the number of children exposed to fluorides from a variety of delivery methods. This interpretation is probably correct.

It is understandable that those of us engaged in research on caries prevention take satisfaction from this demonstration of the success of our efforts. However, it would be short-sighted to fail to recognize that a large and permanent reduction of caries among children (assuming the trend can be sustained) may not be equivalent to the control of this disease but, rather, may inadvertently result in an increase in the incidence of root-surface caries and recurrent coronal caries among older segments of the population. This will occur to the extent that prevention of caries in children increases the risk of caries as these children become adults, and if current population trends continue. We need to ask whether and to what extent teeth are being temporarily saved from caries only to succumb another day.

I will try to outline some possible implications of the changes we are currently seeing in both caries prevalence and population trends that may affect future efforts in research and prevention. For illustrative purposes, I will focus on the disease of root-surface caries, although some of the same considerations are applicable to recurrent coronal caries (as well as to periodontal disease).

A simple epidemiologic risk model will help illustrate the theoretical situation:

$$I = Nt\mu$$

where I = incidence of caries (root-surface caries, for example), N = number of teeth at risk (the 'risk pool'), t = duration of exposure to caries attack, and μ = intensity of caries attack.

We may examine a few of the possible consequences of such a model, by attempting to make some tentative predictions about each of the parameters.

The 'Risk Pool' (N)

From the available evidence of declining caries among children can we make any statements about probable changes in the size of the 'risk pool' as these children reach adulthood? We can, but only crudely and only by accepting several assumptions. Of these, the most crucial is that recent downward trends in caries prevalence will be accelerated or at least maintained. I know of no scientific reason why this should not occur; clearly we have not yet approached the point where further attempts to prevent caries in children will become subject to some biological version of the Law of Diminishing Returns. There are some potentially serious problems of economics and individual behavior which may reverse present trends, but for simplicity these will not be discussed in this paper. Instead my comments will be restricted to consideration of the parameters of the epidemiologic model.

Table I shows some selected data reported for some of the older children examined in recent surveys [1–9], as these seem most relevant to the question of whether, as a result of decreasing caries in childhood, more teeth will be at risk of future disease.

Evidently the decrease in caries at these ages has been substantial. Unfortunately, however, the quality of these data is rather poor. Except for those reported from the US they are derived from examination of relatively small numbers of children, using different diagnostic criteria and, in some instances, are based upon comparisons of results obtained in different geographical locales. Therefore the data do not justify any quantitative statements about the magnitude of the reduction in caries.

Table I. Changes in caries prevalence in selected countries

Country	Reference[1]	Ages	Time period	Caries prevalence (DMFT or DMFS)		Change, %
Denmark	1	military recruits	1972–1982	16.6	11.8	29.0
UK	2	12	1970–1980	8.6	5.6[2]	23.0
Ireland	3	13–14	1961–1980	8.0	4.4	42.0
The Netherlands	4	12	1967–1980	8.0	5.5	31.0
New Zealand	5	12–13	1950–1982	7.9	5.1	35.0
Norway	6	16	1970–1979	~40.0	~18.0[2]	55.0
Scotland	7	11–12	1970–1980	8.1	5.8	28.0
Sweden	8	15	1973–1978	27.7	13.7[2]	51.0
USA	9	16	1972–1980	15.1	9.6[2]	36.0

[1] Source: adapted from references 1–9.
[2] DMFS.

To do so with any reasonable precision will require further sequential surveys of statistically sampled populations of sufficient size that the error of the prevalence estimate is reasonably small.

We may note, however, that to predict changes in the number of teeth that will be at risk of root-surface caries, reductions in coronal caries in children are of interest only insofar as they result in a reduction in tooth mortality. Even a tooth with all surfaces carious or filled will be at risk of root-surface caries if it is still present in the mouth at age 30 or 40. This suggests that changes in the size of the 'risk pool' among adults will be heavily dependent upon changes in the amount and quality of dental care available to children and adolescents in a population, and upon changes in tooth loss due to periodontal disease, as well as on the level of prevention of initial caries lesions. Thus, for prediction of adult caries, we are primarily interested in the components of DMF scores that reflect missing teeth.

Reliable information on recent changes in tooth loss among young adults is difficult to find. Of the studies cited in table I, only three reported data on missing teeth. Table II shows some data on this point from surveys of the US population [10–12]. Using 28 permanent teeth as a base, it appears that in the early 1960s, teenaged children could expect to lose an average of 5.4 more teeth by about age 30. By 1972 this had decreased to fewer than 4 more teeth lost by age 30, thus

Table II. Permanent teeth per person, USA

Age	1963–1965	1972	1980
17	26.9	26.9	27.8
18–24	23.3	27.2	–
25–34	21.5	23.4	–

Source: references 10–12.

substantially increasing the risk-pool for root-surface caries. As there was no evidence for a decline in coronal caries or periodontal disease during the 1960s, the change was presumably due to improved dental care. Whether this trend is still continuing is unknown, as no recent data are available on missing teeth in adults. However, among 17-year-old children, tooth loss due to caries declined sharply during the past decade.

We do have other evidence of high levels of dental care among children. From a recent epidemiologic survey of US children aged 5–17 years, it was estimated that only 37% required any dental treatment [13]. Furthermore, for 17-year-olds, the average number of missing permanent teeth, plus teeth requiring extraction, was only about 22/100 children.

The obvious conclusion is that 'N', the number of teeth at risk of root-surface caries, is slowly increasing and will continue to increase to the extent that present levels of both prevention of coronal caries and restorative treatment are maintained or improved. The rate of this increase cannot be estimated from the data available.

Duration of Exposure (t)

We can be confident that the incidence of caries in root surfaces is some function of the length of time that the tooth is exposed to cariogenic challenge. This is the parameter called 't' in the risk model. The relationship between exposure time and incidence is not necessarily linear, but lacking information to the contrary, it is simplest to assume linearity. To make estimates about future caries incidence in adults we therefore need to know something about the prospective longevity of the population.

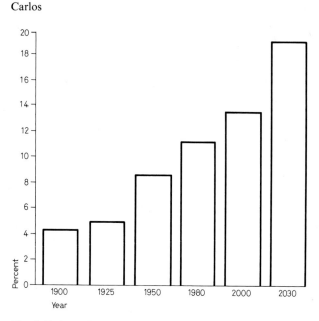

Fig. 1. Estimated percent of population over age 65: USA 1900–2030.

Table III. Average years of life expectancy at age 30, USA

	1960	1970	1980
Males	40.4	40.6	42.6
Females	45.9	47.2	49.2

Figure 1 shows some pertinent data and projections of population changes in the US. Clearly the population is rapidly aging, and this trend is expected to continue. However, the proportionate growth of the older age groups is due, in part, to a decline in the birth rate during recent decades; that is to say that an increase in the average age of a population does not necessarily imply increased duration of exposure to risk of individuals or teeth.

However, as shown in table III, the life expectancy of adults is also increasing. In the US population, a person now aged 30 years, when the risk of root-surface caries probably begins to become measurable, can expect to remain at risk of this disease for 2–4 years longer than a 30-year-old in 1960. With continued advances in research and medical care, this trend also can be expected to continue.

Intensity of Caries Attack (μ)

I intend this final parameter of the risk model to mean the net effect of all biological and environmental factors involved in the etiology of root-surface caries. Presumably these include, at least, the microorganisms which colonize cementum, the substrates required for their growth and pathogenic activity and the resistance of the host to caries initiation. None of these factors is yet well understood. The only reasonable assumption about the intensity of caries attack on root surfaces is that it has not changed recently and will be unchanged for the immediate future.

We do have some information on the end results of this parameter during recent years. Figure 2 shows data from several surveys of the prevalence of root-surface caries conducted in North America during the 1970s [14–18]. Considering that there was no attempt at standard diagnosis in these surveys, as well as the fact that they were based on relatively small samples, the similarity of results is striking. The percentage of persons affected begins to increase rapidly after age 25–30 and is still increasing among persons aged 60 and older. In most surveys, about 70% of those examined at age 65 had some evidence of root-surface caries.

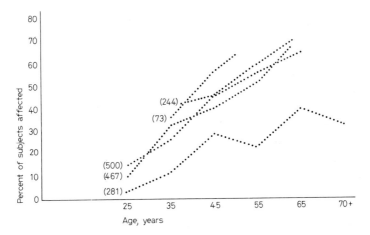

Fig. 2. Prevalence (percent) of root-surface caries by age in 5 surveys in North America. Source: references 14–18.

However, the vagaries of these data do not permit good estimates of disease incidence which, in any case, is confounded by loss of teeth due to periodontal disease; one report indicated that 30% of teeth extracted from adults had root-surface caries. From existing information, the best estimate of incidence of this disease is about 1 surface attacked every 4 years of age, or about 0.25 root-surface lesions per person per year after age 30. This is a *very* tentative estimate!

Discussion

Any attempt to predict future incidence and prevalence of root-surface caries in adult populations is severely hindered by a lack of reliable data on present trends in caries prevalence. The number and consistency of reports from many countries regarding declining levels of coronal caries tend to disguise the fact that the data reported have usually been incomplete, noncomparable and, in some cases, of very doubtful quality. The information we have is sufficient to justify the conclusion that caries is decreasing among children, but it is not adequate to permit meaningful estimates about the size and rate of the decrease. It seems appropriate in this international forum of caries researchers to make a plea for better, more rigorous surveys to detect changes in caries prevalence in adults as well as in children, using comparable diagnostic criteria, and from which results are reported in reasonably standardized formats. We need, in addition, explicit information on changes in tooth mortality from all causes, including periodontal disease. Without these data, it will be impossible to predict whether root-surface caries is, or will become, a public health problem.

I have suggested the simplest of epidemiologic models as a basis for estimating changing patterns of caries among adults. Unfortunately, the parameters of this model cannot, at present, be numerically estimated and even qualitative predictions require some critical and unsupportable simplifying assumptions. Nevertheless, I shall offer a few conclusions:

(1) The number of teeth at risk of root-surface caries, 'N', is slowly increasing. This is partly due to declining coronal caries with associated decreases in tooth loss during childhood and adolescence, but also to improved levels of restorative dental care. The rate of growth of this 'risk pool' will not increase dramatically without a sharp reduction in

the number of teeth lost to periodontal disease. Thus, as successive cohorts of adults reach age 30, I do not foresee during this decade any major increase in the number of teeth becoming at risk of root-surface caries.

(2) Duration of exposure to root-surface caries is a function of duration of adult life. This is increasing in Western countries at the rate of roughly 2 years per decade, and will probably continue at this rate. This will result in increased incidence of root-surface caries.

(3) The intensity of caries attack on root surfaces is the result of interaction among pathogenic and protective ecological factors not yet well defined. The net result, however, is the appearance of, roughly, one new lesion per person for every 4 years of exposure after age 30. This assumes that the current incidence of periodontal disease, with subsequent exposure of cemental surfaces, remains unchanged. In any case, such a statistic is of little use for predictive purposes. Because I have suggested that disease incidence is a function of the size of the 'risk pool', what is needed is a good estimate of the annual incidence of root-surface caries per tooth or per 100 teeth at risk. No such estimates exist today.

I conclude from these circuitous and very general arguments that caries of root surfaces will probably become a gradually increasing problem during the next several decades. Surely the prevalence data now available suggests that this disease already warrants a serious research effort to define its etiology and devise effective methods for prevention. However, I certainly do not expect to see, nor do I advocate, a sudden or major change in research to focus on caries in adults at the expense of continued efforts to prevent coronal caries in younger age groups. The latter problem is far from solved.

Above all, I am seriously concerned about the present lack of high quality comprehensive epidemiological data about caries. A resurgence in epidemiologic research is urgently needed, both to more closely monitor changes in caries patterns among children and to anticipate the emergence of new problems of caries among adults.

References

1   Fejerskov, O.; Antoft, P.; Gadegaard, E.: Decrease in caries experience in Danish children and young adults in the 1970s. J. dent. Res. *61:* suppl., pp. 1305–1310 (1982).

2   Anderson, R.; Bradnock, G.; Beal, J.; James, P.: The reduction of dental caries prevalence in English schoolchildren. J. dent. Res. *61:* suppl., pp. 1311–1316 (1982).

3   O'Mullane, D.: The changing patterns of dental caries in Irish schoolchildren between 1961 and 1981. J. dent. Res. *61:* suppl., pp. 1317–1320 (1982).

4   Kalsbeek, H.: Evidence of decrease in prevalence of dental caries in the Netherlands: an evaluation of epidemiological caries surveys on 4–6 and 11–15-year-old children, performed between 1965 and 1980. J. dent. Res. *61:* suppl., pp. 1321–1326 (1982).

5   Brown, R.: Evidence of decrease in prevalence of dental caries in New Zealand. J. dent. Res. *61:* suppl., pp. 1327–1330 (1982).

6   Fehr, F. von der: Evidence of decreasing caries prevalence in Norway. J. dent. Res. *62:* suppl., pp. 1331–1335 (1982).

7   Downer, M.: Secular changes in caries experience in Scotland. J. dent. Res. *61:* suppl., pp. 1336–1339 (1982).

8   Koch, G.: Evidence for declining caries prevalence in Sweden. J. dent. Res. *61:* suppl., pp. 1340–1345 (1982).

9   Brunelle, J.; Carlos, J.: Changes in the prevalence of dental caries in US schoolchildren, 1961–1980. J. dent. Res. *61:* suppl., pp. 1346–1351 (1982).

10 National Center for Health Statistics: Decayed, missing and filled teeth among persons 1–74 years. United States. Ser. 11, No. 23 (GPO, Washington 1967).

11 National Center for Health Statistics: Decayed, missing and filled teeth among persons 1–74 years. United States. Ser. 11, No. 223 (GPO, Washington 1981).

12 National Caries Program: The prevalence of dental caries in United States children, 1979–1980. NIH publ. No. 82–2245 (1981).

13 National Caries Program: Dental treatment needs of United States children, 1979–1980. NIH publ. No. 83–2246 (1982).

14 Hix, J.; O'Leary, T.: The relationship between cemental caries, oral hygiene status, and fermentable carbohydrate intake. J. Peridont. *47:* 398–404 (1976).

15 Lohse, W.; Carter, H.; Brunelle, J.: The prevalence of root-surface caries in a military population. Milit. Med. *142:* 700–703 (1977).

16 Hazen, S.; Chilton, N.; Mumma, R.: The problem of root caries. 3. A Clinical study (Abstract). J. dent. Res. *50:* 219 (1972).

17 Stamm, J.; Banting, D.: Comparison of root caries prevalence in adults with lifelong residence in fluoridated communities. IADR Abstr. *552:* (1980).

18 Banting, D.; Ellen, R.; Fillery, E.: Prevalence of root surface caries among institutionalized older persons. Community Dent. oral Epidemiol. *8:* 84–88 (1980).

Dr. J.P. Carlos, NIDR, NIH, Bethesda, MD 20205 (USA)

Cariology Today. Int. Congr., Zürich 1983, pp. 33–39 (Karger, Basel 1984)

Dental Caries in Underdeveloped Countries

Aubrey Sheiham

The London Hospital Medical College, London, England

Dental caries is a sugar-dependent infectious disease. Therefore any discussion of the changing patterns of dental caries in underdeveloped countries must consider the changes in sugar consumption. Sugar consumption in all underdeveloped countries is rising. By 1984 their consumption is predicted to exceed the use in industrialized countries, where sugar consumption is falling [27]. Industrialized countries can absorb little more sugar so underdeveloped countries are consuming four-fifths of what they produce. 50 years ago they exported four-fifths of production [31]. In addition to home production, in some underdeveloped countries, sugar is the second largest food item imported. Sugar is one of the first foods to respond to a rise in income in low-income countries and the percentage of sugar consumed in hidden forms rises progressively with rising income and increasing total sugar consumption [28].

The greatest percentage increases in consumption are anticipated in countries which had a per caput consumption of less than 20 kg/year [29]. The biggest users of sugar in underdeveloped countries are the subsidiaries of large multinational food and drink processing companies and include cake and biscuit manufacturers and the soft drink industry. Soft drinks are probably the most important factor in the sharp increase in sugar consumption in countries as diverse as Iran and Venezuela. In Mexico, nearly five bottles of soft drinks are consumed per man, woman and child every week [9].

Increases in Dental Caries

Deteriorating dental health is seen as a necessary consequence of economic growth which in itself is assumed to be a desirable goal for everyone. Yet the extent of the deterioration will reflect the priorities of the society and of policy-makers.

There is no doubt that the prevalence and severity of dental caries is increasing rapidly in underdeveloped countries; of 20 countries where two surveys have been conducted on 12-year-olds some years apart, 15 have recorded marked increases, two (Ghana and China) showed no change and three (Sri Lanka, Argentina, Cuba) have had a decrease in caries [32]. In those countries which have reported increases, the increases in DMFT were from 0.4 to 1.5 between 1966 and 1982 in Uganda, 2.8 to 6.3 in 18 years in Chile, 2.7 to 5.3 in 4 years in Mexico, 0.2 to 2.7 in 19 years in Jordan and 1.2 to 3.6 in 13 years in Lebanon [32]. Further evidence of the increase in caries have been reported by *Barmes* [2] and *Sardo Infirri and Barmes* [17]. *Barmes* [2] described the increased rate of caries in underdeveloped countries as 'absolutely frightening'. He reported changes of 0.1 to 1.7 in 21 years in Kenya, 0.2 to 1.6 in 17 years in Ethiopia and 0.7 to 4.5 in 15 years in Thailand. These changes are frightening when the DMF is converted into treatment needs. *Barmes* [3] estimated that a dentist:population ratio of 1:4,200 would be needed to treat 12-year-olds with a DMF of 3.0. If one dentist and two operating auxiliaries were used the dentist:population ratio would be 1:12,500. A difference in DMF of 0.7 to 3.5 would require an extra 700 dental operators per million children [2]. A level of dental manpower which is impossible to achieve in countries in which the annual per capita expenditure on health is less than 5 US$ the cost of one restoration per child would exhaust the majority of the health budget. What chance is there of treating children in Fiji, for example, where the dental needs are 'At six years of age only 11.4% of children did not need treatment, whilst 48% required one-surface fillings, 73% required two-surface fillings, 16% needed three-surface fillings and 0.5% fillings involving more than three surfaces. 29% of children required extraction of deciduous teeth because of caries' [24].

Sugar and Dental Caries

What is the cause of this frightening increase in dental caries in underdeveloped countries? The consensus view is that refined sugars and in particular sucrose is the principal dietary cause [13, 19, 25]. *Sreebny* [25] found a strong association between the quantity of sugar consumed per person per day on the one hand and the DMF on the other. He found that at levels above 50 g/day the intensity of the caries attack increased. *Schulerud* [18] in Norway and *Takeuchi* [26] and *Shimamura* [21] in Japan had previously shown that the caries pattern changed with increases in sugar consumption. *Takeuchi* [26] found that at a given level of sugar consumption specific teeth were affected differentially.

In underdeveloped countries the first change in the pattern of caries with rising sugar consumption is an increase in the primary teeth [16]. In the permanent teeth pits and fissures are mainly affected at low sugar levels [10]; the second molar being more frequently carious than first molars [1]. With increases in sugar consumption the ratio of first to second molars affected is one – similar to that found in high sugar consuming countries [6]. At the higher sugar levels proximal surface caries becomes more common. These patterns of disease indicate that environmental factors are more important than genetic predisposing factors. They cast further doubt on Jacksons' theory of caries aetiology [22].

In some underdeveloped countries dental caries is a disease of the very young and the middle-aged [20], coronal caries occurring in the young and root caries in the older group [15].

Socio-Demographic Variables

In underdeveloped countries the distribution of caries varies with social class and acculturation, level of urbanization, gender, ethnic group and level of fluoride consumption.

The influence of social class is strong [5]. *Olsson* [14] found that Ethiopian children from more affluent high social class families had four times more caries in primary teeth than poorer children and twice as many permanent teeth with caries. She found that the caries pattern differed by class. Upper class children had more anterior teeth affected and a higher number of both proximal and smooth surface lesions. This pattern of caries was associated with the increased availability of sugar to high income families since the establishment of a national sugar company.

Urbanized populations in underdeveloped countries are more likely to consume refined sugars than those in rural areas. Therefore it is not surprising that caries rates are higher in urban populations. In the Sudan, *Emslie* [4] found seven times more caries in 15- to 19-year-old urban children, where the annual per capita sugar consumption was over 100 lb, than in rural children living in an area where the sugar consumption was below 5 lb/year/person. Similar trends were found in Mozambique [7], Swaziland [8] and South Africa [3].

Females usually had a higher caries rate than males [10]. And there are differences in caries rates in different ethnic groups within a country. In Malaysia, Chinese children had a much higher caries rate than Malays and Indians [11]. Similar trends existed in Singapore despite water fluoridation [12]. In Fiji, Indians also had lower caries rates than Fijians. This difference was mainly due to the differences in the ages of exfoliation of primary teeth and eruption of the permanent teeth [24].

Fluoride levels in water and foods have been shown to be related to caries rates. Studies in underdeveloped countries, some with low levels of sugar consumption, offer an opportunity to assess the effect of fluoride with differing levels of sugar consumption. In an extensive study of populations living on 14 South Pacific islands, *Speake* et al. [23] did not find a clear relationship between enamel fluoride levels and caries prevalence when comparisons were made between islands, yet a significant relationship did exist within island populations. This suggests that where environmental factors were similar, fluoride did have an effect. They found that where sugar levels were high, the influences of fluoride were outweighed by dietary factors. It was possible to develop a predictor chart of caries rates from enamel fluoride levels and sugar consumption levels [23].

Public Health Aspects

The increases in caries in many underdeveloped countries are very rapid. The principal reason for the increase is the increase in consumption of sugar-containing foods, drinks and confections. The conventional methods of preventing caries used in industrialized countries are not appropriate for underdeveloped countries. The cost of fluoride toothpaste, paper cups for fluoride rinses and toothbrushes are beyond the means of the vast majority. Therefore the logical public health strategy is primordial prevention; preventing the emergence of patterns of eating that are known to contribute to caries [33]. The strategy should include a national food and agriculture policy, controls on imports and alternative useful uses of sugar.

To summarize, dental caries is rapidly becoming a severe public health problem in underdeveloped countries. In some countries such as Swaziland, the dental caries rate is as high as in Denmark but the resources are hopelessly inadequate to cope with the treatment of the disease [8]. The increases in dental caries may not appear to be great when compared to the caries rates in industrialized countries but it should be remembered that every increase of 1 in the DMF would require about 200 dental operators per million children. The cost of training and employing such an increase in the dental workforce is considerable and beyond the educational or financial capabilities of many underdeveloped countries.

Increases in dental caries appear to have a well-defined pattern; as the intensity of the disease increases different teeth and tooth sites are affected.

The major factor associated with the increase in dental caries is refined sugar. Therefore if worthwhile efforts are going to be made to control the rising epidemic of dental caries in underdeveloped countries, primordial prevention aimed at controlling the availability of refined sugars and sugar-containing foods, drinks and confections, is needed.

References

1 Akpata, E.S.; Jackson, D.: Caries vulnerability of first and second permanent molars in urban Nigerians. Archs oral Biol. *23:* 795–800 (1978).

2 Barmes, D.E.: Epidemiology of dental disease. J. clin. Periodont. *4:* 80–93 (1977).

3 Barmes, D.E.: Oral health status of children – an international perspective. J. Can. dent. Ass. *12:* 651–658 (1979).

4 Emslie, R.D.: A dental health survey in the Republic of Sudan. Br. dent. J. *120:* 167–178 (1966).

5 Enwonwu, C.O.: Interface of nutrition and dentistry in pre-industrialized tropical countries. Odont. Stom. Trop. *1:* 19–42 (1978).

6 Hirshowitz, A.S.; Rashid, S.A.A.; Cleaton-Jones, P.E.: Dental caries, gingival health and malocclusion in 12 year old urban black schoolchildren from Soweto, Johannesburg. Community Dent. oral Epidemiol. *9:* 87–90 (1981).

7 Hobdell, M.H.; Cabral, J.R.: Dental caries and gingivitis experience of the People's Republic of Mozambique (1978). Odont. Stom. Trop. *3:* 111–126 (1980).

8 Klausen, B.; Fanoe, J.G.: An epidemiologic survey of oral health in Swaziland. Community Dent. oral Epidemiol. *11:* 63–68 (1983).

9   Lappe, F.M.; Collins, J.: Food first. The myth of scarcity, p. 234 (Souvenir Press, London 1980).

10 Legler, D.W.; Al-Alousi, W.; Jamison, J.C.: Dental caries prevalence in secondary schoolchildren in Iraq. J. dent. Res. *59:* 1936–1940 (1980).

11 Ministry of Health, Malaysia: Dental epidemiological survey of adults in Peninsular Malaysia (Dental Division, Kuala Lumpur 1978).

12 Ministry of Health, Republic of Singapore: National dental health survey of school population – 1970 (Dental Branch, Singapore 1973).

13 Newbrun, E.: Sucrose in the dynamics of the caries process. Int. dent. J., Lond. *32:* 13–21 (1982).

14 Olsson, B.: Dental health situation in privileged children in Addis Ababa, Ethiopia. Community Dent. oral Epidemiol. *7:* 37–41 (1979).

15 Powell, R.N.; Cutress, T.W.: Changing patterns of caries prevalence in Tongatapu. Odont. Stom. Trop. *4:* 221–227 (1981).

16 Russell, A.L.: World epidemiology and oral health; in Kreshover, McClure, Environmental variables in oral disease, pp. 21–39 (Am. Ass. Adv. Sci., Washington 1966).

17 Sardo Infirri, J.; Barmes, D.E.: Epidemiology of oral diseases – differences in national levels. Int. dent. J., Lond. *29:* 183–190 (1979).

18 Schulerud, A.: Dental caries and nutrition during wartime in Norway (Fabritius & Sonners, Oslo 1950).

19 Sheiham, A.: Sugars and dental decay. Lancet *i:* 282–284 (1983).

20 Sheiham, A.; Effendi, I.; Noi, B.K.: Assessment of dental needs: pilot studies in Indonesia. Odont. Stom. Trop. *2:* 45–53 (1979).

21 Shimamura, S.: A cohort survey on caries attacks in permanent teeth during a period of approximately 20 kg of annual sugar consumption per person in Japan. J. dent. Hlth *24:* 46–52 (1974).

22 Sofaer, J.A.: Genetics and site attack in dental caries. Comments on Jackson's theory. Br. dent. J. *152:* 267–273 (1982).

23 Speake, J.D.; Cutress, T.W.; Ball, M.E.: The prevalence of dental caries and the concentration of fluoride in the enamel of children in the South Pacific. N.Z. dent. J. *75:* 94–106 (1979).

24 Speake, J.D.; Singh, D.; Ligani, M.: Caries, periodontal disease and the treatment requirements among urban school children in Fiji. Odont. Stom. Trop. *3:* 47–63 (1980).

25 Sreebny, L.M.: Sugar availability, sugar consumption and dental caries. Community Dent. oral Epidemiol. *10:* 1–7 (1982).

26 Takeuchi, M.: On the epidemiological principles in dental caries attack. Bull. Tokyo dent. Coll. *3:* 96–111 (1962).

27 Third World Sugar Forecast. African Business (Jan. 1981).

28 Viton, A.; Pignalosa, F.: Trends and prospects of world sugar consumption. Part I. Mon. Bull. agric. Econ. Statist. *9:* 1–10 (1960).

29 Viton, A.: Pignalosa, F.: Trends and prospects of world sugar consumption. Part II. Mon. Bull. agric. Econ. Statist. *9:* 1–12 (1960).

30 Walker, A.R.P.; Dison, E.; Walker, B.F.; Segal, A.F.: Contrasting patterns of caries profile and dental treatment in pupils of 16–18 years in South African ethnic groups. Community Dent. oral Epidemiol. *10:* 69–73 (1982).

31 World Development Movement: Sugar: crisis in the Third World (London 1980).
32 WHO: Oral health global indicator for 2000. Dental caries levels at 12 years (WHO Oral Health Unit, Geneva 1982).
33 WHO: Prevention of coronary heart disease. Tech. Rep. Ser. 678 (WHO Geneva 1982).
34 Yassin, I.; Low, T.: Caries prevalence in different racial groups of schoolchildren in West Malaysia. Community Dent. oral Epidemiol. 3: 179–183 (1975).

Dr. Aubrey Sheiham, Department of Community Dental Health,
The London Hospital Medical College, Turner Street, London E1 2AD (England)

Cariology Today. Int. Congr., Zürich 1983, pp. 40–48 (Karger, Basel 1984)

Prevention of Dental Disease in Developing Countries

George M. Gillespie

Pan American Health Organization, Washington, D.C., USA

Introduction

In considering the introduction and implementation of preventive programs in oral health in developing countries, it is important to identify certain characteristics which relate to the ability to deliver dental programs as envisaged or designed in more developed countries.

Most notable among these is the per capita income which in many developing countries is less than $500 per year. A review of the World Bank report for 1982 [1] indicates, for example, that in West Africa 13 of the 18 countries identified, in East Africa 10 of the 15, in Middle Asia all 6 identified, and in the Middle East 3 of the 6 identified had per capita incomes less than this level. In Latin America the per capita incomes, with the exception of Haiti, tend to be above this level, even the better-off countries do not have per capita incomes much above $3,000 per year. It is evident therefore, that developing countries have limited capabilities to support continuing programs, particularly in health, which depend on resources more readily available in more affluent and developed countries, some of which also find it hard to continue support for existing health systems.

Developing countries are characterized also by the predominance of the child and adolescent sectors of the population (frequently 40% of the total population) and with a lack of professional and auxiliary dental manpower. Nevertheless, current disease patterns indicate that high levels of dental diseases exist in the populations, such that the matter of conducting dental examinations, other than epidemiological studies, for the purposes of preventive studies would seem of little value [4]. The concept of preventive programs for oral health should therefore concentrate on the enhancement of natural protection [2, 3], provision of added protection against specific disease, procedures to reduce the ability of microorganisms to produce disease, and the modification of behavior patterns to promote oral health and reduce disease.

Current Methods of Prevention

Current methods for the successful prevention of dental caries revolve around the use of fluorides. The first mass preventive measure implemented following the studies by *Dean* and that of the 21 cities in USA was the controlled fluoridation of water supplies. This technique which is now estimated to provide fluoridated water to 300 million persons has proved consistently successful in reducing caries incidence [5]. However, it must be recalled that serious limitations exist to the method in developing countries where treated water is not available to large sectors of the population.

The use of fluoride dentifrices, although expanding rapidly, is now a readily available preventive measure in all countries of the world. Political factors, cost and marketing and distribution problems have limited their use in many countries. Furthermore, the use of toothpaste, rather than traditional or more economical methods, is still a matter for consideration in many cultures.

The opposition and slow implementation of fluoridation prompted the development of alternative approaches to the use of fluorides in developed countries, more specifically, the use of topical fluorides in the form of professionally applied topical application or group applied mouthrinses. Solutions of varying strengths and composition have been utilized to bring fluoride compounds into contact with the tooth surface.

At the present time the results of these approaches are being given considerable attention and credit for the reduction in caries incidence being identified in certain developed countries. Whereas it is worth noting that, apart from water fluoridation, mass applied mouthrinsing for children has been the most readily implemented caries-preventive program, developing countries have utilized manufactured products that are relatively expensive and professional and auxiliary dental manpower.

Fluoride tablet programs have shown great efficacy when conducted in a well-controlled fashion, either on an individual or community basis; however, such tablets are not always readily available and supplies are not constant in many developing countries, quite apart from the relative cost.

In the area of periodontal diseases most emphasis has been placed on treatment of existing disease and the prevention of further recurrence or advancement of the diseases by removal of predisposing factors, such as calculus. Treatment, including if necessary surgical intervention, requires the availability of trained dental personnel, or even a dentist specialized in periodontology, and the currently successful procedures for mechanical removal of calculus require auxiliary personnel trained to perform the appropriate intraoral functions on a frequent basis. It is evident, therefore, that developing countries that are short of dental manpower tend not to have specialized dental manpower. Likewise, such countries often do not have auxiliary personnel trained to perform intraoral functions, let alone in the necessary numbers. Such approaches which have proven effective in reducing the symptoms of disease in developed countries could not be implemented on a large scale in developing countries at this time.

Prevention in the areas of oral cancer, malocclusion, cleft lip and other congenital anomalies depend largely upon the presence of trained personnel to promote such preventive programs and in the availability of professional personnel to treat the disease or correct the deformities. The lack of such personnel in most developing countries signifies that, for the meantime, other approaches will need to be utilized.

Prior to implementation of preventive programs in developing countries it is suggested that the following factors be borne in mind: (1) cultural habits, beliefs and oral hygiene practices; (2) socioeconomic situation; (3) status of existing dental programs and their emphasis; (4) educational level; (5) availability of products and materials; (6) dependence on foreign manufactured materials, products; (7) level of technology required; (8) availability of equipment; (9) currency convertibility; (10) eventual capability to produce materials and products; (11) manpower availability; (12) cost of equipment and materials; (13) maintenance and recurrent program costs; (14) ease of implementation on mass basis, and (15) degree of community organization and participation. It is evident that the most successful long-term programs in most developing countries will make maximum use of national resources, skills and manpower, while reducing costs and dependence on external products and assistance.

Application in Developing Countries

The preceding observations on the most commonly utilized methods for the prevention of the most prevalent dental diseases illustrate that factors of manpower, funds and availability of preventive materials, motivation, and administrators are fundamental to the success of preventive dental programs. In considering the need for preventive programs in developing countries, perhaps the one great determining factor is the need to identify within the particular populations the significance and importance of any preventive procedure [6]. Such a procedure should be one that can be accepted within the cultural behavior patterns of particular populations. For example, the use of an injected vaccine for caries in native populations averse or resistant to any type of injection, the training of dental hygienists for oral prophylactic programs in countries where no awareness exists as to the need to treat or prevent periodontal diseases, and the introduction of toothbrushes and toothpaste to populations accustomed to maintain a good state of oral hygiene through chewstick or natural plants are all preventive approaches that are destined to have little success.

These examples have been provided since in the recent past it has become abundantly apparent that there is an almost universal assumption that all populations accept the toothbrush, toothpaste, dental hygienists, etc. Whereas this assumption no doubt arises because most published dental meetings and seminars tend to involve professionals who have had limited exposure to underdeveloped countries, it is nevertheless to be noted that in a large part of the world such assumptions cannot readily be made. There is also a tendency in area of dental health to assume that a universal mode of dental practice and dental priorities exists. Such an assumption fails to consider that the availability of dental manpower varies from approximately 1 dentist to 500 population in developed urbanized areas to 1 to one million in areas of developing countries. Consequently, different approaches to achieve common objectives need to be devised.

In those parts of the developing world where dental caries presents a problem, or an increasing problem, effective prevention must consider technologies that can be made universally available to the populations at risk. If water supplies reach a majority of the population and the water receives adequate disinfection and treatment, then water fluoridation should be considered. However, thought must be given to the equipment utilized and the ready availability of fluoride compounds. Expensive and complicated machinery imported from industrialized countries should not be considered in favor of simple, more economical equipment that achieves the same objective. The use of saturator cones with sodium silicofluoride and filter beds with fluorspar merit serious consideration in terms of cost, simplicity of operation, and technical scope of available manpower.

Where treated water systems exclude large segments of the population (such as in Latin America where 40% of the population is still without a treated water supply) and where cost and the availability of fluoride compounds are important factors, the fluoridation of salt should be considered as an alternative. With an estimated cost of around 1% of that of water fluoridation (which is in itself cheap as a health preventive measure) and considerable economy in shipping and distribution, yet with benefits comparable to water fluoridation, this approach merits serious consideration in future preventive programs in developing countries. The results of controlled trials and the decision of Switzerland to institute a national program using this vehicle are of great significance in this regard [7, 8].

Limited caries-preventive programs can often be initiated utilizing the approach of mouthrinsing. Such programs which can be directed at a specific population at risk, namely schoolchildren, can readily be implemented since this group is usually captive and controlled. Recognizing the fact that such an approach is not comprehensive for such age-groups, since in developing countries many children may not be enrolled in school, these programs are usually easy to administer and well accepted. A wide variety of personnel, from dental assistants or preventive technicians to schoolteachers, parents and even older grade students, can be utilized to supervise the procedures and such programs are politically attractive since they enable large numbers of people to be identified and covered in a short period of time. In most situations it would appear that the twice monthly mouthrinse with 0.2% sodium fluoride provides the best coverage and use of personnel, while maintaining institutional and individual mouthrinsing. Such programs can easily be combined with supervised oral hygiene or tooth cleaning programs by school personnel.

The use of other vehicles with fluoride, such as fluoride tablets, requires the presence of adequate facilities for the administration and supervision of such a program. However, where such conditions exist, effective caries reductions can be achieved in school populations with daily fluoride intake.

The use of fissure sealants has also been utilized as a preventive measure for dental caries. Such materials can readily and effectively be applied by dental auxiliaries with limited training with notable reduction in dental caries increments; however, the current costs and availability of materials would appear to be limiting their use in countries where manpower is available.

For those who may be sceptical as to the degree to which caries-preventive programs can truly influence the delivery of dental health services, particularly in the public sector, the example of the city of Medellín, Colombia, merits attention. A program of water fluoridation was initiated in 1969, followed by a program of weekly dental education and toothbrushing in school, with an annual supervised self-application of 2% sodium fluoride with a toothbrush over a period of 4 consecutive days. In 1976 a fissure sealant program administered by dental auxiliaries was added. The impact of this combined program has so reduced the increment of dental caries in the school population that schoolchildren now receive dental evaluations and treatment upon school entry and evaluations and treatment prior to school-leaving some 4 years later [9]. The interim caries increment is small and can usually be attended to in 1–2 sessions. Quite apart from the improved oral health and improved cost-benefit of the program, dental health manpower previously utilized for the annual examination and treatment of children now has been effectively utilized to extend population coverage.

In connection with the prevention of periodontal diseases the current approaches to plaque removal in development countries have little application in developing countries [10]. The lack of dental manpower, and specifically dental auxiliary manpower for calculus removal and tooth cleaning, in addition to a general lack of awareness or concern in the populations of the need for such procedures, illustrate that these have limited acceptability at the present time. The use of agents for the removal of plaque, such as chlorhexidine, is dependent upon the availability of such products in the market at an affordable price and on a consistent basis [11, 12].

Prevention of periodontal diseases therefore requires an intensive community effort to make populations aware of the need for oral hygiene and the procedures that they can utilize to facilitate plaque removal. The recent approaches advocated by *Keyes* [13, 14], which also reflect the procedures apparently used effectively by *Van Leeuwenhoek* in the 17th century [15], would seem the most feasible approaches to mass prevention at this time in view of the ready availability of materials and the limited need for dental manpower.

Further studies should be conducted to assess the current ability of traditional oral hygiene practices (such as use of chewsticks, charcoal, toothsticks, plants, roots, etc.) to effect plaque removal or modification to inhibit its dental disease potential. In addition, the widespread nature of periodontal disease and the great volume of the population affected indicates the need for the development of auxiliary personnel capable of instituting simple diagnostic and preventive programs at the community level [16].

General health programs need to involve adequate inclusion of components for the prevention of other oral diseases, such as oral cancer and abnormalities, such as cleft lip and palate. Specific programs need to be implemented to prevent the continuance of certain habits associated with developing countries, such as reverse smoking and tooth mutilation. Other habits which have dietary implications, such as coca chewing with a tendency to produce oral soft tissue hyperplasia, should be included in general diet and nutrition counselling. Wherever possible, diets should be reviewed and the consumption of those substances conductive to plaque formation and dental disease modified. In developing countries, often with consistent dietary habits, change of dietary habits is often impossible, but at least the inclusion of substances into the diet or procedures to modify the effect of cariogenic or other foods should be attemped [17].

The prevention of oral malocclusion is so frequently related to the availability of dental manpower, that such tends to merit limited consideration in the application of preventive programs in most developing countries. Nevertheless, where caries-preventive programs are having an impact, the reduction in tooth morbidity can be considered to be a factor in making preventive programs for maloccusion more accessible to the general population.

Conclusion

The use of mass preventive measures, such as those associated with fluorides, and the implementation of individual or supervised programs of prevention or oral hygiene control have illustrated the feasibility of reducing the prevalence and incidence of dental caries. There is little doubt that in the next decade specific measures for the prevention of dental caries, such as the use of a vaccine for caries or chemotherapeutic or antimicrobial agents for certain periodontal diseases, will further advance the capability to control or prevent such universal dental diseases.

However, the ability to utilize such methods and apply technology in developing countries is dependent upon the ability of the populations involved to accept the procedures recommended within the particular sociocultural and political environment, to make available the necessary ressources to implement the required procedures and to have ready and continuing access to any required technology or proprietary or manufactured products, at a cost that can be supported by the country or population in question.

The process of development has indicated that given the cultural and economic barriers that exist, the successful outcome of prevention of dental diseases in the future will be dependent upon the ability to develop and transfer technology, such that the maximum responsibility is provided to individuals for the simplest and most effective actions to be taken against such diseases.

Any intention or approach to institute a preventive program should first analyze the existing procedures for oral hygiene and treatment of dental disorders, assess their effectiveness and scientific validity prior to instituting new procedures. It is felt that considerable success can be achieved by modifying or encouraging certain existing or traditional oral hygiene practices and by reinforcing the scientific basis of their actions in many countries of the world where it may take time to implement specific dental preventive programs.

References

1   World Bank: Annual report 1982 (World Bank of Reconstruction and Development, Washington 1982).

2   Lehner, T.: Future possibilities for the prevention of caries and periodontal diseases. Br. dent. J. *149:* 318–335 (1980).

3   Lehner, T. et al.: Antibodies to *Streptococcus mutans* and immunoglobulin levels in children with dental caries. Archs oral Biol. *23:* 1061–1067 (1978).

4   Scheiham, A.: Is the six monthly dental examination generally necessary? Br. dent. J. *148:* 94–95 (1980).

5   Strifflen, D.F.; Young, W.O.; Burt, B.A.: Dentistry, dental practice and the community; 3rd ed., pp. 155–256 (Saunders, Philadelphia 1983).

6   Smith, D.F.P.; Brethower, D.; Cabot, D.: Increasing task behavior in a language art program by practicing reinforcement. J. exp. Child Psychol. *8:* 45–62 (1969).

7   Marthaler, T.M.; et al.: Caries preventive salt fluoridation. Caries Res. *12:* 1521 (1978).

8   Mejía, D.R.; Espinal, F.; Velez, H.; Aguirre, S.M.: Use of fluoridized salt in four Colombian communities. VIII. Results achieved from 1964 to 1972. Boln sanit. Panam. *80:* 205–219 (1976).

9   Arango, G.: Personal communication.

10 Davies, G.N.; Downer, M.C.; Holloway, P.J.: The Danish oral health care system for children, and international appraisal (in press, 1983).

11 Ciancio, S.G.: Chemotherapeutics in periodontics. Dent. Clin. N. Am. *24:* (1980).

12 Schiott, C.R.; Loe, H.; Jensen, S.B.; et al.: The effects of chlorhexidine mouthrinses on the human oral flora. J. periodont. Res. *5:* 84 (1970).

13 Keyes, P.H.: Prevención por medios mecánicos y otros medios. Prevención integral en odontología. Ceron *1:* 53–58 (1981).

14 Keyes, P.H.: Prevención pour procedimientos inmunológicos y su perspectiva. Prevención integral en odontología. Ceron *1:* 59–61 (1981).

15 Tal, M.: Periodontal disease and oral hygiene described by Antonio van Leeuwenhoek. J. Periodont. *51:* 668–669 (1980).

16 World Health Organization: Epidemiology, etiology and prevention of periodontal diseases. WHO Techn. Rep. Ser. 621 (World Health Organization, Geneva 1978).

17 Burakoff, R.P.: Dental nutritional guidelines for the 1980's. N.Y. St. dent. J. *47:* 447–448 (1981).

18 Cohen, B.; Bowen, W.H.: Dental caries in experimental monkeys: a pilot study. Br. dent. J. *121:* 269–276 (1966).

19 World Health Organization: Development of indicators, for monitoring progress towards 'Health for All by the Year 2000'. Health for All Series, 4 (World Health Organization, Geneva 1981).

20 World Health Organization: Global strategy for health for all by the year 2000. Health for All Series, 3 (World Health Organization, Geneva 1981).

G.M. Gillespie, DDS, Regional Dental Advisor, PAHO/WHO,
Pan American Health Organization, 525 Twenty-third Street, NW,
Washington, DC 20037 (USA)

Cariology Today. Int. Congr., Zürich 1983, pp. 49–55 (Karger, Basel 1984)

Impact on Research

William H. Bowen

University of Rochester, Department of Dental Research, Rochester, N.Y. USA

The tidal wave of euphoria which greeted the decline in the prevalence of caries has gradually been replaced by a more realistic assessment of what has been accomplished and its consequences for dental research, the practitioner and the general public. Dental caries has not been eliminated nor indeed even brought under control; a reduction in the prevalence by 30% in the Western world is not grounds for complacency although we as a profession are justifiably proud of our accomplishments thus far [*Brunelle and Carlos,* 1982]. It would be flying in the face of reality to believe that the prevalence of dental caries will necessarily continue to decline without any additional efforts. Opinions have been expressed that few challenges [*Leverett,* 1982] remain in caries research and that researchers should abandon cariology and explore other research arenas. I believe that this view is incorrect; the limited, but highly significant, success should entice us to exert even greater efforts to eliminate remaining levels of caries.

Many reasons are offered to explain the declining prevalence of caries in the Western hemisphere [*Bowen,* 1981]. In the United States, where approximately half the population drink fluoridated water, fluoride has undoubtedly played a major role. Nevertheless, significant reductions occurred in areas of the world where water is not fluoridated. Declines in the prevalence of caries have been observed in the Scandinavian countries [*Koch,* 1982] and in Britain [*Anderson* et al., 1982]. Although there is a comprehensive mouth-rinsing program in Scandinavia, this preventive procedure is not widely practiced in Britain. However, fluoride-containing dentifrices now dominate the toothpaste market. Nevertheless, it is difficult to believe that they have had such a major impact because they are used comparatively infrequently in some countries. In addition, they have not been in use in some areas for sufficient duration to explain the observed effects. Furthermore, the usual reduction in caries increment observed in clinical trials of fluoride dentifrices is 20–25%. Several other intriguing possibilities must be examined. For example, there are few individuals who have not been exposed to broad-spectrum antibiotics. The effects on the microbial flora of even short-term exposure to antibiotics are well known. Several studies have shown that patients receiving prophylactic therapy have significantly fewer lesions than untreated cohorts or siblings. Perhaps we are observing a herd immunity. For example the prevalence of other streptococcal diseases such as scarlet fever, rheumatic fever have all declined markedly within the last decade.

It is even conceivable that the public are more dentally conscious than ever before and are more aware of the importance of diet in the etiology of dental caries than heretofore. Indeed in Britain there is evidence that the ingestion of sugars has declined markedly in recent years [*Jervis and Lennon,* 1983].

Although the reasons for the reduction in the prevalence of caries are uncertain, the reduction is nonetheless real. Furthermore, the observed reduction, far from obviating the need for further research, has presented us with an immediate challenge; to determine the reasons for the observed phenomena. There is a clear need for careful epidemiological research, supported by laboratory studies, to explore the reasons for the reduction in caries. A multidisciplined approach is essential if the full potential of any epidemiological study is to be realized.

As a result of the decline in caries prevalence, teeth are being retained longer than before, life expectancy is increasing, and we can therefore expect to observe a changing pattern of oral disease. All the available evidence shows that the prevalence of root surface caries increases with age. Furthermore, the majority of cementum lesions occur on the proximal surfaces of roots thereby making them exceptionally difficult to treat [*Banting* et al., 1980].

Information on the etiology, pathogenesis and methods of prevention of root-surface caries is sparse [*Jordan and Sumney,* 1973]. It appears that a distinctive flora is associated with these lesions and indeed that sucrose ingestion is not essential in the etiology of this disease. Results of investigations carried out by *Schamschula* et al.

[1974] have shown that root-surface caries can develop in some populations even in the complete absence of ingestion of refined carbohydrates.

The pathogenesis of this disease remains obscure. Because of the relatively high organic content of cementum it seems probable that the pathogenesis of root-surface caries differs from that of coronal caries. Research is needed to identify the biochemical changes associated with the initial lesion on cemental caries. Such information could provide avenues for the development of effective methods of prevention.

The use of animal models has contributed greatly to our understanding of coronal caries and has led to means of prevention [*Tanzer*, 1981]. Unfortunately a well-defined animal model to study root surface caries is lacking. Work should proceed to define such a model which will facilitate the evolution of methods for the prevention of root-surface caries.

Recent years have seen a growing interest in the development of remineralizing solutions capable of repairing early enamel lesions. Unequivocal evidence that remineralization of lesions occurs clinically may be found for example in the Turku sugar study [*Scheinin* et al., 1974]. Clearly repair of a carious lesion through remineralization is much more desirable than is the insertion of a restoration. Unfortunately clear guidelines are not available to distinguish those lesions which can be repaired from those that require a restoration. One of the guidelines would undoubtedly include an assessment of the susceptibility of patients to caries. In most instances highly susceptible subjects are not identified until after they have presented themselves at the dental office with numerous lesions. Evidence is available that shows that highly caries prone subjects can be identified by microbiological examination of saliva carried out to estimate the numbers of *Streptococcus mutans* and lactobacilli [*Zickert* et al., 1982a, b]. Microbiological examination of saliva should be as much a part of a dental examination as are radiographs. Persons who are identified as harboring large numbers of these microorganisms have been subjected to a rigorous preventive program with some considerable degree of success [*Zickert* et al., 1982a, b]. However, a large-scale clinical trial is urgently required to determine the effect of rigorous antimicrobial therapy on dental caries. It is imperative that we continue to attempt to develop sophisticated methods of diagnosis which will facilitate the detection of a carious lesion long before cavitation is apparent. Such a development would not only permit the institution of prophylactic treatment in a timely manner, but would probably allow screening of agents with a cariostatic potential in a short period.

The reduction in caries prevalence has increased the difficulty of conducting clinical trials. Frequently many subjects do not develop caries in the course of a trial, increments of caries are small, and as a result large numbers of subjects are required in order to demonstrate a significant effect by an agent with cariostatic potential. Increasing the number of subjects, or prolonging the duration of the trial will add to the costs of conducting the investigation. If clinical trials continue to be conducted in the traditional manner then additional expense may be a major disincentive to the development of cariostatic agents [*König*, 1982].

Although the prevalence of caries is declining in the Western hemisphere there is a growing concern over the upsurge in the developing countries. For the most part the increase appears to be associated with the introduction of Western-type diet [*MacGregor*, 1963]. Many Third World countries frequently lack a sophisticated public health service and therefore the prospects of controlling caries in these situations are poor. Many of the procedures used to prevent caries are based on the assumption that public water supplies are readily available. Attention now needs to be focused on how to deliver preventive measures in developing countries. The fluoridation of a commonly used foodstuff that is centrally produced is an attractive possibility. It appears that salt or sugar [*Marthaler* et al., 1978] could be prime vehicles. However, research is urgently required to determine the optimum dose of fluoride to be added to achieve the desired effect.

It has now been demonstrated unequivocally that dental caries can be prevented in animals by means of vaccination and that immunization can influence the colonization of humans by *S. mutans* [*Bowen*, 1976]. However, the prospects of widespread introduction and acceptance of a vaccine against dental caries in the Western world have declined following the reduction in caries prevalence. Because of increasing prevalence of dental caries, and limited means for its prevention in the Third World, vaccination is a particularly attractive possibility. Every vaccine carries some degree of risk. Because effective means for the prevention of caries are available it appears probable that a caries vaccine would be acceptable in those subjects who are at greatest risk. Many developing countries have active vaccination programs carried out in collaboration with international agencies. The prospect of being able to use a caries vaccine in the Third World should provide a spur to bring the development of a vaccine to a successful conclusion.

Although up to 70% reduction in the prevalence in caries has been reported in areas where water is fluoridated, nevertheless it appears that we are not deriving the maximum potential benefit from the use of fluoride. The protective effect of fluoride is for the most part dependent on the ambient levels of fluoride in the oral cavity. Although it has been established in principle that sustained released fluoride is highly effective in preventing caries in animals, and in raising ambient levels of fluoride in the human mouth [Mirth et al., 1982], further efforts are needed to develop this principle to a level where over-the-counter preparations can be made readily available. It is highly probable that the next major reduction in the prevalence of caries will follow the introduction of readily available sustained release fluoride preparations.

Of all infectious diseases dental caries is unique in that diet plays such a critical role in the expression of the infection. Results from several studies have shown that curbing the frequency of ingestion of carbohydrates has a dramatic effect on the prevalence of caries. Indeed evidence has been presented that shows that this approach is the single most effective method of preventing caries [Granath et al., 1978]. The past several years have seen several methods introduced to determine the cariogenic potential of foods. These have ranged from simplistic in vitro systems to studies in animals and pH measurements in vivo. It is frequently forgotten that all of the tests give information on cariogenic potential and not on cariogenicity of foods per se in humans. The manner and pattern of use will have considerable influence on whether a particular food contributes to the development of caries. There is a need for substantially more investigation into the effect of combination of foods on development of caries. An indication of the importance pattern of ingestion of food can be found in experiments which show the effect of ingestion of cheese after sucrose, in humans and animals [Edgar et al., 1982; Rugg-Gunn et al., 1975]. Epidemiological studies are required that will identify patterns of eating that are associated with high prevalence of caries in humans.

There is growing abundance of evidence showing that a considerable amount of practitioner's time is spent replacing restorations that have fallen prey to secondary caries [Allan, 1977]. Little is known of the factors influencing the development of secondary caries. However, it would appear that if a cavity preparation is 'extended for prevention' that the linear area at risk may be considerably enhanced because the junction between amalgam and enamel is substantially less than perfect. Furthermore, extension of proximal preparations frequently compromises gingival health. With the declining prevalence in caries it is time to evaluate the necessity of routinely adhering to Blacks classic cavity preparations. All too often excess sound tooth structure is removed in the name of a dogma that urgently requires critical reevaluation.

References

Allan, N.: Longitudinal study of dental restorations. Br. dent. J. *143:* 87–89 (1977).

Anderson, R.J.; Bradnock, G.; Beal, J.F.; James, P.M.: The reduction of dental caries prevalence in English schoolchildren. J. dent Res. *61:* 1311–1316 (1982).

Banting, D.W.; Ellen, R.P.; Fillery, E.D.: Prevalence of root-surface caries among institutionalized older persons. Community Dent. oral Epidemiol. *8:* 84–88 (1980).

Bowen, W.H.: Relevance of caries vaccine investigations in rodents, primates and humans: critical assessment. Immunology Abstracts, suppl., Immunologic aspects of dental caries, pp. 11–20 (1976).

Bowen, W.H.: The harvest of research. *60:* 1486–1488 (1981).

Brunelle, J.A.; Carlos, J.P.: Changes in the prevalence of dental caries in US schoolchildren, 1961–1980. J. dent Res. *61:* 1346–1351 (1982).

Edgar, W.M.; Bowen, W.H.; Amsbaugh, S.; Monell-Torrens, E.; Brunelle, J.: Effects of different eating patterns on dental caries in the rat. Caries Res. *16:* 384–389 (1982).

Granath, L.E.; Rootzen, H.; Liljegren, E.; Holst, K.; Kohler, L.: Variation in caries prevalence related to combinations of dietary and oral hygiene habits and chewing fluoride tablets in 4-year-old children. Caries Res. *12:* 83–92 (1978).

Jervis, P.N.; Lennon, M.A.: Sugar consumption in Britain. Department of Child Dental Health, University of Manchester (1983).

Jordan, H.V.; Sumney, D.L.: Root-surface caries: review of the literature and significance of the problem. J. Periodont. *44:* 158–163 (1973).

Koch, G.: Evidence for declining caries prevalence in Sweden. J. dent Res. *61:* 1340–1345 (1982).

König, K.G.: Impact of decreasing caries prevalence: implications for dental research. J. dent. Res. *61:* suppl., pp. 1378–1383 (1982).

Leverett, D.H.: Fluorides and the changing prevalence of dental caries. Science *217:* 26–30 (1982).

MacGregor, A.B.: Increasing caries incidence and changing diet in Ghana. Int. dent J., Lond. *13:* 515–522 (1963).

Marthaler, T.M.; Mejia, R.; Toth, K.; Vines, J.J.: Caries-preventive salt fluoridation. Caries Res. *12:* suppl. 1, pp. 7–14 (1978).

Mirth, D.B.; Shern, R.J.; Emilson, C.; Adderly, D.; Shou-Hua, L.; Gomez, I.; Bowen, W.: Clinical evaluation of an intraoral device for the controlled release of fluoride. J. Am. dent. Ass. *105:* 791–797 (1982).

Rugg-Gunn, A.S.; Edgar, W.M.; Geddes, D.A.M.; Jenkins, G.N.: The effect of different meal patterns on plaque pH in human subjects. Br. dent. J. *139:* 351–356 (1975).

Schamschula, R.; Barnes, D.E.; Keyes, P.H.; Gulbinat, W.: Prevalence and interrelationships of root-surface caries in Lufa, Papua, New Guinea. Community Dent. oral Epidemiol. *2:* 295–304 (1974).

Scheinin, A.; Makinen, K.K.; Ylitalo, K.: Turku sugar studies 1. An intermediate report on the effect of sucrose, fructose and xylitol diets on the caries incidence in man. Acta odont. scand. *32:* 383–412 (1974).

Tanzer, J.: Introduction. Proc. Symp. on Animal Models in Cariology, suppl., pp. xxi–xxii (1981).

Zickert, I.; Emilson, B.G.; Krasse, B.: *Streptococcus mutans,* lactobacilli and dental health in 13–14-year-old Swedish children. Community Dent. oral Epidemiol. *10:* 77–81 (1982a).

Zickert, I.; Emilson, B.G.; Krasse, B.: Effect of caries preventive measures in children highly infected with the bacterium *Streptococcus mutans.* Archs oral Biol. *27:* 861–868 (1982b).

William H. Bowen, BDS, PhD, University of Rochester, Department of Dental Research, 601 Elmwood Avenue, Rochester, NY 14642 (USA)

Saliva

Moderator: J. Mandel, New York, N.Y., USA

Cariology Today. Int. Congr., Zürich 1983, pp. 56–69 (Karger, Basel 1984)

Salivary Flow and Dental Caries

Leo M. Sreebny

Department of Oral Biology and Pathology, School of Dental Medicine, State
University of New York at Stony Brook, Stony Brook, N.Y., USA

'For many years now it has been recognized that the quantity . . .
of saliva has some effect upon the teeth. As to what exactly the effect
is, however, there is considerable divergence of opinion.' This statement
was made by *Pickerill* [1] in Otago, New Zealand, in the year 1912. 70
years later we are still debating the role that the flow of saliva plays in
the pathogenesis of dental caries. That it plays a role there is no doubt.
In the first decade of this century, *Miller* [2] recorded the fact that
individuals with a diminished flow of saliva developed severe, rapidly
spreading carious lesions. Since then, numerous investigators have
demonstrated that severe impairment of salivary secretion, as in irradiation of the glands, tumors, surgical extirpation, hypothyroidism,
Sjogren's syndrome and other conditions, results in a marked increase
in the incidence of caries [3–10]. Similar observations have been made
in experimental animals [11]. *Rosen* et al. [12] showed that extirpation
of the major salivary glands increased caries in caries-resistant rats but
had no effect on caries-susceptible animals; no effect was noted if only
the parotid glands were removed [13, 14]. Accompanying the increase
in caries is a pronounced increase in the number of cariogenic organisms in the oral microflora [15–17].

The situation is quite different when one moves away from conditions wherein salivary flow is severely restricted. Here, despite numerous investigations, it has not been clearly demonstrated that the volume of saliva has a definite relation to caries. (For recent reviews, see
Dawes [18], *Mandel* [19] and *Sweeney* [20]).

Our inability to demonstrate a negative correlation between the
flow of saliva and caries in situations other than those wherein flow is

severely impaired has intrigued and indeed, troubled, many investigators. I do not presume to have the answer to this dilemma, but I
shall, in the course of this presentation, attempt to describe some of the
factors which, I believe, have kept us in limbo.

A major problem arises from the fact that a variety of procedures
have been used to collect the salivary secretions. Contributing to this
variance are – the source of saliva: whole (mixed) saliva or saliva from
the individual salivary glands; the type of saliva: resting or stimulated,
i.e. by mechanical or gustatory agents; the duration of the stimulus, and
the time and method of collection of the specimens. Perhaps of lesser
importance are such factors as the state of hydration of the subjects,
the influence of light and the size of the salivary glands. This methodological potpourri has led to the acquisition of data which are so
diverse, it has been difficult, and in some cases impossible, to compare
one study with another.

Another problem arises from the temporal disjunction which exists
between the collection of saliva and the presence of caries. The existence
of a carious lesion or, indeed, the absence of one, reflects a point in time
which may bear little relation to the flow and composition of saliva
obtained at the time that a particular study is conducted.

The number of subjects examined has also been a problem. A few
quasi-longitudinal studies, e.g. those of *Kerr* [21], have utilized few
subjects; others, like those of *Shannon and Terry* [22], utilized a cross-
sectional approach which involved thousands of individuals. It is
tempting to dismiss those wherein the numbers examined have been few
and to lend credence to those where literally regiments of subjects have
been tested. It has been repeatedly shown, however, that between-
subject variability is greater than within-subject variance. Although one
should rightly question the results obtained from studies with a few
subjects, I should like to remind you that 'safety in numbers' is not a
universal truth. Extreme caution and sense must be used in the interpretation of the data from these different types of investigations.

Finally there is the relationship of saliva to the series of events
which leads to the formation of caries. Caries results from the interaction of organisms in the dental plaque with fermentable carbohydrates
from the diet on a susceptible tooth. Saliva plays an important role in
the pathogenesis of the carious lesion. But it is once removed from the
tooth-plaque locus. It should come as no surprise that significant
relationships between saliva and caries would be more difficult to

obtain than those with events more intimately associated with the site
of the formation of caries.

With respect to the specific issue of salivary flow, I have long felt
that we have been restrictive in our view of how we assess the effect of
the secretion of saliva on dental caries. Perhaps this stems from my love
affair with gardening. Our attitude towards salivary flow is usually
couched in terms which relate to the rate of its entrance into the oral
cavity. This can be compared to the process of irrigation in agriculture.
Any farmer will tell you, however, that the distribution of water to his
plants is but one factor in the success of his irrigation system. Others
involve the addition of fertilizers, the absorption of the irrigating fluid
by the soil and its availability to the plants. With regard to caries, I
propose that salivary flow can conveniently be divided into three
phases: (1) the influx of saliva into the oral cavity; (2) the pooling,
distribution and availability of saliva, and (3) the efflux of saliva from
the mouth. In phase 1, the composition of saliva reflects the composition of the secretions which arise from the ducts of the individual
salivary glands. Contributing to and modifying this ductal secretion,
in phase 2, are the nutrients and other substances which are present in
the foods we eat. In phase 3, the saliva, with its dissolved and suspended
substances, is 'cleared' from the oral cavity.

Phase 1: The Influx of Saliva

The relationship between caries and the rate of flow of saliva has
primarily been investigated for whole saliva and for saliva collected
from the parotid gland. On occasion, studies have also been done with
submandibular saliva. Flow has been measured with and without stimulation.

Parotid Saliva

The most extensive, or should I say exhaustive, study was performed by *Shannon and Terry* [22] with resting, postfasting parotid
saliva. 3,786 male subjects, between 17 and 22 years, were examined.
The subjects were divided into six DMFS groups. The findings showed
that there was a statistically significant inverse relationship between
flow rate and caries susceptibility. The difference in flow between the
caries-free and the caries-active individuals, however, was very small

(0.005 ml/min). This small difference and the high incidence of overlap of flow rate values between the groups led *Shannon and Terry* [22] to question the biologic significance of these findings.

Many other studies with parotid saliva have been conducted; all have failed to show any correlation between flow rates and caries. *Englander* et al. [23] found no significant difference in the flow rate of stimulated parotid saliva between 83 caries-free and caries-rampant subjects. Negative findings were also reported for caries-free and caries-susceptible individuals by *Carter* et al. [24], *Shannon* [25], *Weber* [26] and *Mandel and Zengo* [27].

Submandibular Saliva

By comparison with the parotid gland, few studies have been conducted on submandibular saliva. *Mandel and Zengo* [27] were unable to find significant submandibular gland flow rate differences between 20 caries-resistant and caries-susceptible subjects.

Whole (Mixed) Saliva

The situation is somewhat different with regards to whole saliva. A number of investigators found no significant differences between the rate of flow of resting or stimulated, whole saliva and caries [24, 28–30]. Others have observed an inverse relationship between whole saliva flow and caries experience [31–35].

The relationship of flow rates to caries is further compounded when one considers the matter of the buffer capacity of saliva. Abundant evidence exists which demonstrates that there is a strong negative correlation between the buffering power of whole saliva and caries [1, 36–40]. This relationship has been observed with both resting and stimulated saliva; it is strongest with stimulated saliva [37, 38].

The buffering power of saliva is primarily a function of its bicarbonate content. Its concentration in saliva is positively correlated to the secretory flow rate; so too is salivary pH. It is odd that the secretion-dependent buffering capacity and the pH of saliva have been shown to be significantly and inversely related to dental caries whereas the demonstration of a similar firm relationship between caries and flow rate has remained elusive.

Kleinberg and Jenkins [41] studied the relationship of the rate of flow of resting, whole, saliva to the pH of dental plaques in different areas of the mouth. They observed that there was a significant positive correlation between the rate of flow and the fasting pH of the dental plaque. They showed, moreover, that the higher flow rates of mandibular (submaxillary + sublingual) saliva favored higher plaque pH levels. This was not the case with parotid saliva.

It is clear that, with the exception of the studies that have been performed with the severe interruption of salivary flow, no finite conclusions can be drawn regarding the relationship of the flow of saliva to dental caries. Central to all of the studies are the issues of resting versus stimulated saliva and the type of secretion which should be used.

Resting versus Stimulated Saliva. Becks and Wainwright [42] and recently *Navazesh and Christensen* [43] reported that stimulation decreases the differences in the salivary flow rate among individuals. In the light of these findings, it would appear more prudent to utilize resting rather than stimulated saliva. On the other hand, the caries process occurs during, and immediately following the ingestion of cariogenic foods. It is precisely during this period that saliva is stimulated. This would suggest that stimulated, rather than resting saliva, should be studied.

Whole versus Individual Gland Saliva. With but one exception, none of the many studies with parotid saliva have demonstrated any consistent relationship between flow rate and caries. Likewise, in a study done by *Zengo* et al. [44] on submandibular saliva, no correlation was observed. With resting flow, the parotid gland contributes only about 23% of the total volume of saliva [45]. Since the amount of resting parotid saliva is small (circa 0.05 ml/min) it is not surprising that it has been difficult to correlate any differences between the amount secreted with the prevalence of caries. But even after stimulation, where the contribution of parotid saliva increases to about 50% [18] no association has been found. Only *Shannon and Terry's* [22] massive, but biologically problematic, study showed a slight difference between caries-free and caries-active subjects. It would seem that submandibular saliva, because of its larger contribution to the total volume of saliva, would be the better choice. But in real life, rather than in the sometimes sequestered imagination of scientists, the centerpiece of our concern, the tooth, is bathed in mixed saliva, not by the independent action of saliva from the separate salivary glands. In relating the rate of flow of saliva to caries it would seem more reasonable to study whole, rather than ductal saliva. It is conceivable that small differences in the volume of saliva coupled with but a few percentage differences in the concentration of several ions within it, could account for the differences between resistance or susceptibility to caries.

Phase 2: The Pooling and Availability of Saliva

The salivary glands of man consist of three pairs of large glands – the parotid, submandibular and sublingual glands – and minor glands which are distributed, with the exception of the hard palate and the gingivae, throughout the oral mucosa. The secretions of all of these glands empty into the oral cavity where they are pooled and formed the whole or mixed saliva. This saliva remains in the mouth for a brief period of time and is then swallowed. During this period it lubricates the bolus, i.e. following the ingestion of food, and bathes the teeth, the dental plaque and the oral mucosa.

The whole saliva, however, is not uniformly distributed throughout the mouth. A number of factors contribute to its uneven distribution. Among these are the positioning of the jaws, the division of the mouth into various anatomical compartments, the location of the orifices of the salivary gland ducts and the morphology of the teeth themselves. It is generally recognized that the mandible, especially the area lingual to the anterior teeth retains more saliva than other regions of the mouth. Also, more saliva is available to the smooth surfaces of the teeth than to the deeply fissured and pitted occlusal surfaces.

Deep fissures in teeth are highly susceptible to caries. This, in part is due to the fact that there is an increased retention of food in these areas and to the fact that saliva is not readily available to these restricted regions. In a similar vein, the interproximal areas of tightly apposed teeth are more susceptible to decay and less accessible to saliva than the mesial and distal surfaces of adjacent spaced teeth [48–50].

This distribution of saliva also affects the dental plaque. *Englander* et al. [51] showed that, following a sucrose rinse, there is a greater drop in plaque pH when the availability of saliva is restricted than when saliva is allowed free access to the plaque. *Kleinberg and Jenkins* [41] observed that the fasting pH of the dental plaque for mandibular teeth was higher than that for corresponding maxillary teeth. Moreover, the pH of the plaque in the anterior region of the mandible tended to be higher than that observed in the plaque in the posterior region. They postulated that this was due to the fact that plaques on mandibular, lingual surfaces, as well as those in the anterior region, would be more exposed to saliva than those in other areas of the mouth. It is well known that caries is rarely seen in those areas of the mouth, e.g. the lower incisors, where saliva is abundant. *Kleinberg and Jenkins* [41] also reported that the secretions from the submandibular and sublingual glands had a greater influence on plaque pH than those from the parotid gland. *McNamara* et al. [52], in a study of the composition of human incisor tooth plaques, demonstrated that lactobacilli and *Streptococcus mutans* microorganisms are found more in maxillary incisors than in mandibular approximal plaques. The former site receives less saliva than the latter.

It is evident that in regions of the mouth where the availability of saliva is limited, dental caries, as well as the factors which predispose to caries, are enhanced.

Phase 3: The Efflux of Saliva (Salivary Clearance)

It is widely accepted that dietary carbohydrates play a major role in the pathogenesis of dental caries. Carbohydrate-containing foods which are retained in the mouth, e.g. sticky foods, have the potential to induce high levels of dental decay. Foods which are eliminated or cleared rapidly cause less decay [53]. A number of factors contribute to clearance. Among these are mastication, the flow of saliva and its efflux from the mouth via the process of deglutition.

Limited information is available concerning clearance. The most extensive study was performed by *Swenander-Lanke* [54] in 1957, who showed that individuals differed widely in their ability to clear sugar- and starch-containing foods from the oral cavity. She found moreover, that 10 min after the ingestion of foods, the salivary sugar concentration was an exponential function of the time, i.e. clearance time plotted as a function of the log of the sugar concentration followed a straight line. Although she showed that the mean production of saliva tended to be greater for subjects with a rapid rather than a slow sugar elimination, no statistically significant differences could be observed between the two groups.

Keene et al. [55] could find no differences in the ability of caries-free and caries-active young adults to clear glucose from the oral cavity. On the other hand, *Adorjan and Stack* [56] demonstrated that sugar clearance times were 60% greater in boys with severe caries than in those who were caries-resistant. This distinction could not be shown for girls.

Sreebny et al. [57] showed that sucrose, in solution, was cleared from the saliva in a biphasic manner. Clearance was rapid in phase 1 (0–8 min) and slower in phase 2 (10–20 min). Their findings suggested that the rapid clearance in phase 1 was due to the stimulation of saliva by the sucrose solution; the slow clearance in phase 2 to the resting flow of saliva. Clearance in both phases was linearly related to the log of the sucrose concentration.

Salivary Flow and Dietary Carbohydrates

It has been estimated that the total volume of saliva secreted per day is about 500–620 ml [47]. Virtually no measurable secretion occurs during our daily, hopefully uninterrupted, 7–8 h period of sleep [58]. For most of the remainder of the day, a period of about 15 h, a more or less continuous flow of minimally stimulated basal, or resting, saliva bathes the teeth, the plaque and the oral mucosa. This resting flow contributes about 300 ml to the total volume of saliva. Eating, which occupies about 2 h/day, evokes the secretion of an additional 300 ml of saliva.

Resting saliva contains little carbohydrate but possesses a significant amount of nitrogenous bases. These properties favor the establishment of a plaque oral flora which is more conducive to base, rather than acid, formation [15, 16, 41].

The ingestion of dietary carbohydrates, especially the frequency of their consumption, drastically changes the dynamics of the saliva-plaque system. When dissolved in saliva, the carbohydrates serve as cariogenic substrates for the microorganisms of the dental plaque. However, they also stimulate the flow of caries-protective salivary buffers and nitrogenous compounds because of their physical and gustatory properties. The balance between these factors dictates, to some degree, one's susceptibility or resistance to dental decay.

If the food requires vigorous mastication and/or if it contains potent gustatory stimulants it evokes a copious flow of saliva. If it is in a powdered or liquid form and does not contain strong gustatory agents, it requires little mastication and evokes only a modest flow of saliva [59]. Indeed, it has been shown that powdered and liquid foods induce atrophy of the salivary glands [60].

Stephen [61] was the first to show that, in the presence of a limited, liquid sugar challenge, the plaque pH rapidly falls, often to levels of about pH 5.0. This is then followed by a slow pH rise. If the availability of the substrate is prolonged, as with repeated exposure to sugar, the pH tends to remain low for a protracted period of time and then slowly increases [62]. *Gustafsson* et al. [53] demonstrated that the frequent consumption of solid sugar-containing substances (caramels and toffees) leads to an increase in the incidence of caries. But liquid foods also have the potential to induce decay. *Von der Fehr* et al. [63] demonstrated that rinsing with a 50% sucrose solution, nine times a day, produced incipient carious lesions in a period of 21 days. It is likely that both the frequent intake of the sugar solution coupled with its relative inability to stimulate the flow of saliva contributed to this rapid formation of caries. Evidence also exists that starch, in addition to the mono- and dissacharides, contributes to the development of caries [64–67]. When chewed, starch-containing foods, e.g. bread, tend to be retained on the teeth. As such they have a sustained, rather than a limited ability to provide carbohydrate substrates to the plaque and to stimulate the flow of saliva. In the biphasic Stephan curve, the initial rapid fall in pH represents the cariogenic phase; the slow pH rise, the protective phase. In efforts to correlate the flow of stimulated saliva with caries, salivary samples are usually collected after a poststimulus interval varying between 2 and 15 min, i.e. during the period in which there is a pronounced fall in the plaque pH. There is no a priori reason to believe that this period is sacrosanct; that it alone is critical to our comprehension of the factors which contribute to caries resistance. Indeed, it might be more appropriate to determine the volume of saliva secreted during the protective pH rise phase than during the period in which the pH declines.

Aside from the well-established facts concerning the chewing of paraffin and the use of citric or acetic acids, little is known about the effects of foods on the flow of saliva. It is logical to assume that foodstuffs will differ in their ability to stimulate saliva and therefore differ in their ability to clear carbohydrates from the mouth. A food, for example, which requires vigorous mastication, even though it contains sugar, might evoke an abundant flow of saliva and be eliminated rather quickly. Other foods might prolong clearance; some might clear at the same rate. Indeed, *Swenander-Lanke* [54] showed that a number of starch- and sugar-containing foods which required mastication but which varied greatly in their physical characteristics, had similar clearance rates. In a recent study, *Sreebny* [68] showed that a 25% sucrose and a 25% glucose solution were cleared from saliva at identical rates. Though their saccharide concentrations, on a weight/volume basis, were the same, the sucrose solution is about twice as sweet and its molar concentration is twice that of glucose. The similar clearance rates were attributable to the fact that the sucrose evoked a greater flow of saliva than the glucose.

It is likely that the variable effect of different foods on the flow of saliva exerts a significant effect on their ability to promote caries. This effect might help explain some of the conflicting epidemiologic results which have been obtained regarding the effect of the intake and the frequency of consumption of sugar-containing foods on human dental caries [69]. Indeed, the identification and testing of substances which are present in or could be added to existing foods to promote the flow of saliva would seem to be a profitable area for future research.

It is becoming increasingly evident that the flow of saliva is related to caries resistance. Unfortunately, the evidence is meager and at times conflictual. Much more saliva will have to flow before we fully understand the relationship of flow to the process of dental caries.

References

1   Pickerill, H.P.: The prevention of dental caries and oral sepsis (Baillière, Tindall & Cox, London 1912).
2   Miller, W.D.: A study of certain questions relating to the pathology of teeth. D. Cosmos *46:* 981–1001 (1904).
3   Del Regato, J.A.: Dental lesions observed after roentgen therapy in cancer of the buccal cavity, pharynx and larynx. Am. J. Roentg. *42:* 404–410 (1939).
4   Robinson, H.B.G.: The effect of systemic disease on the caries process – pregnancy, endocrinopathies, osteomalacia, emotional disturbances and others. J. dent. Res. *27:* 113–122 (1948).
5   Frank, R.M.; Herdly, J.; Phillipe, E.: Acquired dental defects and salivary gland lesions after irradiation for carcinoma. J. Am. dent. Ass. *70:* 868–883 (1953).
6   Finn, S.B.; Klapper, C.E.; Volker, J.F.: Intra-oral effects upon experimental hamster caries; in Sognnaes, Advances in experimental caries research, pp. 152–168 (Am. Ass. Adv. Sci., Washington 1955).
7   Silverman, S., Jr.; Chierici, G.: Radiation therapy of oral carcinoma. I. Effect on oral tissues and management of the periodontium. J. Periodont. *36:* 478–484 (1965).

8   Carbone, R.F.; Sweeney, E.A.; Shaw, J.H.: The comparative influence of thyroid imbalance and limited body weight gain on submandibular gland weight, the protein composition of saliva and dental caries in the rat. Archs oral Biol. *11:* 781–792 (1966).

9   Karmiol, M.; Walsh, R.F.: Dental caries after radiotherapy of the oral regions. J. Am. dent. Ass. *91:* 838–845 (1975).

10   Dreizen, S.; Brown, L.; Daly, T.E.; Drane, J.B.: Prevention of xerostomia-related dental caries in irradiated cancer patients. J. dent. Res. *56:* 99–104 (1977).

11   Schwartz, A.; Shaw, J.H.: Studies on the effect of selective desalivation on the caries incidence of albino rats. J. dent. Res. *34:* 239–247 (1955).

12   Rosen, S.; Sreebny, L.M.; Hoppert, C.A.; Hunt, H.R.; Bachem, E.: Studies on salivariectomized Hunt-Hoppert caries-resistant and caries-susceptible rats. J. dent. Res. *37:* 824–831 (1958).

13   Rosen, S.; Hunt, H.R.; Hoppert, C.A.; Sreebny, L.M.; Bachem, E.: Further studies on salivariadenectomized Hunt-Hoppert rats. J. dent. Res. *37:* 54 (1958).

14   Keller, R.F.; Hunt, H.R.; Hoppert, C.A.: Dental caries in caries-susceptible and caries-resistant albino rats *(Rattus norvegicus)* in the absence of secretions of the parotid gland. J. dent. Res. *33:* 558 (1954).

15   Llory, H.; Dammron, A.; Frank, R.M.: Les modifications de la flore buccale aerobic après radiotherapie bucco-pharyrangie. Archs oral Biol. *16:* 617–630 (1971).

16   Llory, H.; Dammron, A.; Gioanni, M.; Frank, R.M.: Some population changes in oral anaerobic microorganisms, *Streptococcus mutans* and yeasts, following irradiation of salivary glands. Caries Res. *6:* 298–311 (1972).

17   Brown, L.R.; Dreizen, S.; Handler, S.; Johnston, D.A.: Effect of radiation induced xerostomia on human oral microflora. J. dent. Res. *54:* 740–750 (1975).

18   Dawes, C.: The effect of diet on salivary secretion and composition. J. dent. Res. *49:* 1263–1272 (1970).

19   Mandel, I.H.: Relation of saliva and plaque to caries. J. dent. Res. *53:* 246–266 (1974).

20   Sweeney, E.A.: Salivary flow and composition in relation to dental caries – methods and problems in studying this relationship in humans and animals; in Kleinberg, Ellison, Mandel, Saliva and dental caries (Information Retrieval Inc., New York 1978).

21   Kerr, A.C.: The physiological regulation of salivary secretions in man (Pergamon Press, New York 1961).

22   Shannon, I.L.; Terry, J.M.: A higher parotid flow rate in subjects with resistance to caries. J. dent. Med. *20:* 128–132 (1965).

23   Englander, H.R.; Mau, L.M.; Hoerman, K.C.; Chauncey, H.H.: Dental caries activity, and the pH, titratable alkalinity and rate of flow of human parotid saliva. J. dent. Res. *37:* 906–911 (1958).

24   Carter, W.J.; Englander, H.R.; Wever, T.B.: Chloride levels in parotid secretion. J. dent. Res. *37:* 902–905 (1958).

25   Shannon, I.L.: Salivary sodium, potassium and chloride levels in subjects classified as to dental caries experience. J. dent. Res. *37:* 401–406 (1958).

26 Weber, T.B.: The rate of flow of constantly stimulated parotid secretion in caries-free and caries-rampant groups. Rep. MR005 (US Naval Training Center, Great Lakes 1960).

27 Mandel, I.H.; Zengo, A.N.: Genetical and chemical aspects of caries resistance; in Mergenhagen, Scherp, Comparative immunology of the oral cavity. DHEW Publ. (NIH) 73–438 (Public Health Service, Bethesda, 1973).

28 White, W.; Bunting, R.W.: A comparison of the chemical composition of stimulated and resting saliva of caries-free and caries-susceptible children. Am. J. Physiol. *117:* 529–532 (1936).

29 Becks, H.; Wainwright, W.W.; Young, D.H.: Does salivary calcium and phosphorous differ significantly in caries-free and caries-active individuals? J. dent. Res. *20:* 171–188 (1941).

30 Ericsson, Y.: Investigations into the relationship between saliva and dental caries. Acta odont. scand. *11:* 179–194 (1954).

31 Trimble, H.C.; Ethrington, J.W.; Losch, P.K.: Rate of secretion of saliva and incidence to dental caries. J. dent. Res. *17:* 299 (1938).

32 Hewat, R.E.T.: Dental caries: an investigation in search of determining factors and its manifestation. N.Z. dent. J. *28:* 45–59 (1932).

33 Cushman, F.H.; Ethrington, J.W.; Thompson, G.E.: Relation of salivary surface tension and rate of flow to dental caries in an adolescent group. J. dent. Res. *20:* 251 (1941).

34 McDonald, R.E.: Human saliva: a study of the rate of flow and viscosity and its relationship to dental caries; thesis Indiana University (1950).

35 Rovelstad, G.H.; Geller, J.H.; Cohen, A.H.: Caries susceptibility tests hyaluronidase activity of saliva and dental caries experience. J. dent. Res. *37:* 306–311 (1958).

36 Hubbell, R.B.: The chemical composition of saliva and blood serum of children in relation to dental caries. Am. J. Physiol. *105:* 436–442 (1933).

37 Karshan, M.: Factors in human saliva correlated with dental caries. J. dent. Res. *18:* 395–407 (1939).

38 Ericsson, Y.: Enamel-apatite solubility. Acta odont. scand. *8:* suppl. 3, pp. 5–139 (1949).

39 DeWar, M.R.: Laboratory methods for assessing susceptibility to dental caries. II. Correlation of results obtained by clinical examination and by standardized laboratory methods. Dent. J. Aust. *22:* 24–35 (1950).

40 Turner, N.C.; Anders, J.T.: Titratable acidity and titratable alkalinity of the saliva of cases with reference to dental caries. J. dent. Res. *35:* 385–390 (1956).

41 Kleinberg, I.; Jenkins, G.N.: The pH of dental plaques in the different areas of the mouth before and after meals and their relationship to the pH and the rate of flow of resting saliva. Archs oral Biol. *9:* 493–516 (1964).

42 Becks, H.; Wainwright, W.W.: The effect of activation on salivary flow. J. dent. Res. *18:* 447–456 (1939).

43 Navazesh, M.; Christensen, C.M.: A comparison of the whole mouth resting and stimulated salivary measurement procedures. J. dent. Res. *61:* 1158–1162 (1982).

44 Zengo, A.N.; Mandel, I.D.; Goldman, R.; Khurana, H.S.: Salivary studies in human caries resistance. Archs oral Biol. *16:* 557–560 (1971).

45 Schneyer, L.H.; Levine, L.K.: Rate of secretion by exogenously stimulated salivary gland pairs in man. J. appl. Physiol. 7: 609–613 (1955).

46 Dawes, C.: Rhythms in salivary flow rate and composition. Int. J. Chronobiol. 2: 253–279 (1974).

47 Jenkins, G.N.: The physiology and biochemistry of the mouth (Blackwell, Oxford 1978)

48 Barr, J.H.: Some characteristics of caries on proximal surfaces of teeth. J. dent. Res. 28: 466–482 (1949).

49 Nevin, R.B.; Walsh, J.P.: Physico-chemical factors in relation to the cause of proximal caries. J. dent. Res. 30: 234–250 (1951).

50 Keene, H.J.; Shklair, I.L.; Hoermann, K.C.: Caries immunity in naval recruits and ancient Hawaiians; in Mergenhagen, Scherp, Comparative immunology of the oral cavity. DHEW Publ. (NIH) 73–438 (Public Health Service, Washington 1973).

51 Englander, H.R.; Shklair, I.L.; Fosdick. L.S.: The effects of saliva on the pH and lactate concentration in dental plaques. I. Caries-rampant individuals. J. dent. Res. 38: 848–853 (1959).

52 McNamara, T.F.; Friedman, B.K.; Kleinberg, I.: The microbial composition of human incisor tooth plaque. Archs oral Biol. 24: 91–95 (1979).

53 Gustafsson, B.; Quensell, C.E.; Lanke, L.S.; Lundquist, C.; Grahen, H.; Bonow, B.O.; Krasse, B.: The Vipeholm Dental Caries Study. Acta odont. scand. 11: 232–363 (1954).

54 Swenander-Lanke, L.: Influence on salivary sugar of certain properties of foodstuffs and individual oral conditions. Acta odont. scand. 15: suppl. 23, pp. 3–156 (1957).

55 Keene, H.J.; Coykendall, A.L.; Lahmeyer, H.A.: Oral glucose clearance time in caries-active and caries-free naval recruits. J. dent. Res. 45: 409 (1966).

56 Adorjan, J.A.; Stack, M.V.: Oral sugar clearance in children. Br. dent. J. 141: 221–222 (1976).

57 Sreebny, L.M.; Chatterjee, R.; Kleinberg, I.: Clearance of sugar from the oral cavity. J. dent. Res. 62: 217 (1983).

58 Schneyer, L.H.; Pigman, W.; Hanahan, L.; Gilmore, R.W.: Rate of flow of human parotid, sublingual and submaxillary secretions during sleep. J. dent. Res. 35: 109–114 (1956).

59 Hall, H.D.; Merig, J.J.; Schneyer, C.A.: Metrecal induced changes in human saliva. Proc. Soc. exp. Biol. Med. 124: 532–536 (1967).

60 Sreebny, L.M.; Johnson, D.A.: Effect of food consistency and decreased food intake on rat parotid and pancreas. Am. J. Physiol. 215: 455–460 (1968).

61 Stephan, R.M.: Changes in hydrogen-ion on tooth surfaces and in carious lesions. J. Am. dent. Ass. 27: 718–723 (1940).

62 DeBoever, J.; Muhlemann, H.R.: The effect of concentrated sucrose solutions on the pH of interproximal plaque. Helv. odont. Acta 13: 27–28 (1969).

63 Fehr, F.R. von der; Loe, H.; Theilade, E.: Experimental caries in man. Caries Res. 4: 131–148 (1970).

64 Volker, J.F.; Pinkerton, D.M.: Acid production in saliva – carbohydrate mixtures. J. dent. Res. 26: 229–232 (1947).

65 Kleinberg, I.: Formation and accumulation of acid on tooth surfaces. J. dent. Res. 49: 1300–1316 (1970).

66   Mormann, J.E.; Muhlemann, H.R.: Oral starch degradation and its influence on acid production in human dental plaque. Caries Res. *15:* 166–175 (1981).
67   Sreebny, L.M.: Cereal availability and dental caries. Community Dent. oral Epidemiol. *10:* 1–7 (1982).
68   Sreebny, L.M.: Unpublished data (1983).
69   Sreebny, L.M.: Sugar and human dental caries. Wld Rev. Nutr. Diet., vol. 40, pp. 19–65 (Karger, Basel 1982).

Prof. Leo M. Sreebny, Department of Oral Biology and Pathology,
School of Dental Medicine, State University of New York at Stony Brook,
Stony Brook, NY 11794 (USA)

Cariology Today. Int. Congr., Zürich 1983, pp. 70–74 (Karger, Basel 1984)

Inorganic Constituents of Saliva in Relation to Caries

C. Dawes

Department of Oral Biology, Faculty of Dentistry, University of Manitoba, Winnipeg, Canada

In 1978, a symposium was held which covered, in a very comprehensive way, the relation of saliva to dental caries [*Kleinberg* et al., 1979]. Only minimal advances have been made since that time in our knowledge of the inorganic constituents of saliva per se. The inorganic constituents of saliva which appear to be particularly related to caries are calcium, phosphate, fluoride, bicarbonate and hydrogen ions. These components are important collectively, rather than individually because their concentrations together determine the degree of saturation of saliva with respect to hydroxyapatite and fluorapatite, of which enamel is composed. However, a complicating factor is that enamel is not a pure apatite but contains a variable content of carbonate and many trace elements. The ion products for hydroxyapatite and fluorapatite are

$$[^aCa^{2+}]^5[^aPO_4^{3-}]^3[^aOH^-] \text{ and } [^aCa^{2+}]^5[^aPO_4^{3-}]^3[^aF^-],$$

respectively, where a is the activity. Since the pCO_2 is relatively constant in saliva and independent of flow rate, the bicarbonate concentration, which increases with flow rate, determines the pH. The relationship is from the Henderson-Hasselbalch equation:

$$pH = pK + \log \frac{[HCO_3^-]}{[H_2CO_3]}$$

where the pK is about 6.1 and $H_2CO_3 = 0.03 \times pCO_2$.

In virtually all samples of saliva the ion product exceeds the solubility product for both hydroxyapatite and fluorapatite and especially for the latter. Thus in order for enamel demineralization to occur in saliva, the pH must be decreased. This then causes a decrease in both $[^aOH^-]$ and $[^aPO_4^{3-}]$. At some so-called critical pH, variously estimated to be between pH 5.5 and 6.5, the enamel will begin to dissolve [Fosdick and Starke, 1939; Ericsson, 1949]. Bicarbonate has an additional role to that of controlling pH. It is a very effective buffer and diffusion of bicarbonate into plaque may be an important mechanism by which stimulated saliva helps to reduce the fall in plaque pH which occurs after carbohydrate consumption [Frostell, 1979; Abelson and Mandel, 1981]. In vivo, of course, caries does not occur at the interface between enamel and saliva but at that between enamel and dental plaque. Thus the composition of the fluid phase of dental plaque rather than that of saliva would appear to be critically important for caries initiation. The concentrations of certain components of plaque fluid were reported by Tatevossian and Gould [1976] to be considerably higher than those in saliva.

We have recently studied the electrolyte content of several plaque fluid samples obtained after pooling plaque from all available sites within the mouths of individual patients a few hours after they had last eaten. The results for four individual samples together with the mean results for analyses of individual electrolytes in a larger number of samples are shown in table I. The findings confirm those of Tatevossian and Gould [1976] and also provide new information on chloride. In calculating the total anion concentration in mEq/l, the pH was assumed to be 7.1 so that the phosphate value in mM/l could be multiplied by 1.5.

There are several surprising and unexplained features of the composition of plaque fluid. Several groups of workers have recently reported that the coefficients for diffusion of various substances through plaque are only slightly less than those through water [Tatevossian, 1979; McNee et al., 1980; Dibdin, 1981; Dibdin et al., 1983]. By what mechanism then is the osmotic pressure in plaque fluid maintained at a value approximately equal to that in plasma (300 mosm/kg) rather than that in unstimulated saliva (about 50 mosm/kg) which is normally in contact with the surface of plaque? The high concentrations of ammonia and organic acids are presumably due to bacterial metabolism of urea and carbohydrate, respectively. However, the concentrations of all other components except chloride are also severalfold higher than those in saliva. Why does water not diffuse into the plaque to

Table I. The composition of plaque fluid (mM/l)

	Complete analysis of individual samples				Mean of separate analyses ± SD	n
	1	2	3	4		
OP, mosm/kg	391	281	244	257	304 ± 48	17
Na	19.0	28.5	27.5	18.7	20.8 ± 4.9	16
K	94.5	79.0	49.5	82.2	78.7 ± 15.0	16
Ca	6.2	4.6	5.6	5.2	5.3 ± 1.6	16
Mg	4.2	2.9	2.9	2.4	4.1 ± 1.4	16
NH_4	43.0	20.6	27.9	34.3	35.6 ± 12.9	11
HCO_3	–	6.4	2.2	–		
Cl	39.4	29.4	32.2	22.8	28.5 ± 5.2	10
PO_4	23.2	12.0	11.6	18.7	20.4 ± 5.9	9
Organic acids	101.5	110.0	106.5	107.0	102.1 ± 9.8	5
Total cations, mEq/l	177.3	143.1	121.9	150.4	153.9	
Total anions, mEq/l	175.7	163.8	158.3	157.8	161.2	

reduce the osmotic gradient or why do the various ions not diffuse out into the surrounding saliva?

Presumably some of the ions such as calcium and phosphate must be bound, otherwise spontaneous precipitation of calcium phosphate salts to form calculus would be expected. This does, of course, occur in many individuals. One possibility which may account for the high concentrations of potassium, magnesium and phosphate and the 'expected' concentration of chloride is that bacteria within the depths of the plaque are continually dying and disintegrating. Potassium, magnesium and phosphate are typically present in high concentrations intracellularly whereas chloride is not.

It should be emphasized that the data shown in table I is for mature plaque. There appears to be no information available about the fluid-phase composition of early plaque or indeed that of plaque from occlusal fissures which is not in contact with gingival crevice fluid. A comprehensive investigation of the factors influencing the composition of plaque fluid would be very appropriate.

At the symposium on Saliva and Dental Caries [*Kleinberg* et al., 1979] there was general agreement that the flow rate of saliva was particularly important with respect to caries because of the rampant caries which occurs in patients with severe xerostomia.

Flow rate would appear to affect caries in two major ways. As the flow rate is decreased, the composition of saliva changes, perhaps the most important effect being a reduction in bicarbonate concentration. This reduces both the buffering capacity of saliva and also, as mentioned previously, its degree of saturation with respect to hydroxyapatite. The other effect of flow rate on caries is that a reduction slows the rate of clearance of sugar from the oral cavity after carbohydrate consumption. In a very recent theoretical analysis of salivary clearance of sugar from the mouth [*Dawes*, 1983], three very important variables were identified. The most important, as might have been expected, was the unstimulated salivary flow rate. However, also very important were the volume of saliva remaining in the mouth after a normal swallow (RESID) and the volume present in the mouth prior to swallowing (VMAX). These latter parameters have previously received no discussion in the literature. Preliminary unpublished studies in this laboratory in collaboration with Dr. *F. Lagerlof* suggest that the value of 0.3 ml for RESID assumed by *Dawes* [1983] in the model, is considerably too low.

In conclusion then, further studies are needed of the interrelationship between the concentrations of the inorganic components of saliva and plaque fluid and of the role of saliva in clearance of sugar from the mouth.

References

Abelson, D.C.; Mandel, I.D.: The effect of saliva on plaque pH in vivo. J. dent. Res. *60:* 1634–1638 (1981).

Dawes, C.: A mathematical model of salivary clearance of sugar from the oral cavity. Caries Res. *17:* 321–334 (1983).

Dibdin, G.H.: Diffusion of sugars and carboxylic acids through human dental plaque in vitro. Archs oral Biol. *26:* 515–523 (1981).

Dibdin, G.H.; Wilson, C.M.; Shellis, R.P.: Effect of packing density and polysaccharide to protein ratio of plaque samples cultured in vitro upon their permeability. Caries Res. *17:* 52–58 (1983).

Ericsson, Y.: Investigations into the calcium phosphate equilibrium between enamel and saliva and its relation to dental caries. Acta odont. scand. *8:* suppl. 3, pp. 1–139 (1949).

Fosdick, L.S.; Starke, A.C.: Solubility of tooth enamel in saliva at various pH levels. J. dent. Res. *18:* 417–430 (1939).

Frostell, G.: The effect of chewing on the pH of dental plaques after carbohydrate consumption. Acta odont. scand. *32:* 79–82 (1979).

Kleinberg, I.; Ellison, S.A.; Mandel, I.D.: Saliva and dental caries. suppl. Microbiology Abstracts, pp. 1–575 (Information Retrieval Inc., New York 1979).

McNee, S.G.; Geddes, D.A.M.; Main, C.; Gillespie, F.C.: Measurements of the diffusion coefficient of NaF in human dental plaque in vitro. Archs oral Biol. *25:* 819–823 (1980).

Tatevossian, A.: Diffusion of radiotracers in dental plaque. Caries Res. *13:* 154–162 (1979).

Tatevossian, A.; Gould, C.T.: The composition of the aqueous phase in human dental plaque. Archs oral Biol. *21:* 319–323 (1976).

C. Dawes, BDS, PhD, Department of Oral Biology, Faculty of Dentistry, University of Manitoba, Winnipeg R3E OW3 (Canada)

Cariology Today. Int. Congr., Zürich 1983, pp. 75–88 (Karger, Basel 1984)

Antimicrobial Activity of the Secretory Innate Defense Factors Lactoferrin, Lactoperoxidase and Lysozyme[1]

Roland R. Arnold[a,b], James E. Russell[a], Sara M. Devine[a], Michael Adamson[a], Kenneth M. Pruitt[c]

[a]Department of Oral Biology, School of Dentistry, and [b]Department of Microbiology and Immunology, School of Medicine, University of Louisville, Louisville, Ky.; [c]Division of Molecular Biology, University of Alabama in Birmingham, Medical Center, Birmingham, Ala., USA

Introduction

Saliva contains a variety of factors including secretory IgA (SIgA), lactoferrin (LF), lysozyme and lactoperoxidase, which could contribute to the regulation of the dental plaque flora. The independent effects of the purified components on selected isolates of the oral flora have been the subjects of investigation of several laboratories. An understanding of the antimicrobial potential of these molecules is essential to our understanding of the host-parasite relationships that exist at surfaces bathed by secretions. In examining the individual aspects of these factors, it is important not to lose sight of the environment in which they operate. It is apparent that these components occur concurrently in secretions and they may influence the activity of one another. The purpose of this paper is to characterize the activity of several of these secretory glycoproteins on *Streptococcus mutans* and explore several potential interactions between these factors that may be expressed in situ.

[1] This work was supported in part by Public Health Service grant DE 05722 from the National Institute for Dental Research. Dr. *Adamson* was supported by Public Health Service National Research Service Award DE 05323.

Antimicrobial Abilities of LF

LF is a member of the transferrin group of molecules, which are unique in nature in their coordinate binding of metallic ions and anions [1, 2]. There is preferential binding of ferric ion with a bicarbonate anion at two independent sites on the molecule each with an affinity of approximately 10^{36} [3]. LF is synthesized by acinar epithelial cells of virtually all mucosal surfaces and is found in the specific granules of polymorphonuclear leukocytes [4, 5]. A biological function for LF has been attributed to its high affinity for iron and its consequent deprivation of this essential metal from invading microorganisms [reviewed in 6]. The importance of this bacteriostatic (iron-reversible) function is suggested by the association of bacterial iron-chelating molecules with virulence and the enhancement of infectivity by simultaneous challenge with iron [reviewed in 6].

LF is also capable of a bactericidal effect on *S. mutans,* as well as a variety of other microorganisms [7, 8] that is distinct from simple iron deprivation. Although iron saturation of purified LF eliminates this activity, exogenous iron (either as Fe^{3+}, Fe^{2+}, hematin or ferritin) does not block LF killing of *S. mutans* when introduced into the reaction mixture [9]. *S. mutans* is dependent on iron for growth, however, it can be maintained in the absence of iron for periods to 72 h without significant loss in viability. This is in contrast to the rapid loss in viability (within 15 min at 37 °C) observed with LF treatment [10]. Furthermore, *S. mutans* can grow in iron-depleted medium containing iron-saturated LF [9], suggesting that *S. mutans* is not only not susceptible to LF stasis, but is capable of using LF-associated iron.

Bactericidal Activity of Purified Colostral LF

Subsequent studies have been directed at characterizing the mechanism of action and the conditions that modulate LF-mediated killing of *S. mutans.* For these studies LF is purified from the decaseinated whey of human colostrum and early milk by heparin affinity chromatography [11] to a fidelity equivalent to that obtained by the more involved ion exchange and molecular sieve procedures previously employed [12]. LF is deferrated (apo-LF) by dialysis against 0.04 *M*

EDTA–0.2 M phosphate–0.04 M acetate buffer (pH 4.6) followed by exhaustive dialysis against deionized, distilled water [13].

S. mutans strain NCTC 10449 is grown to early exponential phase in Todd-Hewitt broth at 37 °C, washed in distilled water and incubated at 1×10^7 CFU equivalents with various concentrations of apo-LF in 1 ml. Viability is determined by plating serial dilutions on trypticase soy agar containing 1% sucrose. As can be seen in figure 1, there is a concentration dependent cidal kinetics with killing detected at each of the dilutions tested. The effect of reducing the relative concentration of apo-LF is an increase in the lag period before initiation of death. Increasing the concentration above an optimum of 1.2×10^{-6} M (100 μg/ml) for 1×10^7 CFU does not detectably influence the kinetics of killing at 37 °C, which is characterized by a lag of 15 min prior to the

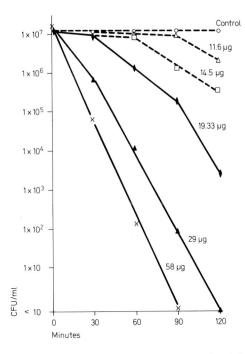

Fig. 1. Effects of LF concentrations on the viability of S. mutans NCTC 10449. Washed suspensions of exponential phase bacteria (1×10^7 CFU/ml) were treated at 37 °C with increasing concentrations (as μg/ml) of purified, iron-free human LF. Control contained 58 μg/ml iron-saturated LF.

initiation of exponential death [10]. It is important to note that there is significant killing (80% reduction in recoverable CFU) by 2 h with 11.6 μg/ml (1.5×10^{-7} M) (fig. 1). This level is in the concentration range of LF in parotid saliva and cidal activity can even be detected with tenfold less apo-LF over a longer time period (data not shown).

Effects of Increased Temperature on Killing

Previous studies have indicated that temperature influences the bactericidal activity of apo-LF on S. mutans, with no death detected at 2 °C, detectable activity at 4 °C and intermediate killing at 22 °C [10]. Recent studies have indicated that increasing the temperature of treatment to 39 or 41 °C has pronounced effects on apo-LF killing of various enteric bacteria [manuscript submitted]. Likewise elevating the temperature enhanced apo-LF killing of S. mutans (table I). There is a significant difference between the rate of killing observed at 37 °C and that at 39 °C. The most pronounced effect appears at 15 min where there is greater than 97% reduction in viable CFU at 39 °C. There was no detectable difference between the effects at 39 and 41 °C. This temperature effect may have biological implications for febrile responses.

Effects of Iron and Glucose Deprivation on LF Susceptibility

The iron-chelating properties of LF have been well characterized and the potential involvement of iron binding in the cidal mechanism would be logical. Although exogenous iron does not block LF killing, it is possible that the iron was not introduced in a proper form to be competitive with bacterial-associated iron. It is possible that the cidal mechanisms of LF involve active removal of essential iron from the cell, therefore bacteria deprived of iron would be predicted to be more sensitive to LF killing. S. mutans was serially passaged in PD medium depleted of iron [9] or glucose until the bacteria were no longer capable of growing. These bacteria were maintained for 18 h at 37 °C without growth in these media. Control cultures were grown to an equivalent number of CFU/ml in complete PD medium. Cells were washed and resuspended in mineral salts, and tested for LF susceptibility. The rate of killing of iron-deprived *S. mutans* was consistently reduced when compared to controls (table II). In contrast, bacteria maintained under glucose-free conditions were more readily killed by LF. Previous studies have suggested that an initial event in LF activity is an inhibition of glucose utilization [9]. These data suggest that LF mechanism may

Table I. Effects of increasing temperature on the bactericidal activity of LF[1] on *S. mutans* NCTC 10449

Incubation temperature	Exp.	Time of apo-LF exposure, min				
		0	15	30	60	120
37 °C	I	98[2]	64	0.58	0.20	0.028
	II	112	NT[3]	NT	5.01	0.11
39 °C	I	88	2.2	0.12	0.04	0
	II	102	NT	NT	0.01	0
41 °C	II	110	NT	NT	0.04	0

[1] Apo-LF at 25 µg with 1×10^7 CFU equivalents/ml of mineral salts.
[2] Percentage recoverable CFU.
[3] Not tested.

Table II. Effects of iron deprivation and glucose deprivation in partially defined media (PD) on susceptibility of *S. mutans* NCTC 10449 to the bactericidal activity of LF

Medium	Exp.	Time at 37 °C, min		
		0	60	120
Complete PD	I	93.3[2]	0.0068	0
	II	117.5	0.013	0.00023
PD (–Fe)	I	107.2	0.32	0.0035
	II	103.4	0.55	0.0059
PD (–Glu)	I	97.7	0	0
	II	101.7	0	0

[1] Apo-LF at 43 µg with 1.0×10^7 CFU equivalents/ml.
[2] Percentage recoverable CFU.

involve effects on carbohydrate utilization and or energy reserves, rather than iron depletion.

LF Activity in Secretions

Evidence from several areas suggests that LF must gain access to the bacterial cell surface and likely to the cytoplasmic membrane for expression of the cidal effect. Increased extracellular carbohydrate polymers (e.g. glucan for S. mutans and pneumococcal polysaccharide capsule) increase the resistance of these bacteria to LF [8]. Likewise, wild type strains of Salmonella typhimurium are resistant to LF, but mutants with progressive deletions in carbohydrate side chains in LPS are increasingly sensitive to LF, as are wild type strains pretreated with EDTA [manuscript submitted]. In addition purified SIgA with antibody activity to S. mutans can block LF killing [12]. Recent studies indicate that the cytoplasmic membrane of S. mutans becomes leaky to ATP following exposure to LF [unpublished observations].

Although LF is present in human parotid saliva and milk whey at concentrations that should be bactericidal the majority of native samples from normal individuals tested do not kill S. mutans. This could be due to iron saturation, improper bicarbonate/citrate ratios [14, 15], SIgA blocking [12] or calcium-mediated tetramer formation. The latter would result in a molecular complex greater than 300,000 daltons that would not be expected to penetrate the cell wall. That this may block LF killing is suggested by the observation that dialysis against Ca^{2+} blocks the bactericidal capabilities of this molecule [unpublished observations].

Of numerous normal human milk whey samples tested only two have been found that were capable of killing S. mutans. Both were early colostral samples and subsequent samples from the same mothers failed to kill. Experiments were designed to determined what was responsible for the lack of killing in saliva and whey (table III). Test samples were added in 200-μl volumes to a final volume of 1 ml containing 1×10^7 CFU of S. mutans NCTC 10449. Viability was determined after 1 h at 37 °C. The early whey sample resulted in greater than a 99% reduction in CFU; whereas, the later whey (day 5) was noncidal (table III). The cidal activity of the early whey could be eliminated by dialysis against iron (implicating LF as the cidal component) and was blocked by the

Table III. Viability as % recoverable CFU of *S. mutans* 10449 after incubation for 1 h at 37 °C with various admixtures of LF, SIgA, colostral whey and parotid saliva

	Mineral salts	SIgA[1]	Whey (day 5)	Parotid saliva
LF (70 µg/ml)	0.08 (89)[2]	107	111	70.1 (6.76)[3]
Early whey (day 2)	0.32 (72)[2]	118	98 (96.5)[3]	NT
Mineral salts	100	100	96.2 (99.7)[3]	93.3 (70.1)[3]

[1] Bacteria preincubated with 1 mg purified SIgA were washed and resuspended in mineral salts prior to testing.
[2] Dialysis against 100 mM Fe(NH$_4$)$_2$SO$_4$ followed by exhaustive dialysis against deionized, distilled water.
[3] Dialysis against EDTA-PO$_4$-acetate buffer followed by exhaustive dialysis against deionized, distilled water.

presence of the noncidal milk. The inability of the day 5 whey to kill was not simply due to inactive LF as dialysis procedures to remove Fe^{3+} and Ca^{2+} failed to render this sample cidal and LF purified from noncidal milk was fully capable of killing *S. mutans,* but not in the presence of whey (table III). SIgA purified from noncidal milk was capable of blocking *S. mutans* killing by LF and whey. That this was not a nonspecific protein effect was suggested by the fact that SIgA-coated bacteria were not susceptible to LF mediated killing (table III). SIgA may also contribute to the blocking effects of parotid saliva; however, unlike the whey, dialysis of saliva against EDTA-phosphate-acetate buffer reduced the observed inhibition of LF (table III). The lower concentrations of salivary IgA (approximately 40 µg/ml, log$_2$ agglutinin titer of 5) may not be adequate kinetically to completely block LF killing, as is observed with whey (approximately 1 mg/ml SIgA, log$_2$ agglutinin titer of 10).

Both whey samples had detectable SIgA antibody activity (agglutinin and indirect immunofluorescence) reactive with *S. mutans,* however the epitope specificity was not determined. The oral streptococci, including *S. mutans,* are likely perceived as normal flora by the host immune system. All the oral streptococci tested were sensitive to LF killing [8]. In addition, levels of antibodies reactive with the oral flora are consistently elevated in salivary IgA relative to that in the serum immunoglobulins [16]. This may suggest an additional function for SIgA, one of selecting for normal flora by protecting against other antimicrobial factors. Such a regulatory function has additional validity when one considers that LF killing of certain enterics requires the presence of synergistic SIgA [manuscript submitted] and that the presence of SIgA (either purified, in whey or in saliva) does not block LF killing of *Legionella pneumophila* [manuscript in preparation]. These data suggest a dual function of synergism and antagonism for LF that may be involved in the selection for normal flora and against potential pathogens. The shift from killing of *S. mutans* in early whey to blocking in later samples may suggest a shift in epitope specificity (nonblocking or synergistic to antagonistic) as the normal flora is being established.

Antimicrobial Effects of the Salivary Peroxidase System

An antibacterial system consisting of peroxidase (LPO) enzyme and the cofactors hydrogen peroxide (H_2O_2) and thiocyanate (SCN^-) has been demonstrated in saliva [17] and milk [18, 19]. In human saliva, LPO catalyzes the oxidation of SCN^- to produce hypothiocyanite ($OSCN^-$) and hypothiocyanous acid (HOSCN) which are in acid-base equilibrium [20, 21]. Inhibition of metabolism is attributed to oxidation of essential bacterial sulfhydryls to the sulfenyl or disulfide oxidation state [22, 23]. This inhibition is generally reversible by the addition of reducing agents such as 2-mercaptoethanol (2-ME) or dithiothreitol. Antibacterial activity is greater at lower pH [18] presumably due to the ability of the uncharged HOSCN to diffuse across the cell membrane and attack essential intracellular enzymes [24]. The salivary glands concentrate SCN^- from blood and the concentration of SCN^- in human saliva ranges from 0.1 to 5 mM [25]. The H_2O_2 production in saliva has been attributed to leukocytes [26] and to oral streptococci and lactobacilli [27]. Although H_2O_2 has not been measured directly in saliva, there is an accumulation of detectable amounts of $OSCN^-$ [28]. It is generally agreed that H_2O_2 is the rate-limiting component for this system in vivo and is primarily dependent on the metabolism of certain catalase-negative oral bacteria (primarily streptococci and lactobacilli) in the presence of oxygen [29]. Therefore the anaerobic conditions that exist in plaque may offer bacteria an escape from this system, though they may have increased susceptibility to LPO after anaerobic growth [30].

Synergistic Inhibition of S. mutans *Metabolism by Lysozyme and Lactoperoxidase*

Although all *S. mutans* are catalase-negative and release detectable amounts of H_2O_2, only a few release amounts of sufficient quantity to be inhibited by LPO and SCN^- in the absence of added H_2O_2 [31]. In the present study, *S. mutans* NCTC 10449 harvested in early exponential phase were exposed to 0.3 mg/ml hen egg white lysozyme (muramidase activity equivalent to that in saliva) and 0.3 mg/ml purified bovine LPO (Sigma Chemical Co.) in 370 μM KSCN and 150 mM NaCl for periods to 1 h. The treated bacteria were suspended in 2.0 ml unbuffered saline and pH was maintained at 6.5 by automatic titration of bacterial acid with 2.0 mM NaOH using a Radiometer pH stat system. Acid production was stimulated by the addition of 100 μl glucose solution to give a final concentration of 1%. The rate of acid production was measured as the slope of the curve of volume of added base versus time from the recorder tracing. Acid production was expressed as nmol $\times$ min^{-1} $\times$ ml^{-1} $\times$ abs. units^{-1} as previously described [32]. When glucose was added to untreated cells or to cells incubated in the absence of any of the three components, acid production began immediately. However, cells incubated with lysozyme, LPO and SCN^- for 1 h did not produce acid until after the addition of 2-ME to 0.24 mM (table IV). The percentage inhibition of acid production was calculated by comparing acid production rates following addition of

Table IV. Rates of acid production[1] by *S. mutans* NCTC 10449 following incubation with lysozyme[2], lactoperoxidase and SCN^-[2]

Duration of incubation, min	Glucose rate[3]	2-ME rate[4]	% inhibition
15	34.6	38.9	11
30	25.0	41.8	40
60	0.5	29.8	98

[1] Expressed as nanomoles acid produced per minute.
[2] Hen egg white lysozyme (300 µg/ml), bovine lactoperoxidase (300 µg/ml) and KSCN (370 µM)..
[3] Glucose added to 1% to 2-ml volumes containing bacterial aliquots collected at the various times after incubation as indicated.
[4] 2-ME added to 40 µM 5 min after glucose addition.

glucose to that attained following 2-ME addition. The complete inhibition of acid production and the rapid recovery with 2-ME suggest that bacteria in the presence of lyzozyme, LPO and SCN$^-$ may be slowly generating H_2O_2 that reacts to form OSCN$^-$. To test this hypothesis, catalase (40 μg/ml) was added to bacterial suspensions containing LZ-LPO-SCN. Addition of catalase at the beginning of incubation reduced the inhibition to only 23%; however, with addition of catalase 1 min before addition of glucose (at the end of the 1 h incubation) metabolism was inhibited just as in the absence of catalase (95% inhibition). Apparently catalase added at the beginning of the incubation could compete with LPO for the H_2O_2 as it was being generated, thus reducing the amount of OSCN$^-$ generated. These data suggest that the bacteria are induced to generate H_2O_2, even in the absence of exogenous glucose, at sufficient levels to form enough OSCN$^-$ to inhibit metabolism.

The mechanism of action of lysozyme in the phenomenon described here is not clear. Since lysozyme under the conditions employed had no effect on the acid production or viability of *S. mutans* NCTC 10449, there may be a synergistic interaction of lysozyme with lactoperoxidase and thiocyanate. *Thomas* et al. [31] reported a direct relationship between the amount of H_2O_2 released by various strains of *S. mutans* and their inhibition by LPO and SCN$^-$ in the absence of added H_2O_2. It appears that the factor that determines whether a given strain will be inhibited by LPO and SCN$^-$ alone is the balance between the rate of peroxide production via NADH oxidase and the rate of peroxide destruction by bacterial peroxidases [30, 31]. Lysozyme could increase bacterial peroxide generation either directly or through interference with bacterial peroxidase. Such synergism might explain the enhanced inhibition observed when nonmetabolizing *S. mutans* are incubated with saliva in the absence of added cofactors [unpublished observations].

Other Potential Interactions between Salivary Constituents

As suggested above, the interaction between secretory antibodies and innate defense factors may be important modulators of their respective antibacterial activities. In this regard specific antibodies have been reported to enhance the antibacterial properties of transferrin and LF [33, 34]. In addition colostral antibodies have been shown to lyse bacterial cells only in the presence of complement (C) and lysozyme

[35]. However, several studies have indicated that the bactericidal events of antibody and C are independent of lysozyme [36, 37] or lysozyme is required only for cytolysis by the alternative C pathway [36]. Recent studies by *Tenovuo* et al. [38] have indicated that IgA (either as SIgA or myeloma IgA1 or IgA2) but not IgG or IgM significantly enhanced the inhibition of *S. mutans* metabolism by the LPO system. In addition, LF, especially in the iron-saturated form, caused a substantial enhancement of the peroxidatic activity of LPO [38]. LPO is surface active and adsorbs in active form to hydroxyapatite [39], salivary sediment [40] and various strains of streptococci [41]. LPO and SIgA concentrate in dental plaque fluid to 19.8 and 210 mg/dl respectively [42]. The major portion of this IgA is intact SIgA [43]. LF concentrations in human whole saliva range from 15 to 46 μg/ml [42] which is far below the concentration reported for LPO synergism [38]. It has been reported that most oral microorganisms are not lysed nor killed by lysozyme [44]. However, recent studies by *Iacono* and co-workers [45, 46] have reported variable effects of lysozyme on *S. mutans* depending on the strain used and the ionic conditions of incubation. They present evidence that the bactericidal or bacteriostatic effects of lysozyme are not necessarily equated with its lytic ability [45]. Evidence suggests that lysozyme may act on the cell membrane disrupting its function as a permeability barrier; furthermore, the lytic process appears to be enhanced by the presence of chaotropic ions [45]. Interestingly SCN^- was the most effective ion in this series and because of its charge density $OSCN^-$ would be predicted to be a better chaotropic agent. The SCN^- required for this effect is far in excess of the salivary concentration; however, local generation of the $OSCN^-$ at the bacterial surface may effectively concentrate the chaotrope at its target surface.

It is apparent that there are numerous possible interactions between the various salivary constituents representing a complex array of permutations. These are at best only poorly understood and require considerable attention in the future if we are to understand the regulation of microflora at mucosal surfaces.

References

1   Masson, P.L.; Heremans, J.F.: Metal combining properties of human lactoferrin (red milk protein). I. The involvement of bicarbonate in the reaction. Eur. J. Biochem. 6: 579–584 (1968).

2   Schlabach, M.R.; Bates, G.W.: The synergistic binding of anions and Fe^{3+} by transferrin: implications for the interlocking site hypothesis. J. biol. Chem. *250:* 2182–2188 (1975).

3   Aisen, P.; Leibman, A.: Lactoferrin and transferrin: a comparative study. Biochim. biophys. Acta *257:* 314–323 (1973).

4   Masson, P.: La lactoferrine (Arscia, Brussels 1970).

5   Leffell, M.S.; Spitznagel, J.K.: Association of lactoferrin with lysozyme in granules of human polymorphonuclear leukocytes. Infect. Immunity *6:* 761–765 (1972).

6   Bullen, J.J.; Rogers, H.J.; Griffiths E.: Role of iron in bacterial infection; in Arber, Current topics in microbiology and immunology, vol. 80, pp. 1–36 (Springer, Berlin 1978).

7   Arnold, R.R.; Cole, M.F.; McGhee, J.R.: A bactericidal effect for human lactoferrin. Science *197:* 263–265 (1977).

8   Arnold, R.R.; Brewer, M.; Gauthier, J.J.: Bactericidal activity of human lactoferrin: sensitivity of a variety of microorganisms. Infect. Immunity *28:* 893–898 (1980).

9   Arnold, R.R.; Russell, J.E.; Champion, W.J.; Brewer, M.; Gauthier, J.J.: Bactericidal activity of human lactoferrin: differentiation from the stasis of iron deprivation. Infect. Immunity *35:* 792–799 (1982).

10 Arnold, R.R.; Russell, J.E.; Champion, W.J.; Gauthier, J.J.: Bactericidal activity of lactoferrin: influence of physical conditions and metabolic state of the target microorganism. Infect. Immunity *32:* 655–660 (1981).

11 Blackberg, L.; Hernell, O.: Isolation of lactoferrin from human whey by a simple chromatographic step. FEBS Lett. *109:* 180–184 (1980).

12 Cole, M.F.; Arnold, R.R.; Mestecky, J.; Prince, S.; Kulhavy, R.; McGhee, J.R.: Studies with human lactoferrin and *S. mutans,* in Stiles, Proc. of Microbial Aspects of Dental Caries, 1976. Microbiology Abstracts, No. 2, pp. 359–373 (Information Retrieval, Washington 1977).

13 Mazurier, J.; Spik, G.: Comparative study of the iron-binding properties of the human transferrins. 1. Complete and sequential iron saturation and desaturation of the lactotransferrin. Biochim. biophys. Acta *629:* 399–408 (1980).

14 Griffiths, E.; Humphreys, J.: Bacteriostatic effect of human milk and bovine colostrum on *Escherichia coli:* importance of bicarbonate. Infect. Immunity *15:* 396–401 (1977).

15 Bishop, J.C.; Schanbacher, F.L.; Ferguson, L.C.; Smith, K.L.: In vitro growth inhibition of mastitis-causing coliform bacteria by bovine apolactoferrin and reversal of inhibition by citrate and high concentrations of apolactoferrin. Infect. Immunity *14:* 911–918 (1976).

16 Arnold, R.R.; Mestecky, J.; McGhee, J.R.: Naturally-occurring secretory immunoglobulin A antibodies to *Streptococcus mutans* in human colostrum and saliva. Infect. Immunity *14:* 355–362 (1976).

17 Hamon, C.B.; Klebanoff, S.J.: A peroxidase-mediated *Streptococcus mitis* dependent antimicrobial system in saliva. J. exp. Med. *137:* 438–450 (1973).

18 Hogg, D.M.; Jago, G.R.: The antibacterial action of lactoperoxidase. The nature of the bacterial inhibitor. Biochem. J. *117:* 779–790 (1970).

19 Bjorck, L.; Rosen, C.-G.; Marshall, V.; Reiter, B.: Antibacterial activity of the lactoperoxidase system in milk against pseudomonads and other gram-negative bacteria. Appl. Microbiol. *30:* 199–204 (1975).

20 Aune, T.M.; Thomas, E.L.: Accumulation of hypothiocyanite ion during peroxidase-catalysed oxidation of thiocyanate ion. Eur. J. Biochem. *80:* 209–214 (1977).

21 Hoogendoorn, H.; Piessens, J.P.; Scholtes, W.; Stoddard, L.A.: Hypothiocyanite ion; the inhibitor formed by the system lactoperoxidase-thiocyanate-hydrogen peroxide. Caries Res. *11:* 77–84 (1977).

22 Mickelson, M.N.: Antibacterial action of lactoperoxidase-thiocyanate-hydrogen peroxide on *Streptococcus agalactiae*. Appl. environ. Microbiol. *38:* 821–826 (1979).

23 Thomas, E.L.; Aune, T.M.: Lactoperoxidase, peroxide, thiocyanate antimicrobial system: correlation of sulfhydryl oxidation with antimicrobial action. Infect. Immunity *20:* 456–463 (1978).

24 Thomas, E.L.: Lactoperoxidase-catalyzed oxidation of thiocyanate: equilibria between oxidized forms of thiocyanate. Biochemistry *20:* 3273–3280 (1981).

25 Tenovuo, J.; Makinen, K.K.: Concentration of thiocyanate and ionizable iodide in saliva of smokers and non-smokers. J. dent. Res. *55:* 661–663 (1973).

26 Colonius, P.E.B.: The leukocyte count in saliva. Oral Surg. *11:* 43–46 (1958).

27 Kraus, F.W.; Nickerson, J.F.; Perry, W.I.; Walker, A.P.: Peroxide and peroxidogenic bacteria in human saliva. J. Bact. *73:* 727–735 (1957).

28 Thomas, E.L.; Bates, K.P.; Jefferson, M.M.: Hypothiocyanite ion: detection of the antimicrobial agent in human saliva. J. dent. Res. *59:* 1466–1472 (1980).

29 Whittenbury, R.: Hydrogen peroxide formation and catalase activity in the lactic acid bacteria. J. gen. Microbiol. *35:* 13–26 (1964).

30 Carlsson, J.; Iwami, Y.; Yamuda, T.: Hydrogen peroxide excretion by oral streptococci and effect of lactoperoxidase-thiocyanate-hydrogen peroxide. Infect. Immunity *40:* 70–80 (1983).

31 Thomas, E.L.; Pera, K.A.; Smith, K.W.; Chwang, A.K.: Inhibition of *Streptococcus mutans* by the lactoperoxidase antimicrobial system. Infect. Immunity *39:* 767–778 (1983).

32 Tenovuo, J.; Mansson-Rahemtulla, B.; Pruitt, K.M.; Arnold, R.: Inhibition of dental plaque acid production by the salivary lactoperoxidase system. Infect. Immunity *34:* 208–214 (1981).

33 Rogers, H.J.; Synge, C.: Bacteriostatic effect of human milk on *Escherichia coli:* the role of IgA. Immunology *34:* 19–24 (1978).

34 Rogers, H.J.: Ferric iron and the antibacterial effects of horse 7S antibodies to *Escherichia coli* 0111. Immunology *30:* 425–431 (1976).

35 Adinolfi, M.; Glynn, A.A.; Lindsay, M.; Milne, C.M.: Serological properties of IgA antibodies to *Escherichia coli* present in human colostrum. Immunology *10:* 517–525 (1966).

36 Schreiber, R.D.; Morrison, D.C.; Podach, E.R.; Muller-Eberhart, H.J.: Bactericidal activity of the alternative complement pathway generated from 11 isolated plasma proteins. J. exp. Med. *149:* 870–885 (1979).

37 Martinez, R.J.; Carroll, S.F.: Sequential metabolic expression of the lethal process in human serum treated *E. coli:* role of lysozyme. Infect. Immunity *28:* 735–745 (1980).

38 Tenovuo, J.; Moledoveanu, Z.; Mestecky, J.; Pruitt, K.M.; Rahemtulla, B.-M.: Interaction of specific and innate factors of immunity: IgA enhances the antimicro-

bial effect of the lactoperoxidase system against *Streptococcus mutans*. J. Immun. *128:* 726–731 (1982).

39 Pruitt, K.M.; Adamson, M.: Enzyme activity of salivary lactoperoxidase adsorbed to human enamel. Infect. Immunity *17:* 112–116 (1977).

40 Tenovuo, J.; Valtakoski, J.; Knuuttila, M.: Antibacterial activity of lactoperoxidase adsorbed by human salivary sediment and hydroxyapaptite. Caries Res. *11:* 257–262 (1977).

41 Pruitt, K.M.; Adamson, M.; Arnold, R.: Lactoperoxidase binding to streptococci. Infect. Immunity *25:* 304–309 (1979).

42 Cole, M.F.; Hsu, S.D.; Baum, B.J.; Bowen, W.H.; Sierra, L.I.; Aquirre, M.; Gillespie, G.: Specific and nonspecific immune factors in dental plaque fluid and saliva from young and old populations. Infect. Immunity *31:* 998–1002 (1981).

43 Taubman, M.A.: Immunoglobulins of human dental plaque. Archs oral Biol. *19:* 439–446 (1974).

44 Gibbons, R.J.; de Stoppelar, J.D.; Harden, L.: Lysozyme insensitivity of bacteria indigenous to the oral cavity of man. J. dent. Res. *45:* 877–881 (1966).

45 Iacono, V.J.; McKay, B.J.; Di Rienzo, S.; Pollock, J.J.: Selective antibacterial properties of lysozyme for oral microorganisms. Infect. Immunity *29:* 623–632 (1980).

46 Cho, M.-I.; Holt, S.C.; Iacono, V.J.; Pollock, J.J.: Effects of lysozyme and inorganic anions on the morphology of *Streptococcus mutans* BHT: electron microscopic examination. J. Bact. *151:* 1498–1507 (1982).

R.R. Arnold, PhD, Department of Oral Biology,
Emory University School of Dentistry, Atlanta, GA 30322 (USA)

Cariology Today. Int. Congr., Zürich 1983, pp. 89–97 (Karger, Basel 1984)

Role of Antibodies in Saliva: Facts and Extrapolations

P. Brandtzaeg

Laboratory for Immunohistochemistry and Immunopathology,
The National Hospital, Rikshospitalet, Oslo, Norway

Relation between Salivary Immunoglobulins and Dental Caries Susceptibility

The oral microbiota is under continuous influence of two principal immunoglobulin (Ig) classes: secretory IgA and IgG. The former is synthesized as IgA dimers by immunocytes present in major and minor salivary glands [*Brandtzaeg*, 1977; *Korsrud and Brandtzaeg*, 1980]; these dimers show specific affinity for secretory component which is produced by serous-type glandular elements [*Korsrud and Brandtzaeg*, 1982] and acts as an epithelial Ig receptor [*Brandtzaeg*, 1981a]. Small amounts of pentameric IgM is normally transported through the salivary glands by the same mechanism. Most salivary IgG reaches the oral cavity through the gingival crevice and is mainly derived from serum [*Brandtzaeg* et al., 1970], although a fraction of the crevicular IgG (10–20%) may originate in local plasma cells when the gingiva is inflamed [*Brandtzaeg*, 1972].

Reliable and reproducible measurements of salivary IgA are extremely difficult to achieve; variables such as stimulation of flow rate, concentration and storage of the samples, and method of quantitation may significantly influence the results [*Brandtzaeg* et al., 1970]. In addition comes a substantial variation in individual concentrations of secretory IgA over time [*Brandtzaeg* et al., 1970; *Gahnberg and Krasse*, 1981]. It is not surprising, therefore, that discrepant reports have been published as to the relation of salivary IgA levels and dental decay. Nevertheless, the balance of evidence indicates that there is an inverse relationship between caries susceptibility and the output of salivary IgA in children and young adults (table I). In older individuals it seems that the continuous presence of active caries is associated with increased

Table I. Relation between high caries activity and salivary IgA level

Authors	Subjects studied		Type of fluid	IgA level	Correlation between DS or DMF and IgA
	n	age, years			
Whole saliva					
Lehner et al. [1967]	30	20–24	S, CF, C	lowered (conc.)[1]	ND
Shklair et al. [1969]	15	17–21	no information	normal (conc.)	ND
Everhart et al. [1972]	22	10–19	US, CF	ND	negative (DS/SR)[1]
	40	20–29	US, CF	ND	negative (DMF/conc.)
	15	30–39	US, CF	ND	positive (DS/SR and DMF/conc.)[1]
Serre et al. [1972]	55	15–74	US, CF	ND	positive (DS/conc.)
Sims [1972]	24	approximately 22	US, CF C	normal	ND
Everhart et al. [1977]	48	3–7	US, CF	ND	negative (DMF/conc. and DMF/SR)[2]
Parotid fluid					
Shklair et al. [1969]	20	17–21	S, C	increased	ND
Zengo et al. [1971]	40	adults	S	lowered	ND
Serre et al. [1972]	55	15–74	S	ND	no correlation
Ørstavik and Brandtzaeg [1975]	27	22–33	S	ND	negative (DMF/SR)[1]
Challacombe [1976]	96	18–25	S	ND	negative (DMF/SR)[1]
Stuchell and Mandel [1978]	26	20	S	lowered (conc.)[1]	ND
Submandibular secretion					
Zengo et al. [1971]	40	adults	S	lowered (conc.)[1,3]	ND
Stuchell and Mandel [1978]	34	20	S	lowered (conc.)[1]	ND

DS = Decayed surfaces; DMF = decayed, missing or filled teeth; S = stimulated; CF = centrifuged; C = concentrated; ND = not determined; US = unstimulated; SR = secretion rate (µg IgA/min/gland).
[1] Statistically significant ($p < 0.05$).
[2] Statistically significant only when IgA was considered together with oral hygiene in multiple correlation analysis.
[3] The levels of both IgA and albumin were significantly raised in the caries-resistant control group.

concentrations of salivary IgA [*Everhart* et al., 1972], perhaps because of a persistent microbial stimulation of the secretory immune system without any beneficial effect on established dental lesions. An increased antigenic load due to active caries may likewise result in raised levels of serum IgG [*Challacombe*, 1976] and IgG antibodies to *Streptococcus mutans* [*Challacombe*, 1980].

Recent studies in immunodeficient patients have supported the notion that susceptibility to caries is inversely related to the activity of the salivary-gland immune system [*Legler* et al., 1981]. Subjects totally lacking both secretory IgA and secretory IgM show marked elevation of caries incidence, whereas those who compensate for their IgA deficiency by producing substantial amounts of secretory IgM usually show normal susceptibility to dental decay [*Arnold* et al., 1977].

Relation between Salivary Antibodies and Dental Caries Susceptibility

Since the original observation that certain oral bacteria become coated with IgA in vivo [*Brandtzaeg* et al., 1968], several studies have been carried out to map the antibody activities of salivary IgA. Naturally occurring secretory IgA antibodies to *S. mutans* have been found not only in saliva, but also in colostrum and tears [*Arnold* et al., 1976; *Burns* et al., 1982], indicating generalized dissemination of specific B cells from the site of stimulation [*Brandtzaeg,* 1983]. Particularly high titres of such antibodies have been found in secretions from the minor salivary glands [*Krasse* et al., 1978]. *Challacombe* [1978] and *Huis in 't Veld* et al. [1978] found no clear correlation of caries experience with salivary IgA titres to *S. mutans* in adults, whereas *Everhart* et al. [1978] reported an inverse relationship in young children.

Difficulties in obtaining consistent results may partly be ascribed to the fact that whole bacterial cells have been used in most assays; IgA shows affinity for streptococci unrelated to antibody specificity [*Christensen and Oxelius,* 1975]. In addition, there is evidence suggesting that the magnitude of salivary antibody titres to *S. mutans* may be considerably influenced by immune responses elicited through exposure to cross-reacting antigens [*Bammann and Gibbons,* 1979]. The use of better defined microbial antigens may afford more valid results. *Challacombe* et al. [1973] reported a substantial IgA antibody titre to partially purified glucosyltransferase to be present in parotid fluid from most adults; the titre was significantly decreased in those with active caries. Nevertheless, this result has been questioned because IgA-producing cells specific for glucosyltransferase could not be revealed in human parotid glands [*Brandtzaeg*, 1976]. Recently, *Bolton* [1981] found significantly higher levels of salivary IgA antibodies to glycerol-teichoic acid in subjects free of active caries than in those with one or more active lesions. This result is in keeping with the notion that there is an inverse relation between the activity of the salivary gland immune system and caries susceptibility, but does not necessarily indicate that *S. mutans* is the principal immunogen eliciting antibodies to teichoic acid.

The way salivary IgA antibodies to microbial antigens may reduce caries susceptibility is only partly understood. Experimentally induced salivary antibodies to glucosyltransferase in the rat can inhibit the enzyme activity and reduce caries activity [*Smith* et al., 1979; *Taubman and Smith*, 1977]. Some inhibition of *S. mutans* colonization has been indicated, but seems to be easier to obtain by immunization with whole bacterial cells (table II). It is possible that IgA antibodies through bacterial agglutination enhance elimination of *S. mutans* from the oral cavity or interfere with bacterial adherence to the enamel. However, no conclusive results to this end have been obtained by testing adherence of *S. mutans* to hydroxyapatite [*Gahnberg* et al., 1982; *Kilian* et al., 1981], whereas the adherence of *Streptococcus sanguis* in similar experiments is enhanced by IgA antibodies bound to the hard surface [*Kilian* et al., 1981; *Liljemark* et al., 1979]. It is clear that IgA is only one of several salivary factors that influence dental plaque formation in a very complex and individually variable way [*Gahnberg* et al., 1982].

Results of Vaccination against Dental Caries

The results of vaccination experiments that have been analyzed in terms of salivary antibody responses are summarized in table II. Subcutaneous immunization with killed *S. mutans* cells and Freund's incomplete adjuvant has been conclusively shown by *Lehner* and his colleagues to give about 70% reduction of caries in deciduous teeth of rhesus monkeys. They have been able to repeat this result by subcutaneous immunization with purified protein antigens from *S. mutans* mixed with Freund's incomplete adjuvant or aluminium hydroxide [*Lehner* et al., 1980b]. The effect of the subcutaneous vaccine is ascribed to the bactericidal and opsonizing properties of serum-derived IgG antibodies reaching the enamel surface through the crevicular fluid [*Lehner* et al., 1975, 1978b; *Scully,* 1980]. The same workers have reported human studies indicating that relatively increased serum levels of IgG antibodies to *S. mutans* are associated with enhanced resistance to caries [*Challacombe,* 1980; *Lehner* et al., 1978a]. *Lehner* [1982] recently carried out extensive work to dissect immunoregulatory mechanisms involved in systemic immune responses to purified streptococcal antigens.

Subcutaneous immunization of monkeys has elicited little or no secretory IgA response. Conversely, in the rodent model several routes of vaccination have successfully afforded induction of salivary IgA antibodies (table II). It is noteworthy, however, that a concomitant IgG response was observed in serum and saliva in all those experiments where a biological effect was obtained in terms of enhanced caries resistance and reduced colonization of *S. mutans.* It cannot be exluded, therefore, that the results were mediated by complement-activating IgG antibodies to *S. mutans* rather than by specific IgA. Nevertheless, passive transfer of lacteal secretions containing IgG or IgA antibodies indicated that either isotype can afford protection against caries when delivered to saliva [*Michalek and McGhee,* 1977].

The experimental immune responses observed in primates apparently differ from those in rodents [*Ciardi* et al., 1978]. Unlike the situation in rats and hamsters, a consistent salivary IgA titre to *S. mutans* has not been obtained by application of peroral or enteral killed vaccines in monkeys. Such immunization in man has elicited salivary IgA antibodies in 2 of 3 experimental series (table II). The biological effects of the antibodies thus induced remains questionable, however. In the one human study where inhibited colonization of *S. mutans* was noted, concomitant induction of serum IgG antibodies took place. Passive transfer of IgG through the crevicular fluid, therefore, might have explained the observed results as discussed above for the rodent model.

Applicability and Acceptability of a Caries Vaccine in Man

Vaccination against infectious diseases is a highly valued principle of preventive medicine. According to some authors, dental caries fulfills the criteria of an infectious disease and, therefore, should be liable to

Table II. Identified IgA and IgG antibodies and their suggested biological effects after immunization with S. mutans antigens

Authors	Species	Immunization variables			Salivary antibody[1]		Serum antibody[1]	Reduction[2]
		immunogen	route	adjuvant	IgA	IgG	IgG	S. mutans caries
Taubman and Smith [1974]	rats	S. mutans (killed)	s.c.	FCA	+	±	+	+
Emmings et al. [1975]	irus monkeys	S. mutans (killed)	s.c.	GTF	–	–	+	
		S. mutans (killed)	s.c. + i.d.	GTF	+	±/+	+	
Evans et al. [1975]	irus monkeys	S. mutans (killed)	s.c. + i.d.	GTF	+	±/+	+	+
McGhee et al. [1975]	rats	S. mutans (killed)	s.c.	FCA	+		+	+
Michalek et al. [1976, 1978]	rats	S. mutans (killed)	peroral	none	+	±	±	+
Lehner et al. [1977]	rhesus monkeys	S. mutans (killed)	s.c.	FIA	(±)[3]		+	+
Taubman and Smith [1977]	rats	GTF	s.c.	FCA	+	+	+	±
Mestecky et al. [1978]	man	S. mutans (killed)	enteral	none	+	–	(±)[3]	
Challacombe and Lehner [1980]	rhesus monkeys	S. mutans (killed)	s.m.	FIA	+	±	+	
		S. mutans (killed)	s.c.	FIA	±	±	+	
		S. mutans (killed)	enteral	none	+	–	–	
		S. mutans (live)	peroral	none	+	–	±	

Reference	Animal	Antigen	Route	Adjuvant					
Lehner et al. [1980a]	rhesus monkeys	S. mutans (live)	peroral	none	+	+	+	−	±
	monkeys	S. mutans (killed)	s.c.	FIA	±	±	+	+	+
Smith et al. [1980]	hamsters	GTF	peroral	none	+	+	+	±/+	
Linzer et al. [1981]	irus monkeys	S. mutans (killed)	i.d.	GTF	+	−	+	+	
		S. mutans (killed)	peroral	none	−	−	−	−	
		S. mutans (killed)	s.c.	FIA	−	−	+	+	
Walker [1981]	irus monkeys	S. mutans (killed)	s.c. + s.m.	AH	−	±	+	+	
		S. mutans (killed)	i.d.	none	+	+	+	+	
		S. mutans (killed or live)	enteral	none	(±)³	(±)³	(±)³		
Cole et al. [1981, 1982]	man	S. mutans (killed)	enteral	none	+	+	+		
Gahnberg and Krasse [1983]	man	S. mutans (killed)	peroral	none	(+)³		+/±		

s.c. = Subcutaneous; FCA = Freund's complete adjuvant; GTF = glucosyltransferase; i.d. = intraductal (parotid); FIA = Freund's incomplete adjuvant; s.m. = submucosal (oral); AH = aluminium hydroxide.

¹ Results of isotype-specific antibody titration were conclusive (+) or uncertain (±).

² Biological effects (numerical reduction of S. mutans and inhibition of caries activity) were significant (+) or tentative (±).

³ No increase compared with preimmunization titre.

control by an appropriate vaccine – primarily directed against *S. mu-*
tans [*Lehner,* 1978, 1982]. However, this notion is probably in its
essence not fully acceptable for two reasons. Firstly, although *S. mutans*
seems to be the principal microbial factor in the development of dental
decay [*McGhee and Michalek,* 1981], other bacteria may turn out to be
important as well. Secondly, the term 'infectious' implies spontaneous
spread or communicability of disease. This feature is distinctive from
transmissibility which implies capacity to be spread under appropriate
circumstances. Only the latter is true for dental decay. The term 'infective disease' – introduced more than 30 years ago [*Rosebury,* 1952] –
may thus be applied more appropriately to caries, since it is caused by
the indigenous or commensal oral microbiota. As in other endogenous
microbial diseases, significant factors other than the infective agent are
involved in the pathogenesis of tooth decay.

From an immunological point of view, it is important to realize
that dental caries is an infective rather than an infectious disease. It is
well known that continuous exposure of lymphoepithelial tissues to a
particular antigen may result in a state of systemic hyporesponsiveness
[*Brandtzaeg,* 1981b]. Such a gradual development probably explains
why only low antibody titres are normally found to dietary constituents
and commensal microorganisms. High levels of circulating antibodies
to such antigens can only be elicited by a subcutaneous or submucosal
vaccine that is potentiated through, for example, admixture with
Freund's incomplete adjuvant or aluminium hydroxide. However,
these depot-forming adjuvants are prone to induce granulomas which
may develop into unacceptable local reactions. Intraductal immunization to enhance parotid IgA titres is clearly unacceptable, even without
the inclusion of an adjuvant because of inflammatory reactions impair-
ing the secretory function of the gland.

Peroral and enteral application of live or killed *S. mutans* vaccines
is probably inefficient, because preexisting low levels of 'natural' secretory antibodies lead to rapid elimination of the introduced organisms
– thereby preventing stimulation of lymphoepithelial tissues [*Walker,*
1981]. *S. mutans* does not adhere well to mucosal surfaces, and basic
research is currently carried out to evaluate certain orally administered
adjuvants that may enhance the secretory immune response to this
organism [*Kiyono* et al., 1982].

It follows from the above discussion that the simplest and most
promising current approach to caries vaccination seems to be sub-

cutaneous immunization. Nevertheless, certain potential hazards caused by circulating IgG antibodies must be seriously considered. Firstly, systemic immunization with *S. mutans* in rabbits elicits antibodies that cross-react with human and monkey heart and kidney tissues and induce pathological alterations in the same organs of the immunized animals [*Hughes* et al., 1980; *Nisengard* et al., 1983]. If a subcutaneous *S. mutans* vaccine were to be applied in man, therefore, the possibility of autoimmune disease exists as a reality. Secondly, both in vitro [*Brandtzaeg and Tolo,* 1977a] and in vivo [*Lim and Rowley,* 1982] studies have shown that systemic immunization may result in increased mucosal penetrability for unrelated antigens. It is thus possible that systemic sensitization to a single oral antigen or microbe may jeopardize gingival protection against other plaque antigens. Although no untoward effects have been reported after parenteral vaccination with *S. mutans* in monkeys, it is well known that man is more liable to develop periodontitis; IgG antibodies apparently play a role in the pathogenesis of this disease [*Brandtzaeg and Tolo,* 1977b; *Tolo and Brandtzaeg,* 1982].

In conclusion, a subcutaneous *S. mutans* vaccine is afflicted with potential hazards that definitely render its application in man unacceptable at present. Adverse side effects may be avoided, if methods will become available for successful peroral or enteral stimulation of secretory immunity without the concomitant induction of high levels of circulating IgG antibodies. Almost 100 years have elapsed since *Sanarelli* [1892] reported tentative effects of salivary antibodies on microorganisms. Nevertheless, much more has to be learned about the regulation of the secretory immune system [*Brandtzaeg,* 1983] before the hope for a useful and safe caries vaccine based on induction of salivary IgA antibodies can be scientifically nourished.

References

A complete reference list for the information included in this review can be found in: Brandtzaeg, P.: The oral secretory immune system with special emphasis on its relation to dental caries. Proc. Finn. dent. Soc. *79:* 71–84 (1983).

Prof. P. Brandtzaeg, Institute of Pathology,
The National Hospital, Rikshospitalet, N-Oslo 1 (Norway)

Cariology Today. Int. Congr., Zürich 1983, pp. 98–108 (Karger, Basel 1984)

Specific Functional Salivary Proteins

Donald I. Hay

Department of Biochemistry, Forsyth Dental Center, Boston, Mass., USA

Introduction

The mouth represents a unique multifunctional interface with the body's external environment. Since it acts as an airway and an entry point for fluids and solid food, its surfaces are exposed to a wide range of environmental insults. The degree of exposure, and the vulnerability of oral surfaces and tissues to infection and damage, seems likely to be greater than that experienced by the surfaces and structures of any other body orifice. Considering this complexity and vulnerability, it is not surprising to find that salivary proteins are involved in a wide range of protective systems, the importance of which becomes apparent when salivary function is lost.

Many of the protective systems are identical to those found elsewhere in the body, such as the secretory immunoglobulin and the nonspecific antibacterial systems. Other systems appear to be unique to the mouth, such as the system which maintains the saliva in a state of supersaturation with respect to calcium phosphate salts, and so provides a protective and reparative environment for the teeth. It also seems highly likely, considering the large number of salivary proteins which, as yet, have no known function, that there are other protective systems which remain to be discovered.

In this paper, salivary proteins will be considered from a functional point of view, with emphasis being placed both on recent advances in knowledge and on areas which require further clarification. To provide a framework for this discussion, oral functions in which salivary proteins play a role are summarized in table I.

Table I. Oral functions of salivary proteins

---

1 Antibacterial activity
    Specific, e.g., immunoglobulins
    Nonspecific, e.g., lysozyme, lactoperoxidase, lactoferrin, vitamin B_{12}-binding protein, growth-inhibiting proteins
    Effects on microbial adherence and aggregation which affect bacterial colonization, e.g., various glycoproteins

2 Protection of soft tissues
    Lubrication and protection from dehydration, e.g., mucins
    Possible protection against viral infections
    Possible protection against carcinogens
    Possible role in wound healing, e.g., growth factors and growth factor potentiators

3 Maintenance of a protective environment for tooth mineral; statherin and the proline-rich phosphoproteins
4 Digestion, e.g., amylase in humans and other enzymes in nonhuman species
5 pH control in plaque; sialine
6 Possible role in taste; gustin
7 Possible role in gastrointestinal physiology

Understanding these functions requires (1) identification of the proteins and possible cofactors responsible for each of the biological activities; (2) knowledge of the structures of the proteins at the molecular level; (3) an understanding of the relationships between molecular structure and function; (4) knowledge of possible modulation of activity of the active proteins by other salivary constituents; (5) information on variations of activity in health and disease; (6) identification of the glandular and cellular source of the proteins concerned; (7) an understanding of their biosynthesis, and (8) knowledge of the genetic factors involved in the expression of the biological activities.

Antibacterial Activity

Regulation of microbial colonization and growth constitutes a major function of saliva. The importance of this activity is emphasized by the fact that all three of the subtopics in this area (table I) are dealt with in separate papers at this conference. Although an understanding of the roles of the secretory immune system and nonspecific factors such as lactoferrin, lysozyme and lactoperoxidase are well advanced, there are still many questions relating to salivary antibacterial activity which remain poorly understood or even unexplored. For instance, the concept of 'nutritional immunity' [41, 42] has been considered in relation to lactoferrin and iron [4]. Are there other systems in saliva designed to deprive bacteria of nutrients? What, for instance, is the function of the vitamin B_{12}-binding protein [26]. Is it fully saturated with B_{12} in the saliva, or does it bind this important bacterial nutrient and make it unavailable. Do any oral organisms overcome nutrient deprivation by the host by synthesizing siderophores or enterochelins, which compete with lactoferrin for iron, as do some *Escherichia coli* [5] and Neisseria [43] species? It seems likely that much remains to be learned in this area. A recent report [6], for instance, indicates the existence of as yet uncharacterized salivary proteins which inhibit microbial growth. These anionic proteins appear to be distinct from known specific and nonspecific immune factors and exhibit their activity under conditions of minimal nutrition, a condition likely to be encountered in the oral cavity.

During the last decade, considerable attention has been given to salivary proteins which are considered to enhance or decrease specific bacterial adherence to oral surfaces, particularly to the teeth, or to aggregate bacteria with the latter process possibly leading to deletion of organisms from the mouth. Generally, salivary glycoproteins of moderate to high molecular weight have been considered to be important in these activities, but the identification and structure determination of the specific proteins responsible for these activities in humans is only just beginning to advance.

The nature of the proposed bacteria-protein interactions in attachment and aggregation have been said to involve electrostatic, ion mediated, lectinlike, or hydrophobic interactions between the bacterial surface and salivary protein. Determination of the actual forces involved, and their relative contributions to these interactions, requires a detailed understanding of the structure of the proteins concerned. Significant advances have been made in this direction and recently reviewed [39]. These authors emphasize the phenomenal diversity of structures which may be created from the five monosaccharides commonly present in glycoproteins. For instance, three different amino acids can give rise to only six tripeptides, but three different sugars can yield 1,056 isomeric trisaccharides. Although only a few of the possible intermolecular linkages have been found to occur naturally, a great diversity of structures can still occur. Tertiary and higher structure arrangements can give rise to molecular domains with specific properties. Additional complexity arises from minor variations in structure of the carbohydrate side chains, described as microheterogeneity. It is not clear whether this variation in structure is deliberate and plays a role in function or whether it represents incomplete synthesis or post-synthetic degradation.

In addition to variations in the detailed structure of the carbohydrate side chains, the chains themselves may be distributed in various ways along the protein backbone. Some glycoproteins are uniformly glycosylated. In others, nonglycosylated or 'naked' sections of the protein backbone may occur. Because such naked sections often contain a large proportion of the cysteinyl and hydrophobic residues, they probably confer further special properties on the molecule and provide sites for additional specific interactions. The net effect of these structural features, which are only touched on here, is to produce a molecule with an exceptional range of properties, some of which are important in other functions described below.

Protection of the Soft Tissues

Lubrication and Hydration

The soft tissues of the oral cavity have to be kept moist and lubricated, otherwise tissue will be damaged by abrasion, and infection and ulceration may result. It is obvious that mucous secretions possess exceptional lubricating properties, compared to other fluids. Effective lubrication requires formation between moving surfaces of fluid layers with high film strength, a property which is associated with elongated or highly expanded molecular structures, rather than a globular form. These features are exhibited by mucin molecules and have been recently discussed [39]. As noted above, a typical mucin has a protein backbone with carbohydrate side chains attached. This type of structure leads to an open, random coil structure, often stabilized by the presence of negatively charged groups such as acyl neuraminic acids or sulfate on the side chains. Intermolecular interactions through disulfide bond formation, hydrophobic and ionic bonds, and complexing with other proteins, yield large, three-dimensional molecular networks. Because of their structure, these will act as effective lubricants. Also, again as a consequence of their molecular properties, particularly those associated with presence of carbohydrate and ionic groups, they will bind and entrain large amounts of water and so maintain mucous surfaces in a hydrated state. It is also important to note that many of the compositional and structural features of mucins confer on these molecules substantial resistance to proteolysis, an important property considering the environment in which they act.

Possible Protection against Viruses and Carcinogens

The fact that mucins, possibly complexed with other salivary proteins, form highly adherent viscous films over mucous surfaces suggests other protective functions. Several investigators have noted interactions between viruses and glycoproteins [9, 13, 19, 32]. Presumably, virus particles have to come into contact with cell surfaces to effect infection. It seems likely that a mucin layer, particularly one possessing appropriate functional groups or complexed with other specific molecules [39], could bind virus particles and so prevent or greatly reduce the possibility of infection. A similar mechanism could act to protect the mucosal surfaces from carcinogens. Experiments in which salivary flow was reduced pharmacologically or the salivary glands were removed surgically gave evidence for increases in penetration of oral tissues by carcinogens [1, 40] or increases in malignancy [38]. Also, at least one study [29] has shown that saliva inactivates specific carcinogens, when these are assayed in the Ames test, but the details of possible mechanisms by which these protective effects are achieved are not known.

The extreme complexity of mucin structure and behavior and the variety of functions in which mucins participate make research in this area particularly challenging. Nonetheless, substantial progress is being made, both with respect to salivary mucins in general [21] and in relation to isolation, structure, and function studies of human and other primate salivary mucins [22]. Beyond this remain questions related to the role of mucins in pellicle formation, a structure which not only strongly influences bacterial colonization, but also provides considerable protection for the teeth against enamel demineralization [44]. Also, the formation and significance of biologically active associations between mucins and other proteins, such as mucin-immunoglobulin [10] and mucin-lysozyme complexes [7], are intriguing observations, with work so far indicating an additional level of mucin function.

Possible Role in Wound Healing

The discovery of specific growth factors such as epidermal and nerve growth factors as secretory products in several nonhuman salivas [14] led to the suggestion that these may play some role in the unusually rapid healing of injured oral mucosal tissues. This speculation received little subsequent support, because growth factors were not found to be present at significant concentrations as secretory products in salivas of humans or many other species, and it seemed more likely that growth factors would act through the circulatory system rather than in the oral cavity. Nonetheless, recent work [37] has shown that combinations of epidermal growth factor and recently discovered transforming growth factors [8, 30] from porcine salivary glands offer a practical approach to enhancing wound healing. The possibility that similar effects occur *in vivo* seems worth considering.

Maintenance of a Protective Ionic Environment for the Teeth

The stability and protection of enamel mineral *in vivo* is critically dependent on the state of saturation of saliva with respect to the calcium phosphate salts which form the teeth. Most investigators concluded that human saliva is supersaturated with respect to hydroxyapatite and dental enamel, a property which provides considerable protection for the teeth [16]. This conclusion stemmed from experimental studies of saliva [11, 15] and clinical studies which showed that a large fraction of early carious lesions recalcify, both in children [2] and adults [12]. Recent studies of the state of supersaturation of saliva with respect to calcium phosphate salts have shown these secretions to be significantly more supersaturated than previously thought [16]. Although the supersaturated state of the saliva explains the source of the thermodynamic driving forces which protect dental enamel and which provide the mechanism for recalcification, there is obviously an anomaly in that calcium phosphate salts do not precipitate from saliva, either spontaneously or by seeded growth onto the teeth.

The absence of latter process appears to contravene basic physical chemical principles, that is, how can saliva recalcify subsurface lesions, yet not form mineral on the teeth? This anomaly is particularly striking considering that processes favorable for the teeth, such as repair of early lesions, occur in the mouth, but that undesirable processes, such as spontaneous precipitation, or unwanted mineral formation on the teeth, do not normally occur. This anomaly was resolved by the discovery of two types of specific inhibitors of calcium phosphate precipitation in human and other mammalian salivas [17]. One of these was a small, tyrosine-rich phosphopeptide, named statherin [33], the other was a group of anionic proline-rich phosphoproteins [17]. The presence of these molecules in saliva explains how recalcification can occur in a selective manner. Thus, in early subsurface lesions, which retain a surface layer of sound enamel, calcium and phosphate ions enter and recalcify the lesion. The inhibitors, because of their size, cannot pass through the surface enamel. Presumably, if the surface enamel layer is sufficiently demineralized and is penetrated by the inhibitors, repair will no longer be possible. The formation of dental calculus, which requires the prior formation of dental plaque, can be rationalized in a similar manner. In this case, the inhibitors, even if they are initially present, will be degraded by the plaque microflora. Calculus formation may then occur, because calcium and phosphate may enter the plaque, but the inhibitors will be physically excluded or degraded.

This selectively controlled protective system for the enamel seems to have a sound logical and experimental base [18], but significant questions remain. An essential feature of the system is that in order to act, the inhibitory molecules must adsorb to the tooth surface. Extensive in vitro studies of adsorption of the inhibitors onto hydroxyapatite have been conducted [28], but little is known of their behavior in vivo. The proline-rich proteins have been shown to be present on the tooth surface, using immunochemical methods [25], but there are questions with respect to their long-term survival [3]. Also, questions still remain with respect to the molecular basis for their activity. Results obtained so far show that the entire statherin molecule is required to inhibit spontaneous precipitation of calcium phosphates, but the inhibitory activity of the proline-rich proteins resides in their thirty-residue aminoterminal segments, with no known function for the remainder of the molecule, which forms as much as 80% of the larger of these proteins.

Digestion

In humans, the only digestive enzyme in saliva is amylase which produces maltose and glucose as end products of starch digestion [31].

Other enzymes such as proteases and ribonucleases occur in salivas of other species. There seems no doubt, considering the high amylase concentration and activity in human saliva, that digestion of starches will be initiated in the mouth, and this will continue in the stomach until the enzyme is inactivated by gastric secretions. It also seems obvious that amylase will aid in clearing the teeth of carbohydrate debris. It is less clear why amylase occurs in tears, nasal and bronchial secretions, milk, serum, urine, and in the secretions of the male and female urogenital tracts [18]. The observation that the growth and survival of 13 strains of *Neisseria gonorrhoeae* are inhibited by salivary amylase [27], the widespread distribution of this enzyme in the body, and its synthesis alongside other macromolecules with antibacterial activity suggest a possible antibacterial role for this enzyme.

pH Control of Plaque

Several salivary factors act to help neutralize acids produced as the end products of bacterial glycolysis in plaque. Bicarbonate and other buffer anions from saliva diffuse into plaque. Urea, also present in saliva, is metabolized by the plaque microflora to give ammonia which increases plaque pH. Recent studies [23, 24] have identified additional agents. These are arginine- or lysine-containing peptides which are readily transported into bacterial cells. When present at sufficiently high concentrations, they reduce or nearly prevent the decrease in pH which occurs when oral bacterial mixtures such as plaque and salivary sediment are incubated with glucose [36]. A peptide having the structure NH_2-Gly-Gly-Lys-Arg-COOH, named sialine, has been found to be particularly effective. In systems containing saliva sediment or plaque preparations and glucose, which normally exhibit a pH decrease from about 7 to below 5 when incubated, sialine, present at a concentration of 0.33 mM, maintained the pH at above 5.5 At 3.33 mM, sialine kept the pH above 6.5. Peptides containing arginine and lysine will be amongst the proteolytic degradation products of salivary proteins, a large fraction of which are basic and rich in these amino acids. These may play a role in controlling plaque pH, and there is the possibility that sugar-rich cariogenic foods could be supplemented with peptides such as sialine.

Possible Role in Taste and Gastrointestinal Physiology

A zinc-binding protein, gustin, has been isolated from human parotid saliva [34]. Since individuals with hypogeusia (taste deficiency) exhibit low gustin levels, averaging one fifth normal values, and zinc deficiency has been associated with hypogeusia, it has been proposed that gustin is important in mediating taste sensation [35]. The mechanism by which it acts still has to be revealed, but it seems conceivable that gustin could interact with and activate receptors on taste buds.

There remain a large number of salivary gland products with proposed or possible functions in gastrointestinal physiology. As an example, urogastrone has been identified using immunological methods in secretory granules in human submandibular gland acinar cells [20]. This material has been shown to inhibit gastric acid serection and also to stimulate cell proliferation and regeneration of the intestinal mucosa, a surprising diversity of function. Problems such as these, and the presence in saliva of many other proteins with no known function [18], indicate that there are many challenging problems in this area.

References

1   Adams, D.: The effect of saliva on the penetration of fluorescent dyes into the oral mucosa of the rat and rabbit. Archs oral Biol. *19:* 505–510 (1974).

2   Backer-Dirks, O.: Post-eruptive changes in dental enamel. J. dent. Res. *45:* 503–511 (1966).

3   Bennick, A.; Chau, G.; Goodlin, R.; Abrams, S.; Tustian, D.; Madapallimattam, G.: The role of human salivary acidic proline-rich proteins in the formation of acquired dental pellicle *in vivo* and their fate after adsorption to the human enamel surface. Archs oral Biol. *28:* 19–28 (1983).

4   Bezkorovainy, A.: Anti-microbial properties of iron-binding proteins. Adv. exp. Med. Biol. *135:* 139–154 (1981).

5   Bullen, J.J.; Rogers, H.J.; Leigh, L.: Iron binding proteins in milk and resistance to *Escherichia coli* in infants. Br. med. J. *i:* 69–75 (1972).

6   Cowman, R.A.; Baron, S.S.; Fitzgerald, R.J.; Danziger, J.L.; Quintana, J.A.: Growth inhibition of oral streptococci in saliva by anionic proteins from two caries-free individuals. Infect. Immunity *37:* 513–518 (1982).

7   Creeth, J.M.; Bridge, J.L.N.; Horton, J.R.: An interaction between lysozyme and mucous glycoproteins. Biochem. J. *181:* 717–724 (1979).

8   DeLarco, J.E.; Todaro, G.J.: Growth factors from murine sarcoma virus-transformed cells. Proc. natn. Acad. Sci. USA *75:* 4001–4005 (1978).

9   DiGirolamo, R.; Liston, J.; Matches, J.: Ionic bonding, the mechanism of viral uptake by shellfish mucus. Appl. environ. Microbiol. *33:* 19–25 (1977).

10   Edwards, P.A.W.: Is mucus a selective barrier to macromolecules. Br. med. Bull. *34:* 55–56 (1978).

11   Ericsson, Y.: Enamel-apatite solubility. Acta odont. scand. *8:* suppl. 3, pp. 1–139 (1949).

12   Fehr, F.R. von der; Loe, H.; Theilade, J.: Experimental caries in man. Caries Res. *4:* 131–148 (1970).

13   Gottschalk, A.; Bhargava, A.S.; Murty, V.L.N.: Submaxillary gland glycoproteins; in Gottschalk, Glycoproteins: their compositions, structure and function; 2nd ed., pp. 810–829 (Elsevier, Amsterdam 1972).

14   Greene, L.A.; Shooter, E.M.: The nerve growth factor: biochemistry, synthesis and mechanism of action. Annu. Rev. Neurosci. *3:* 353–402 (1980).

15   Gron, P.: Saturation of human saliva with calcium phosphates. Archs. oral Biol. *18:* 1385–1392 (1973).

16   Hay, D.I.; Schluckebier, S.K.; Moreno, E.C.: Equilibrium dialysis and ultrafiltration studies of calcium and phosphate binding by human salivary proteins. Implications for salivary supersaturation with respect to calcium phosphate salts. Calcif. Tissue int. *34:* 531–538 (1982).

17   Hay, D.I.; Moreno, E.C.; Schlesinger, D.H.: Phosphoprotein inhibitors of calcium phosphate precipitation from salivary secretion. Inorg. Perspect. Biol. Med. *2:* 271–285 (1979).

18   Hay, D.I.: Human glandular salivary proteins; in Lazzari, Handbook of experimental aspects of oral biochemistry (CRC, Cleveland, in press).

19   Heineman, H.S.; Greenberg, M.S.: Cell-protective effect of human saliva specific for Herpes simplex virus. Archs, oral Biol. *25:* 257–261 (1980).

20   Heitz, P.U.; Kasper, M.; Noorden, S. van: Polak, J.M.; Gregory, H.; Pearse, A.G.E.: Immunohistochemical localisation of urogastrone to human duodenal and submandibular glands. Gut *19:* 408–413 (1978).

21   Herp, A.; Wu, A.M.; Moschera, J.: Current concepts of the structure and nature of mammalian salivary mucous glycoproteins. Mol. cell. Biochem. *23:* 27–43 (1979).

22   Herzberg, M.; Levine, M.J.; Ellison, S.A.; Tabak, L.A.: Purification and characterization of monkey salivary mucin. J. biol. Chem. *254:* 1487–1494 (1979).

23   Kleinberg, I.; Kanapka, J.A.; Craw, D.: Effect of saliva and salivary factors on the metabolism of the mixed oral flora; in Stiles, Loesche, O'Brien, Microbiology abstracts. Proc. Microbial Aspects of Dental Caries, vol. II, pp. 433–464 (Information Retrieval, London 1976).

24   Kleinberg, I.; Kanapka, J.A.; Chatterjee, R.; Craw, D.; D'Angelo, N.; Sandham, H.J.: Metabolism of nitrogen by the oral mixed bacteria; in Kleinberg, Ellison, Mandel, Microbiology abstracts. Proc. Saliva and Dental Caries, pp. 357–377 (Information Retrieval, London 1979).

25   Kousvelari, E.I.; Baratz, R.S.; Burke, B.; Oppenheim, F.G.: Immunochemical identification and determination of proline-rich proteins in salivary secretions, enamel pellicle, and glandular tissue specimens. J. dent. Res. *59:* 1430–1438 (1980).

26   Kumar, S.; Rathi, M.; Meyer, L.M.: Studies on vitamin B_{12} binding proteins in human saliva. Proc. Soc. exp. Biol. Med. *151:* 212–214 (1976).

27 Mellersh, A.; Clark, A.; Hafiz, S.: Inhibition of *Neisseria gonorrhoeae* by normal human saliva. Br. J. vener. Dis. *55:* 20–23 (1979).

28 Moreno, E.C.; Kresak, M.; Hay, D.I.: Adsorption thermodynamics of acidic proline-rich human salivary proteins onto calcium apatites. J. biol. Chem. *257:* 2981–2989 (1982).

29 Nishioka, H.; Nishi, K.; Kyokane, K.: Human saliva inactivates mutagenicity of carcinogens. Mut. Res. *85:* 323–333 (1981).

30 Roberts, A.B.; Anzano, M.A.; Lamb, L.C.; Smith, J.M.; Sporn, M.B.: New class of transforming growth factors potentiated by epidermal growth factor: isolation from non-neoplastic tissues. Proc. natn. Acad. Sci. USA *78:* 5339–5343 (1981).

31 Roberts, P.J.P.; Whelan, W.J.: The mechanism of carbohydrase action. Biochem. J. *76:* 246–253 (1960).

32 Rolla, G.; Jonsen, J.: A glycoprotein from human sublingual saliva with virus neutralizing and calcium binding capacities. Acta path. microbiol. scand., suppl. *187:* pp. 96–97 (1967).

33. Schlesinger, D.H.; Hay, D.I.: Complete covalent structure of statherin, a tyrosine-rich acidic peptide which inhibits calcium phosphate precipitation from human parotid saliva. J. biol. chem. *252:* 1689–1695 (1977).

34 Shatzman, A.R.; Henkin, R.I.: Metal-binding characteristics of the parotid salivary protein gustin. Biochim. biophys. Acta *623:* 107–118 (1980).

35 Shatzman, A.R.; Henkin, R.I.: Gustin concentration changes relative to salivary zinc and taste in humans. Proc. natn. Acad. Sci. USA *78:* 3867–3871 (1981).

36 Singer, D.L.; Chatterjee, R.; Denepitiya, L.; Kleinberg, I.: A comparison of the acid-base metabolisms of pooled human dental plaque and salivary sediment. Archs oral Biol. *28:* 29–35 (1983).

37 Sporn, M.B.; Roberts, A.B.; Shull, J.H.; Smith, J.M.; Ward, J.M.; Socek, J.: Polypeptide transforming growth factors isolated from bovine sources and used for wound healing *in vivo.* Science *219:* 1329–1331 (1983).

38 Stormby, D.R.; Wallenius, R.: Effect of reduced salivation on oral tumor induction in hamsters by 9,10-dimethyl-1,2-benzanthracene. Odont. Revy *15:* 186–191 (1964).

39 Tabak, L.A.; Levine, M.J.; Mandel, I.D.; Ellison, S.A.: Role of salivary mucins in the protection of the oral cavity. J. oral pathol. *11:* 1–17 (1982).

40 Wallenius, R.: Experimental oral cancer in the rat with special reference to the influence of saliva. Acta path. microbiol. scand., suppl. 180, pp. 1–91 (1966).

41 Weinberg, E.D.: Iron and susceptibility to infectious diseases. Science *184:* 952–956 (1974).

42 Weinberg, E.D.: Iron and infection. Microbiol. Rev. *42:* 45–66 (1978).

43 Yancey, R.J.; Finkelstein, R.A.: Siderophore production by pathogenic *Neisseria* spp. Infect. Immunity *32:* 600–608 (1981).

44 Zahradnik, R.T.; Propas, D.; Moreno, E.C.: *In vitro* enamel demineralization by *Streptococcus mutans* in the presence of salivary pellicles. J. dent. Res. *56:* 1107–1110 (1977).

Donald I. Hay, PhD, Department of Biochemistry,
Forsyth Dental Center, 140 Fenway, Boston, MA 02115 (USA)

Cariology Today. Int. Congr., Zürich 1983, pp. 109–118 (Karger, Basel 1984)

Further Information on the Composition of the Acquired Enamel Pellicle

Kristen Hannesson Eggen, Gunnar Rölla

Department of Pedodontics and Caries Prophylaxis, Dental Faculty,
University of Oslo, Norway

Introduction

The physiological role of the pellicle is thought to involve protection of the enamel against bacteria and bacterial products (acids), reduction of the friction between the teeth and the surrounding soft tissues, and possibly in providing a matrix for remineralization.

The mechanisms by which proteins adsorb to hydroxyapatite are well established; basic proteins adsorb to the exposed phosphate groups in the surface of the mineral, whereas acidic proteins adsorb to calcium ions adsorbed to the surface (fig. 1). It has been assumed that salivary proteins adsorb to tooth enamel by the same mechanisms. However, there is only scant experimental evidence to support this assumption. Much research has been performed on the composition and formation of the acquired enamel pellicle during the last two decades [*Leach* et al., 1967; *Armstrong*, 1967; *Belcourt* et al., 1974; *Sønju and Rölla*, 1973; *Hay*, 1969; *Bennick and Cannon*, 1978]. Two major approaches have been used: (1) to remove the protein film directly from teeth in vitro or in vivo with subsequent chemical analysis, or (2) to purify individual proteins from saliva and examine their affinity for hydroxyapatite in vitro; proteins which exhibit high affinity for hydroxyapatite are assumed to possess high affinity for enamel in vivo and are considered as likely contributors to the protein film formed on teeth (i.e. the acquired enamel pellicle).

Both approaches have limitations. The average amino acid composition of the pellicle obtained by method 1 does not allow any conclusions as to how many or which proteins are present in the pellicle.

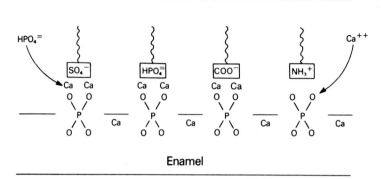

Fig. 1. A diagrammatic representation of the current concept of the mechanism involved in protein adsorption to hydroxyapatite [*Rölla* et al., 1982]. Basic proteins (right) are adsorbed to the surface proper (which is negatively charged). Such proteins can be desorbed by calcium ions (arrow). Acidic proteins are adsorbed to the counter ions (i.e. calcium) present on the surface of the mineral. Such proteins can be desorbed by phosphate ions (arrow).

These experiments have, however, shown that a selective adsorption of salivary proteins occurs; the amino acid composition of the hydrolyzed pellicle is clearly different from that of hydrolyzed whole saliva. It has also been shown that bacterial molecules are not a major component of the pellicle film.

Method 2 can establish the affinity of a homogeneous protein to hydroxyapatite. One cannot, however, be certain that the same mechanisms are involved in pellicle formation, as discussed above, and the competitive aspects of adsorption which will be an important point in vivo with the numerous salivary proteins available is not easy to mimic in vitro.

The experiments presented in the present paper describe *solubilization* of salivary proteins adsorbed to hydroxyapatite in vitro and to human teeth in vivo, and subsequent chromatography of the dissolved proteins in different column chromatography systems [*Eggen and Sønju*, 1981; *Eggen*, 1982; *Eggen and Rölla*, 1982]. The aim was to compare the chromatographic properties of the proteins from the two sources. Several salivary proteins were identified in the pellicle by immunological techniques. The chemical composition of a purified protein component obtained from human teeth in vivo was compared with the

composition of purified proteins with high affinity for hydroxyapatite
or for calcium ions described in the literature.

*Solubilization of Proteins Adsorbed to Hydroxyapatite
(Bio-gel HTP) when This Mineral Is Exposed to
Clarified Whole Saliva in vitro*

Hydroxyapatite which had been exposed to whole saliva was obtained and the mineral phase was dissolved in EDTA and the protein
preparation obtained dialyzed against a buffer. The technical details
have been published elsewhere [*Eggen*, 1981]. The solubilized adsorbed
proteins were then subjected to gel filtration, to ion exchange chro-

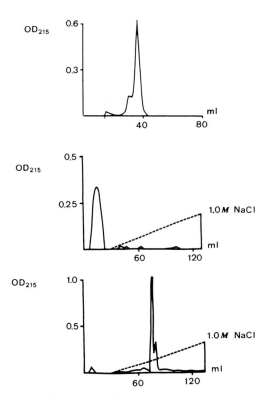

Fig. 2. Chromatography of proteins recovered from the surface of hydroxyapatite
which had been exposed to whole saliva. Gel filtration on agarose (top); ion-exchange
chromatography on CM-Sephadex (middle); ion exchange-chromatography on DEAE-
Sephadex (bottom).

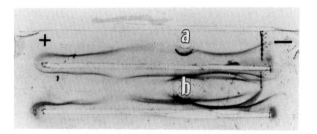

Fig. 3. Immunoelectrophoresis of serum (*a*) and whole saliva (*b*) against an antiserum against saliva-coated hydroxyapatite. At least two anionic antigens and several cationic antigens are evident. Two serum proteins cross-react with the antiserum.

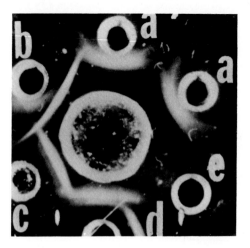

Fig. 4. Gel precipitation of proteins recovered from saliva coated hydroxyapatite reacted against specific antisera. a = Antiserum against saliva-coated hydroxyapatite; b = antialbumin; c = anti-IgA; d = anti-IgG; e = anti-IgM.

matography on a negatively charged column (Sephadex CM) and finally on a positively charged column (Sephadex DEAE). The results are shown in figure 2. It can be seen that the proteins obtained after treatment with EDTA and dialysis behaved as one component in gel filtration, whereas ion-exchange chromatography separated this component into one major anionic component and several minor peaks of cationic, anionic and neutral nature. In an additional experiment, a suspension of saliva-coated hydroxyapatite was used as antigens in rabbits. The antiserum exhibited 6–8 different precipitation lines

against whole saliva and the following proteins were identified by use
of specific antisera: IgA, IgG, lysozyme and albumin (fig. 3, 4). The
presence of glucosyltransferase in the pellicle was demonstrated by
inhibition of an enzyme preparation from a strain of *Streptococcus
mutans*. *a*-Amylase was identified directly in the recovered proteins by
the use of a starch substrate and iodine. The technical details of this
part of the study have been published elsewhere [*Rölla* et al., 1983a].

The two studies described above thus showed that a major anionic
component is present in the salivary proteins which adsorb to hydroxyapatite in vitro. Several minor components are also present in the
material. Several of these were identified by immunological techniques.

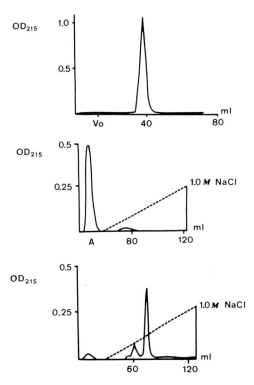

Fig. 5. Chromatography of proteins recovered from human teeth in vivo (the 2-hour
pellicle). Gel filtration on agarose (top); CM-Sephadex (middle), and DEAE-Sephadex
(bottom).

Solubilization of Proteins Adsorbed to Human Teeth in vivo
(the 2-Hour Pellicle)

The results of chromatography of proteins solubilized in EDTA after scraping of pellicle material from teeth in vivo are presented in figure 5. It can be seen that the pellicle material behaved very similarly to the proteins obtained from hydroxyapatite in vitro (fig. 2). One major component was seen after gel filtration, and the major component was anionic and was eluted at the same molarity of sodium chloride as the corresponding peak obtained from hydroxyapatite in vitro. The presence of IgA, IgG and lysozyme in the pellicle was demonstrated by Elisa technique (fig. 6). a-Amylase was demonstrated by the use of a starch substrate and iodine, and the presence of glucosyl-transferase by incubation of pellicle material with ^{14}C-sucrose. Radioactive glucan was demonstrated through the use of the paper disc method employing 75% ethanol to precipitate polysaccharide. Further details are given in a recent publication [*Rölla* et al., 1983c].

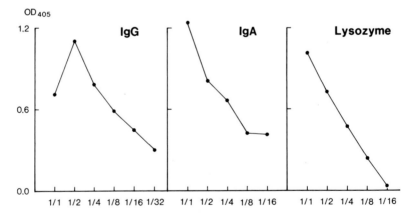

Fig. 6. Results of Elisa of pellicle material obtained by chromatography on CM-Sephadex (fig. 6). The left curve represents optical density at different dilutions of pellicle material reacted with antiserum against human IgG; the middle curve shows a similar sample reacted against an antiserum against human IgA, and the right curve shows reaction against antihuman lysozyme. The antisera were used in a 1:400 dilution. The antisera were from rabbits and were obtained from Dako.

Tentative Identification of the Major Anionic Component in the Acquired Enamel Pellicle

The amino acid composition of several proteins with high affinity for hydroxyapatite is shown in figure 7. It can be seen that the component isolated from teeth and from hydroxyapatite has a composition similar to a phosphoprotein isolated by *Boat* et al. [1974]. The other proteins have a clearly different amino acid composition. The amino acid composition of the anionic peaks from hydroxyapatite and the pellicle material is given in table I. The chemical composition of the phosphoprotein described by *Boat* et al. [1974] is included for comparison.

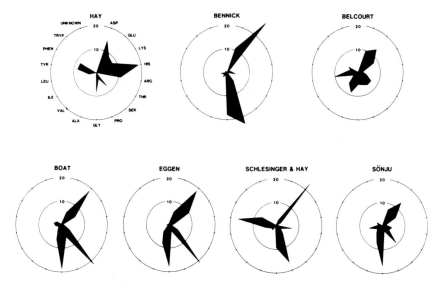

Fig. 7. Diagrams of amino acid composition of selected saliva proteins with high affinity for hydroxyapatite. It is apparant that the purified anionic component from the 2-hour pellicle (Eggen) has a composition very similar to a phosphoprotein described by *Boat* et al. [1974]. The other proteins show no similarity with the pellicle component. The lower right diagram in the figure represents the amino acid composition of the total pellicle [*Sønju and Rölla*, 1973]. The diagrams are prepared according to the method of *Robinson* et al. [1975].

Table I. The amino acid composition of the major anionic component which adsorbs to hydroxyapatite in vitro (HA), to human teeth in vivo (2-hour pellicle) and of the calcium-binding protein of *Boat* et al. [1974]

mol/100 mol	HA	2-hour pellicle	*Boat* et al. [1974]
Asp	6.9	5.6	5.4
Glu	16.5	18.8	18.9
Lys	11.3	9.9	6.6
His	2.3	2.8	0.8
Arg	1.3	1.4	2.0
Thr	4.3	4.6	3.6
Ser	20.2	20.2	22.0
Pro	3.4	3.0	5.7
Gly	17.3	17.5	18.2
Ala	8.9	8.6	6.6
Val	3.3	3.9	2.8
Ile	1.9	0.8	1.7
Leu	2.3	2	2.9
Tyr	–	–	3.6
Phen	0.8	2	2.7

Discussion

The experiments described above showed that the pattern of protein uptake by hydroxyapatite and by teeth in vivo is very similar. The mechanisms involved are thus probably the same. The presence of a major anionic component with an amino acid composition like *Boat* et al.'s [1974] phosphoprotein support this concept because this is a protein with very high affinity for calcium; a property which is considered essential in the present concept of affinity of interaction between anionic proteins and hydroxyapatite (fig. 1). It may seem surprising that none of the other phosphoproteins described with high affinity for hydroxyapatite were found in the pellicle. These proteins all have clearly identified special features in their amino acid composition and should thus be easily identified (fig. 7). It appears possible that *Boat's* phosphoprotein acts in two steps: (1) it is adsorbed to the surface and (2) it precipitates and forms a layer of protein [*Bettleheim,* 1971; *Boat* et al., 1974]. Another observation which supports the significance of *Boat's* phosphoprotein in the pellicle is that the major amino acids in this protein (serine, glycine and glutamic acid) can be readily identified in crude pellicle material obtained from teeth before dialysis or frac-tionation [*Belcourt* et al., 1974]. Whether the major anionic component of the pellicle is homogeneous or if it consists of a family of closely related proteins is not known at present. However, the criteria of homogeneity published by *Boat* et al. [1974] are strong and the com-ponent in the present study appears as one peak in chromatography on DEAE (fig. 2, 5), and presumably as one precipitation line against an antipellicle serum in the studies described above [*Rölla* et al., 1983a]. *Shomers* et al. [1982] have recently reported the presence of a family of cysteine-containing phosphoproteins in saliva. These may well be re-lated to *Boat's* phosphoprotein; they cross-react immunologically; the amino acid compositions are, however, markedly different.

Saliva-coated hydroxyapatite is often used as a 'target' to study bacterial adherence to teeth in vitro. The present data show that im-munoglobulins, lysozyme, amylase, albumin and glucosyltransferase are available in the pellicle. These proteins clearly provide a number of potential binding mechanisms for bacteria, which are not usually con-sidered in these types of studies. Care should thus be taken in the interpretation of data from such studies. The potential role of glucosyl-transferase in sucrose-enhanced colonization of bacteria in vitro and in vivo has been discussed in two recent papers [*Rölla* et al., 1983b, c].

References

Armstrong, W.G.: The composition of organic films formed on human teeth. Caries Res. *1:* 87–103 (1967).

Belcourt, A.; Frank, R.M.; Houver, G.: Analyse des acides aminés de la pellicule exogène acquise et des protéines à l'émail superficiel chez l'homme. J. Biol. buccale *2:* 161–180 (1974).

Bennick, A.; Cannon, M.: Quantitative study of the interaction of salivary acidic proline rich proteins with hydroxyapatite. Caries Res. *12:* 159–169 (1978).

Bettleheim, F.A.: On the aggregation of a calcium precipitable from human submaxillary saliva. Biochim. biophys. Acta *23b:* 702–705 (1971).

Boat, T.F.; Wiesman, U.N.; Pallavicini, J.C.: Purification and properties of a calcium-precipitable protein in submaxillary saliva of normal and cystic fibrosis subjects. Pediat. Res. *8:* 531–539 (1974).

Eggen, K.H.: Interaction between human saliva and various hydroxyapatite surfaces; in Frank, Leach, Surface and colloid phenomena in the oral cavity. Methodological aspects, pp. 227–238 (IRL Press, London 1982).

Eggen, K.H.; Rölla, G.: Gel filtration, ion exchange chromatography and chemical analysis of macromolecules present in the acquired enamel pellicle (2 hour pellicle). Scand. J. dent. Res. *90:* 182–188 (1982).

Eggen, K.H.; Sønju, T.: Solubilization of the two hour pellicle collected from human teeth in vivo; in Rölla, Sønju, Embery, Tooth surface interactions and preventive dentistry, pp. 95–103 (IRL Press, London 1981).

Hay, D.I.: Some observations on human saliva proteins and their role in the formation of the acquired enamel pellicle. J. dent. Res. *48:* 806–810 (1969).

Hay, D.I.; Moreno, E.C.: Macromolecular inhibitors of calcium phosphate precipitation in human saliva. Their roles in providing a protective environment for the teeth; in Kleinberg, Ellison, Mandel, Saliva and dental caries, pp. 45–58 (IRL Press, Washington 1979).

Leach, S.A.; Chritchley, A.B.; Kolindo, A.B.; Saxton, C.A.: Salivary glycoproteins as components of the enamel integuments. Caries Res. *1:* 104–111 (1967).

Mayhall, C.W.: Concerning the composition and source of the acquired enamel pellicle of human teeth. Archs oral Biol. *15:* 1327–1341 (1970).

Robinson, C.; Lowe, N.R.; Weatherell, J.A.: Amino acid composition distribution and origin of 'tuft' protein in human and bovine dental enamel. Archs oral Biol. *20:* 29–42 (1975).

Rölla, G.; Ciardi, J.E.; Bowen, W.H.: Ionic exchange reactions on hydroxyapatite surfaces studied by the use of radioactive counterions (^{45}Ca and ^{32}PO$_4$) in Frank, Leach, Surface and colloidal phenomena in the oral cavity. Methodological aspects, pp. 203–212 (IRL Press, London 1982).

Rölla, G.; Ciardi, J.E.; Bowen, W.H.: Identification of IgA, IgG, lysozyme, albumin, α-amylase and glucosyl transferase in the protein layer adsorbed to hydroxyapatite from whole saliva. Scand. J. dent. Res. *91:* 186–190 (1983a).

Rölla, G.; Ciardi, J.E.; Schulz, S.A.: Adsorption of glycosyltransferase to saliva coated hydroxyapatite. Possible mechanism for sucrose dependant bacterial colonization of teeth. Scand. J. dent. Res. *91:* 112–117 (1983b).

Rölla, G.; Ciardi, J.E.; Eggen, K.H.; Bowen, W.H.; Afseth, J.: Free glucosyl and fructosyltransferase in human saliva and adsorption of these enzymes to teeth in vivo; in Doyle, Ciardi, The chemistry and biology of glucosyltransferases (IRL Press, Washington 1983c).

Shomers, J.P.; Tabac, L.A.; Levine, M.J.; Mandel, I.D.; Ellison, S.A.: Characterization of cystein-containing phosphoproteins from human submandibular sublingual saliva. J. dent. Res. *61:* 764–767 (1982).

Sønju, T.; Rölla, G.: Chemical analysis of the acquired pellicle formed in two hours on cleaned teeth in vivo. Caries Res. *7:* 30–37 (1973).

Kirsten H. Eggen, MD, Department of Pedodontics and Caries Prohylaxis, Dental Faculty, University of Oslo, N-Oslo (Norway)

Diet

Moderator: E. Newbrun, San Francisco, Calif., USA

Cariology Today. Int. Congr., Zürich 1983, pp. 119–124 (Karger, Basel 1984)

Nutrition and Diet in a Changing Society

Arnold E. Bender

Department of Food Science and Nutrition, Queen Elizabeth College, University of London, England

During the past two or three generations two major changes have taken place in the diets of all industrialised communities: (1) the provision of adequate supplies of food at all times, and (2) replacement of traditional home-prepared foods by a vast range of processed foods.

Food Technology

Until the beginning of this century, famines were common in all countries and the amount of food available to most people was very limited. One result was widespread deficiency diseases such as pellagra and scurvy (and beriberi in rice-eating communities) as well as general undernutrition and malnutrition. As recently as 1928, there were 10,000 deaths from pellagra in the southern part of the United States and this deficiency disease persisted in Italy until the 1930s. In Great Britain, there was widespread malnutrition among the unemployed and lower-paid in the 1930s.

The enormous improvements in one generation are due to a variety of factors, mainly economic, together with increased efficiency of agricultural production and the developments of the twin subjects of nutrition and food science. The former enables us to identify and rectify some of the deficiencies and the latter has made available a very much greater variety of foods at all times of the year.

Many of these improvements date only from the end of the 1945 war when several developments took place at the same time which reinforced and supplemented one another. Post-war reconstruction led to virtually full employment so that people were able to buy what they wanted while spending a steadily decreasing proportion of their disposable income on food (the proportion fell from about 50 to 20–30%).

Social change resulted in more housewives going to work so that not only was there more money available in the family but a desire for less bondage to the kitchen and so greater demands for processed and particularly convenience foods. This occurred at the time that food technology was making rapid strides leading to large-scale production and preservation of food together with the developments in packaging, distribution and storage throughout all countries of the industrialised world. Marketing methods, as exemplified by supermarkets, also played a rôle.

In the home these changes were reinforced by the introduction of refrigerators, freezers and microwave ovens – all helping to reshape our food habits.

The availability of a wider variety of foods leads to less dependence on the staple food and inevitably to an improved diet. Food technology also permits the enrichment of foods and the preparation of therapeutic diets and special foods for infants. Improved methods of processing intended to inflict less change in texture, flavour and colour also result in less damage to the nutrients, even if this was not the original intention of the improved processing methods.

Such changes, however, are paralleled by less beneficial changes since the 'new' foods replace traditional foods and this has led to an increased consumption of sugar, fats and alcohol. These are at best empty calories and at worst are implicated in a variety of modern diseases. A wide variety of foods permits unwise selection so that while, in general, a wider variety provides a better diet it can also lead to a poorer diet.

Processed Foods

Processed foods as such are frequently compared unfavourably with home-prepared foods but this is only partly true. Losses of nutrients during manufacture are often in place of those that take place in the home rather than additional; they may be less if processing is adequately controlled compared with domestic preparation.

The composition of some of the common manufactured foods appears to be nutritionally poor. For example, biscuits contain up to 35% sucrose and 30% fat, while cakes contain up to 40% sucrose and 25% fat. They certainly bear a great deal of blame for dental decay as well as being of poor nutritional value, but similar recipes are used in home-made biscuits and cakes.

It is difficult to make generalisations as may be exemplified by a comparison between a traditional breakfast cereal, muesli, and a modern large-scale factory-produced product such as corn flakes. The former is usually regarded as a fibre-rich 'health-giving' food compared with the latter but four brands of muesli were shown to contain 26% sucrose compared with 7% in corn flakes, and only 7% dietary fibre compared with 11% in corn flakes (Standard British Food Composition Tables). Both products, in fact, are factory-made and comparison could be made instead, between factory corn flakes and home-prepared muesli based on 'better' ingredients. Such comparison would be valid only if the traditional home-prepared cereal were replaced by an inferior processed food but even then a difference between two foods may not affect the diet as a whole. In all such comparisons it is necessary to take account of the part played by the foods in question in the diet as a whole. Since major changes have taken place any comparison between individual foods provides little evidence of nutritional changes due to processing.

Processed foods are also criticised for their contribution to the intake of sodium and again it is difficult to generalise since this applies only to a limited number of foods. Clearly, those preserved by salting such as olives, bacon and other meat products are very high in sodium content; bacon contains 2,000 mg sodium per 100 g, salt beef, and canned and processed meats of various types and smoked fish contain 1,000 mg. A search of the food composition tables shows only a few other foods with a high sodium content; when haricot beans are canned, the sodium content is increased from 15 to 480 mg, when carrots are canned sodium is increased from 23 to 280 mg, peas from a 'trace' to 200–300 mg and sweet corn from 1 to 310 mg/100 g. But these appear to be the only foods in which the sodium content is markedly increased by the processor. The greater part of the dietary sodium, apart from salt-cured foods, is added during cooking and at the table. The consumer habits rather than processing as such bear the greater part of the blame in this respect.

Snack Foods

There appears to be a discrepancy between dental dietary advice offered (at least in some parts of Great Britain) and that offered by nutritionists. One of the greater changes that has taken place in the diets of some people is the habit of snacking in place of structured meals. Two snack foods that are extremely popular are salted peanuts (49% fat and 440 mg sodium per 100 g) and potato crisps or chips (36% fat and 550 mg sodium). Since sugary foods in prolonged contact with teeth are a major cause of dental decay the dental educators designated sugary snack foods as 'bad' and suggested as 'good' ones, salted peanuts and potato crisps. As discussed below, these two foods would be regarded as bad by the nutritionist so it is clearly necessary for the two professions to work together.

Natural Foods

There has been a growth in demand for what are thought of as 'natural' foods together with the use, where necessary, of 'natural' additives rather than synthetic ones.

One reason may possibly be rebellion against regimentation of modern society, epitomised by multiplication of regulations, international business and manipulation by the media. It is fostered by those who find the appeal of so-called health foods highly profitable and also by the manufacturers of branded foods who make use of this appeal. This last point is epitomised by the struggle for sales between the manufacturers of butter – who claim that this is a natural food – and those of margarine – who claim that it is made from natural materials.

This trend away from processed or manufactured towards 'natural' products varies considerably in different countries and different sections of the community. In France, for example, there is much less reliance on factory-processed foods than there is in Great Britain; it is the middle class rather than the working class who have both the inclination and the money to spend on anything other than mass-produced cheap foods; such trends are taken up almost as a religious movement by certain sections of the community. The claims and counter claims have reached such proportions in the United States that it must be impossible for the ordinary person to distinguish between fact and fancy. There are said to be a score of organisations, ranging from Government agencies and the 'Better Business Bureau' to publicly-minded academics, who attempt to provide the true facts of foods and diets and an equal or greater number of organisations who are misleading the public.

Nutritional Goals

Evidence of varying reliability has come to light in recent years implicating food in a number of diseases of modern society – coronary heart disease, diabetes, diverticular disease and other bowel disorders, and certain types of cancer. The evidence is far from clear and there is much controversy but a number of desirable changes have been suggested – so-called nutritional goals.

Leaving aside arguments as to whether these are all acceptable there are two points to be made. Firstly, people are reluctant to change their food habits and, secondly, the manufacturer has already made foods available which permit these nutritional changes without having to change dietary habits.

Each of the goals has its appropriate food already available:

(1) 'Overweight people should lose their surplus'. There are a number of low-energy foods (so-called slimming foods) and other preparation such as energy-controlled meal-replacers on the market.

(2) 'Reduce total fat intake, especially saturated fats and consume more polyunsaturated fatty acids'. There are substitutes for meat made from vegetable proteins which can be fat-free or polyunsaturated fats can be used in their manufacture. These products illustrate the fact that the substitute food must be at least as attractive as the one it replaces if it is to be accepted. Partly skimmed milk, low-fat bread spreads and polyunsaturated margarines are all available.

(3) 'Reduce sugar consumption'. There are several new artificial sweeteners being made available.

(4) 'Eat whole grain cereals rather than white bread'. This does not appear to be acceptable and people prefer white bread. The problem has been solved by making white bread with added bran – containing even more bran than whole grain bread.

(5) 'Reduce alcohol consumption'. There are low-alcohol beers and alcohol-free wines.

(6) 'Reduce salt intake'. Unfortunately, all substitutes for salt lack the preferred flavour and here we can only offer advice to the consumer.

So in our changing society we can observe a number of contrary changes in nutrition. The mass production of foods has replaced many traditional foods with both advantage and potential disadvantages. The trend towards manufactured foods is partly rejected by some sections of the community. The blame laid at the door of the food manufacturer for the detrimental effects of increased intake of sugar and fats and reduced intake of dietary fibre can be converted into praise since he is carrying out the task in which nutritional advice is failing.

Incidentally, all the dietary goals discussed above are open to argument and controversy with the single exception that prolonged contact between sucrose and the teeth leads to dental decay. Here, also, the manufacturer can aid the dental health adviser. If people will not refrain from eating sweets they can be made with sugar-alcohols which do not ferment.

There may well be considerable advantage to be gained by combining the forces of the public health adviser with the commercial sales of these relatively beneficial foods instead of, or perhaps as well as, attempting the difficult task of advising people to change their food habits.

Prof. Dr. Arnold E. Bender, Department of Food Science and Nutrition, Queen Elizabeth College, University of London, Campden Hill Road, London W8 7AH (England)

Cariology Today. Int. Congr., Zürich 1983, pp. 125–135 (Karger, Basel 1984)

Influence on Caries of Trace Metals Other than Fluoride

M.E.J. Curzon

Department of Oral Biology, Eastman Dental Center, Rochester, N.Y., USA

In many parts of the world, substantial differences in caries prevalence occur between populations resident within the same geographic location and with similar fluoride levels. In many of these areas evidence has shown that variations in trace element intake from food and/or water may be implicated. It has not, as yet, been possible to obtain evidence of sufficient strength to establish conclusive causal relationships between individual trace elements and caries prevalence. However, the multitude of studies indicating associations of trace metals to caries prevalence in both man and animals provides enough evidence to substantiate the thesis that a number of trace metals do affect the caries process. It is some of these studies concerning a selected number of trace metals that will be discussed here.

Trace Metals and Caries

Copper

Inferential studies using associations of copper in water supplies to dental caries indicate that the metal is related to increased caries [*Ludwig* et al., 1970; *Adkins and Losee*, 1970]. Animal experiments have been limited and shown either no effect [*McClure*, 1948; *Shaw*, 1950] or a reduction in caries [*Hein and Shaffer*, 1951; *Hein*, 1953].

More importantly, recent research has indicated a strong anti-plaque and anti-bacterial effect of copper. Significant reductions in acid production in plaque have been shown by $CuSO_4$ [*Afseth* et al., 1980]. As copper has been used as an inhibitor of the growth of organisms, such as anti-fouling on ships, it is not surprising that it should have marked effects on oral bacteria. A very recent report has shown a promising anti-plaque and anti-caries effect of copper [*Afseth* et al., 1983] both topically and in drinking water.

Lithium

Lithium in recent years has been associated with low caries prevalence. Research in Papua-New Guinea on the variables associated with low caries in Sepik River tribesmen showed a statistically strong association of lithium in saliva solids with low caries prevalence [*Schamschula* et al., 1978]. Further work by the same team of researchers has also demonstrated similar associations for lithium in school children in Australia [*Schamschula* et al., 1981]. These findings are worth further investigation, as they are in some degree supported by the association of low caries to trace metals in drinking water noted by *Curzon* et al. [1970] in Ohio (USA). In the latter study, there was high lithium in the water of the low caries towns.

Animal studies on lithium and caries are entirely equivocal with both increases, decreases and no effect being noted in rats. The most recent studies have again shown a trend towards a reduction in caries by lithium, but without any statistically significant results [*Curzon*, 1982].

Molybdenum

Molybdenum and dental caries has been excellently reviewed by *Jenkins* [1983]. In a very comprehensive investigation of the difference in caries rates between children resident in the adjacent towns of Napier and Hastings (New Zealand), a major association of the low caries level in Napier was with molybdenum. No other environmental differences between the two towns were identified except that Napier was situated on highly alkaline soils of recent marine origin [*Ludwig* et al., 1960]. However, it must also be pointed out that analysis of human teeth collected in the towns did not show differences in molybdenum content which would be expected.

Using the 'teart' pastures (areas of toxic molybdenum in soils and vegetation) of a district in Somerset, England, *Anderson* [1969] showed children resident in these areas to have a lower caries prevalence than in a control low molybdenum area. Analysis of tooth, urine and milk pooled samples yielded results showing higher levels of molybdenum in all samples collected from the molybdenosis area.

A similar finding of low caries in an area of alkaline soils and high available molybdenum has been reported from South Africa [*Pienaar and Bartel,* 1968]. However, no such effect was found in an area of molybdenosis in California [*Curzon* et al., 1971].

Although research in the 1960s seemed to indicate a relationship of caries to molybdenum, animal studies have been equivocal and no further work has been attempted since that time. This may be because of the complex chemistry of molybdenum which has many valencies, and it has not been possible to sort out the effects of different molybdenum salts on *in vivo* and *in vitro* production of caries. If molybdenum does reduce caries the mechanism is still unknown.

Selenium

In areas where trace elements are present at high levels, such as in soils, water, and foods, there may be an increased intake of such elements by man. *Tank and Storvick* [1960] showed that urinary levels of selenium in children living in seleniferous areas of the N.W. United States averaged 0.21 ppm, compared with 0.05 ppm Se in children in a nearby low selenium area. Variations in selenium content of human enamel have also been shown to vary, and related to caries prevalence [*Hadjimarkos and Bonhurst,* 1959]. Levels of selenium intake by children in these areas reflected local soil selenium, originating, in all probability, from ingestion of locally produced foods such as dairy products. Thus, foods of animal origin may also show variations in trace element composition.

Urinary levels of selenium related to increased caries experience in the N.W. United States were described by the investigations of *Hadjimarkos* [1965] and in many subsequent reports. Supporting evidence for *Hadjimarkos'* hypothesis that selenium is associated with high caries comes from the *Tank and Storvick* [1960] study cited above. *Ludwig and Bibby* [1969] also demonstrated a positive association of selenium and caries in high and low selenium areas in parts of Oregon, Montana, and South Dakota, USA.

A possible interaction of fluoride and selenium has been tested but none of the studies reported to date have indicated any such action. This may be because the two elements are principally located in different parts of the tooth: fluoride in the mineral portion of enamel where it may affect dissolution and remineralization, and selenium in the protein matrix fraction. In the latter case, it has been suggested that selenium, in high concentrations, may disorganize protein matrix formation [*Shearer*, 1983]. As this forms the framework on which calcification of the enamel subsequently takes place, disorganization by the selenium could lead to a defective tooth enamel. Adequate levels of selenium would promote good enamel formation and a negative relation of the element in enamel to dental caries has been shown [*Curzon and Crocker*, 1978].

Selenium has already been demonstrated as essential by its uptake into the glutathione peroxidase enzymes. Conversely, selenium inhibits other enzymes including succinic dehydrogenase which is an enzyme present in the ameloblast – the cell responsible for enamel matrix formation. Disorganization of enamel formation by inhibition of essential enzymes could also be a mechanism of action of selenium associated with increased caries prevalence. Recently, it has been shown that selenium offsets the deleterious effects of cadmium in increasing dental caries [*Shearer*, 1983]. As with a number of trace elements, the role of selenium in dental caries is a complex one involving the interaction with other elements.

Strontium

Strontium was identified as being in very high levels in the drinking water supplies of a number of caries-free recruits inducted into the United States Navy [*Losee and Adkins*, 1969] originating from a small area of N.W. Ohio. An epidemiologic study in the same area found a 35.7% lower mean caries rate DMFS in 12–14 year olds in high strontium towns than in a control low strontium town, which has recently been shown to still be so [*Curzon*, 1983]. This difference was greater than could be accounted for by levels of fluoride alone and was related to significantly higher levels of boron, lithium and particularly strontium. A number of other reports have indicated an association between strontium and low caries [*Lödrop*, 1953; *Curzon* et al., 1978; *Barmes*, 1969].

Reports have associated high strontium in enamel [*Vrbic and Stupar*, 1980] and in plaque [*Curzon and Spector*, 1983] with low dental caries and a number of recent animal studies have also shown caries in rats to be inhibited by strontium in the drinking water [*Ashrafi* et al., 1980].

Because of its close similarity to calcium, strontium can replace up to four of the ten calcium ions in human enamel apatite, which may bring about changes in the physical properties of the enamel apatite [*LeGeros* et al., 1977]. As the early lesion is a process of acid dissolution, the resistance of enamel apatite to such dissolution is important. *Dedhiya* et al. [1974] studied the incorporation of strontium and/or fluoride in synthetic apatites. When used in combination, the effect of the strontium and fluoride in reducing dissolution was far greater than fluoride alone. A recent finding is that there is a reduction in carbonate content of apatite by incorporation of strontium [*Featherstone* et al., 1980]. Furthermore, strontium appears to play a role in the remineralization process [*Featherstone and Shariati,* 1983] where optimum concentrations of strontium are necessary for rapid remineralization.

Vanadium

Vanadium is another trace element associated with low caries prevalence based on early epidemiologic studies of *Tank and Storvick* [1960]. These authors reported that the relationship they found between the metal and dental caries was also affected by the fluoride levels in the same water supplies. So here again a fluoride-trace element interaction was suggested. Further epidemiologic studies on dental caries related to trace element content of drinking water by *Sandor and Denes* [1972] recorded low frequencies of dental caries where water concentrations of vanadium were high. Thus, low levels of caries were also found to be related to increased levels of calcium and magnesium as well as total water hardness.

High concentrations of vanadium have been found to stimulate growth of *A. viscosus* [*Beighton and McDougall,* 1981]. However, *Gallagher and Cutress* [1977] found acid production of streptococci and actinomyces inhibited by vanadium. Although more than 12 animal experiments have been completed on vanadium and dental caries, the results are unclear with both reductions and increases reported.

Zinc

Zinc has attracted attention in recent years, no doubt because of its major role in health but also because of studies showing a beneficial effect of the metal on caries. Epidemiologic data for a relationship of zinc to dental caries is sparse, compared with other trace elements discussed so far. In extensive trace element studies in Papua-New Guinea [*Schamschula* et al., 1978], zinc did not show any associations with caries. *Helle and Haavikko* [1977] have demonstrated a negative correlation of zinc with caries, whereas *Adkins and Losee* [1967] could not find such a correlation. Similarly, zinc concentrations in enamel have not been related to caries [*Curzon and Crocker*, 1978].

Evidence of an effect of zinc on caries is more substantial from animal studies where results have generally shown a reduction in caries [*Sortino and Palazzo*, 1971; *Steinman and Leonora*, 1975]. This effect is, however, very dependent on the zinc concentrations of the basal diet, and whether animals were zinc deficient during early growth [*Al-Hayali* et al., 1981]. The role of zinc during the period of tooth development is therefore of some importance but requires much more research to identify the mechanism of action involved.

Zinc occurs in high concentrations in plaque [*Schamschula* et al., 1977] and all samples seem to contain substantial levels. It is not clear if the presence of such amounts of zinc in plaque will modify dental caries. However, an effect of zinc on oral bacteria has been shown where $ZnSO_4$ depressed growth of *S. mutans*, initial plaque formation and inhibition of acid production [*Bates and Navia*, 1979]. Other researchers have shown similar results with zinc and zinc fluoride combinations [*Izaguirre-Fernandez*, 1982]. *Muhlemann and Schmid* [1982] have reported substantial reductions in plaque values in rats using zinc with fluoride and hexetidine in an organoleptically acceptable mouthwash. This significant finding shows promise.

It has also been suggested that zinc may play a role in rehardening of enamel during the remineralization phenomenon [*Featherstone* et al., 1982]. Such an action would require high and constant levels of zinc at the enamel surface as are to be found in plaque. Our knowledge of the role of zinc on dental caries is still far too limited. The probable beneficial role of zinc and its action in plaque and enamel requires much further research.

Other Trace Elements

These have also been studied but limitations of space preclude a detailed discussion of them here. Readers are referred to the recent review of *Curzon and Cutress* [1983] for a discussion of a number of other trace elements and dental disease. Trace metals which have not been mentioned so far, but for which there is some slight evidence for an effect on dental caries include titanium, chromium, iron, cobalt, nickel, arsenic, yttrium, zirconium, niobium, tin, barium, gold and bismuth. However, the data are in most cases sparse and equivocal.

Possible Mechanisms of Trace Metals Action on Caries

If trace metals influence susceptibility to dental caries it would seem quite possible that they do so by altering the resistance of the enamel itself, or by altering intra-oral environment. Such influences might include changes in the morphology of teeth, either in overall size, fissure pattern, or fissure depth, or alternatively affect the enamel structure itself and in particular the character of the apatite crystals. Changes in these crystallites could affect the initiation of enamel dissolution.

Exposure to fluorides has been suggested as leading to small changes in the morphology of the teeth of both man and experimental animals. The extensive researches of *Kruger* [1958] with the trace elements boron, fluoride, copper, manganese, and molybdenum have indicated that trace elements other than fluoride may affect tooth dimensions as well as fissure morphology and depth. Similar findings have also been reported by *Castillo-Mercado and Bibby* [1972] using yttrium, cadmium, and strontium.

Changes in apatite composition and properties can result from a high substitution of fluorine, lead, strontium, magnesium, tin, and copper, especially in the surface layers of the enamel. The presence of these elements will affect the solubility of the enamel surface, thereby influencing susceptibility to dissolution. As described above, strontium has recently attracted attention for such effects upon enamel dissolution and subsequent remineralization. Thus, in theory, the incorporation of some trace metals in the enamel apatite, either during apatite formation or, perhaps more importantly, during remineralization, may materially affect the subsequent caries history of the tooth.

It may also be expected that variations in the intake of different trace metals will be reflected in the composition of saliva and especially of the dental plaque. *Hardwick and Martin's* [1967] studies suggest that trace elements may accumulate in plaque at surprisingly high levels. That accumulation in this way may influence susceptibility to caries is suggested by the findings of *Bowen and Eastoe* [1967] who showed that acid production on caries-susceptible tooth surfaces in monkeys was reduced following treatment with solutions containing 60 mg/l molybdenum. Other studies by *Bowen* [1972] showed that selenium and vanadium concentrations in plaque were related to caries in monkeys.

Furthermore, the trace elements discussed herein could well affect the physiology and metabolism of the oral bacteria. Evidence is already at hand showing that fluoride has a number of actions in this regard and it would not be surprising if other trace elements had a similar effect.

Conclusion

During the past 30 years evidence from human, animal and laboratory studies has accumulated to indicate that trace metals, besides or in combination with fluoride, affect dental caries. Some of these elements such as strontium, lithium and vanadium have been shown to be associated with low caries. On the other hand, a larger number of trace elements including cadmium, lead, manganese, and barium increase caries. For a third group, zinc, iron, sulfur and yttrium, there is insufficient evidence of an effect on dental caries, and more research is needed on them. Selenium appears to be associated with increased caries when present in high concentrations but at adequate levels is important for good enamel matrix formation. The metals zinc and copper have recently been shown to show promise as antiplaque agents and therefore may be of some benefit as anti-caries agents. Strontium and zinc may play an important role in remineralization of enamel after initial demineralization.

References

Adkins, B.L.; Losee, F.L.: A study of the covariation of dental caries prevalence and multiple trace element content of water supplies. N.Y. St. dent. J. *36:* 618–622 (1970).

Adler, P.: Experiments with albino rats on the protective effect of water-borne molybdenum. Proc. 4th ORCA. Odont. Rev. suppl., pp. 48–53 (1957).

Afseth, J.; Oppemann, R.V.; Rolla, G.: The in vivo effect of glucose solutions containing Cu^{++} and Zn^{++} on the acidogenicity of dental plaque. Acta odont. scand. *38:* 229–233 (1980).

Afseth, J.; Amsbaugh, S.M.; Monell-Torrens, E.; Bowen, W.H.; Dahl, E.; Rolla, G.: Effect of Cu in drinking water or in mouthwashes on caries in rats. Abstr. 1026, AADR Ann. Session, Cincinnati 1983.

Al-Hayali, R.; Hsieh, H.S.; Navia, J.M.: Gestational and postnatal dietary zinc and dental caries. J. dent. Res. *60:* 401 (1981).

Anderson, R.J.: The relationship between dental conditions and the trace element molybdenum. Caries Res. *3:* 75–87 (1969).

Ashrafi, M.H.; Spector, P.C.; Curzon, M.E.J.: Pre- and post-eruptive effects of low doses of strontium on dental caries in the rat. Caries Res. *14:* 341–346 (1980).

Barmes, D.E.: Caries etiology in Sepik villages – Trace element micronutrient and macronutrient content of soil and food. Caries Res. *3:* 44–59 (1969).

Bates, D.; Navia, J.M.: Chemotherapeutic effect of zinc on *Streptococcus mutans* and rat dental caries. Archs oral Biol. *24:* 799 (1979).

Beighton, D.; McDougall, W.A.: The influence of certain added water-borne trace elements on the percentage bacterial composition of tooth fissure plaque from conventional Sprague Dawley rats. Archs oral Biol. *26:* 419 (1981).

Bowen, W.H.: The effects of selenium and vanadium on caries activity in monkeys *(M. irus)*. J. Irish dent. Ass. *18:* 83 (1972).

Bowen, W.H.; Eastoe, J.E.: The effect of sugar solution containing fluoride and molybdate ions on the pH of plaque in monkeys. Caries Res. *1:* 130–136 (1967).

Castillo-Mercado, R.; Bibby, B.G.: Trace element effects on enamel pigmentation, incisor growth and molar morphology in rats. Archs oral Biol. *18:* 629–635 (1973).

Curzon, M.E.J.: An experimental study of lithium and dental caries in the rat. Archs oral Biol. *27:* 573–576 (1982).

Curzon, M.E.J.: Combined effect of trace elements and fluorine on caries. Changes over 10 years in NW Ohio (USA). J. dent. Res. *62:* 96–99 (1983).

Curzon, M.E.J.; Adkins, B.L.; Bibby, B.G.; Losee, F.L.: Combined effect of trace elements and fluorine on caries. J. dent. Res. *49:* 526 (1970).

Curzon, M.E.J.; Crocker, D.C.: Relationships of trace elements in human tooth enamel to dental caries. Archs oral Biol. *23:* 647–653 (1978).

Curzon, M.E.J.; Cutress, T.W.: Trace elements and dental disease (John Wright, Littleton 1983).

Curzon, M.E.J.; Kubota, J.; Bibby, B.G.: Environmental effects of molybdenum on dental caries. J. dent. Res. *50:* 74–77 (1971).

Curzon, M.E.J.; Spector, P.C.: Strontium concentrations of human plaque and surface enamel. J. dent. Res. (in press, 1983).

Curzon, M.E.J.; Spector, P.C.; Iker, H.P.: An association between strontium in drinking water supplies and low caries prevalence. Archs oral Biol. *23:* 647–653 (1978).

Dedhiya, M.G.; Young, F.; Higuchi, W.I.: Mechanism of hydroxyapatite dissolution. The synergistic effects of solution fluoride, strontium and phosphate. J. physiol. Chem. *78:* 1273–1279 (1974).

Featherstone, J.D.B.; et al.: Acid reactivity of carbonated-apatites with strontium and fluoride substitutions. J. dent. Res. (submitted, 1983).

Featherstone, J.D.B.; Nelson, D.G.A.: Effect of F, Zn, Sr, Mg and Fe on the structure of synthetic carbonated apatites. Aust. J. Chem. *33:* 2363–2368 (1980).

Featherstone, J.D.B.; Shariati, M.: Dependence of remineralization on concentration of calcium, strontium and zinc. Abstr. 163, AADR Annual Session, Cincinnati 1983.

Gallagher, I.H.C.; Cutress, T.W.: The effect of trace elements on the growth and fermentation by oral streptococci and actinomyces. Archs oral Biol. *22:* 555 (1977).

Hadjimarkos, D.M.: Effect of selenium on dental caries. Archs envir. Hlth *10:* 893–899 (1965).

Hadjimarkos, D.M.; Bonhorst, C.W.: Selenium content of human teeth. Oral Surg. *12:* 113–116 (1959).

Hardwick, D.L.; Martin, C.J.: A pilot study using mass spectrometry for the estimation of the trace element content of dental tissues. Helv. odont. Acta *11:* 62–70 (1967).

Hein, J.W.: Effect of copper sulfate on initiation and progression of dental caries in the Syrian hamster. J. dent. Res. *32:* 654 (1953).

Hein, J.W.; Shafer, W.G.: Further studies on the inhibition of experimental caries by sodium copper chlorophyllin. J. dent. Res. *30:* 510 (1951).

Helle, A.; Haavikko, K.: Macro- and micromineral levels in deciduous teeth from different geographical areas correlated with caries prevalence. Proc. Finn. dent. Soc. *73:* 87 (1977).

Izaguirre-Fernandez, E.J.: Trace element effects on oral bacterial physiology; thesis, University of Rochester, Rochester, N.Y. (1982).

Jenkins, G.N.: Molybdenum; in Curzon, Cutress, Trace elements and dental disease (John Wright, Littleton 1983).

Kruger, B.J.: Effect of trace elements on experimental dental caries in albino rats. Aust. dent. J. *3:* 236–247 (1958).

LeGeros, R.Z.; Miravite, M.A.; Quirologico, G.B.; Curzon, M.E.J.: The effect of some trace elements on the lattice parameters of human and synthetic apatites. Calcif. Tissue Res. *22:* 362–367 (1977).

Lödrop, H.: The low rate of dental decay in Bonn and Rhein and the conclusions that can be drawn from it. Den Norske Tannl. Tid. *63:* 35–50 (1953).

Losee, F.L.; Adkins, B.L.: A study of the mineral environment of caries resistant Navy recruits. Caries Res. *3:* 23–31 (1969).

Ludwig, T.G.; Adkins, B.L.; Losee, F.L.: Relationship of concentrations of eleven elements in public water supplies to caries prevalence in American school children. Aust. dent. J. *15:* 126–132 (1970).

Ludwig, T.G.; Bibby, B.G.: Geographic variations in the prevalence of dental caries in the USA. Caries Res. *3:* 32–43 (1969).

Ludwig, T.G.; Healy, W.B.; Losee, F.L.: An association between dental caries and certain soil conditions in New Zealand. Nature Lond. *186:* 695–696 (1960).

McClure, F.J.: Observations on reduced caries in rats. V. Results of various modifications of food and drinking water. J. dent. Res. *27:* 34–40 (1948).

Muhlemann, H.R.; Schmid, R.: Effects of topical hexetidine and zinc fluoride on caries incidence, plaque formation, molar surface dissolution rate and fluoride content in the rat. Abstr. 54, 29th ORCA Congr., Annapolis 1982.

Pienaar, W.J.; Bartel, E.E.: Molybdenum content of vegetables and soils in the Vredendal and Langkloof areas. J. dent. Res. S. Afr. *23:* 242–244 (1968).

Sandor, T.; Denes, I.: Caries es az ivoviz nyomelemci. Or Hetil. *113:* 1062–1064 (1972).

Schamschula, R.G.; Adkins, B.L.; Barmes, D.E.; Charlton, G.; Davey, B.G.: Caries experience and the mineral content of plaque in a primitive population in New Guinea. J. dent. Res. *56:* special issue C62 (1977).

Schamschula, R.G.; Adkins, B.L.; Barmes, D.E.; Charlton, G.; Davey, B.G.: WHO Study of Dental Caries Etiology in Papua-New Guinea. WHO Publ. No. 40 (World Health Organisation, Geneva 1978).

Schamschula, R.G.; Cooper, M.H.; Agus, H.M.; et al.: Oral health in Australian children using surface and artesian water supplies. Comm. Dent. Oral Epidemiol. *9:* 27–31 (1981).

Shaw, J.H.: Ineffectiveness of sodium copper chlorophyllin in prevention of experimental dental caries. N.Y. State dent. J. *16:* 503–505 (1950).

Shearer, T.R.: Selenium; in Curzon, Cutress, Trace elements and dental disease (John Wright, Littleton 1983).

Sortino, G.; Palazzo, H.: Zinco e carie sperimentale nel ratto. Riv. Ital. Stomatol. *26:* 509 (1971).

Steinman, R.R.; Leonora, J.: Effect of selected dietary additives on the incidence of dental caries in the rat. J. dent. Res. *54:* 570–577 (1975).

Tank, G.; Storvick, C.A.: Effect of naturally occurring selenium and vanadium on dental caries. J. dent. Res. *39:* 473 (1960).

Vrbic, V.; Stupar, J.: Dental caries and the concentration of aluminum and strontium in enamel. Caries Res. *14:* 141–147 (1980).

Dr. M.E.J. Curzon, Department of Child Dental Health,
University of Leeds, Clarendon Way, Leeds (UK)

Cariology Today. Int. Congr., Zürich 1983, pp. 136–146 (Karger, Basel 1984)

Can Foods be Ranked According to Their Cariogenic Potential?

Charles F. Schachtele, Mark E. Jensen

Microbiology Research Laboratory, School of Dentistry, University of Minnesota, Minneapolis, Minn., USA

Introduction

The ingestion of foods containing fermentable carbohydrate initiates a sequence of events which can result in the demineralization of tooth enamel and eventually the formation of carious lesions. We take the position that with the advances that are being made in biodental research it is likely that we will eventually be able to establish a scientifically sound ranking system for the cariogenic potential of foods. A combination of tests based on sound methodology will be required for the development of such a system. Due to the critical role of diet in caries the utilization of appropriate tests for developing foods with reduced or no cariogenic potential is a worthwhile goal.

A portion of the interactions which lead to caries involves conversion of dietary carbohydrate to bacterial plaque acids. By measuring acid production by plaque following exposure to various foods one might obtain data related to disease potential. The technology to monitor changes in human dental plaque pH has evolved to a point where we can begin to address the issue of whether this measurement can be used to separate foods based on their cariogenic potential and, most importantly, what additional studies are needed to allow development of an acceptable food evaluation protocol.

Various methods have been used to monitor changes in the pH of human dental plaque. The techniques have recently been reviewed and their strengths and weaknesses discussed [1]. Due to the site-specific nature of caries development, a strong argument can be made for the utilization of methods for monitoring acid production at caries-prone sites in the dentition. Appropriate methodology was presented from Zurich [2], and other investigators have recently developed similar technologies [3–6]. Briefly, by placing the ion-sensitive surface of microelectrodes, where they simulate proximal tooth surfaces and allowing plaque to accumulate, it becomes possible to monitor changes in hydrogen ion levels as a consequence of plaque metabolism. Wire telemetry is normally used to transmit pH data out of the oral cavity for analysis. In carefully controlled studies employing solutions of sucrose and human subjects with defined oral characteristics it has been possible to demonstrate the outstanding reproducibility of data generated in different laboratories using telemetry from interproximal sites in the human dentition [1].

After a series of studies the scientists in Switzerland concluded that foods could be placed into two categories based on their acidogenic potential in humans [7]. Most foods fell into the acidogenic category, since they caused the interproximal plaque pH to rapidly fall to close to 4.0. In contrast, several types of foods including certain meats, nuts, and cheeses could be placed in a nonacidogenic category, since they did not cause significant decreases in plaque pH [8]. In general, studies with rodent model systems have supported these observations when caries development was studied as a consequence of diets containing acidogenic and nonacidogenic foods [9–12].

By using a telemetry system similar to that employed in Switzerland we have confirmed that most foods that contain fermentable carbohydrate cause marked decreases in interproximal plaque pH within 30 min after ingestion [6]. Since these foods cause rapid decreases in interproximal pH to close to 4.0, our capacity for distinguishing between various acidogenic foods, as has been done in the rat model [11], appeared to be limited. However, since our previous studies with sucrose [13] demonstrated that the sequestering of high concentrations of acid at interproximal sites might take 120 min or longer, it seemed reasonable that long-term telemetry might allow us to distinguish between different acidogenic foods. The availability of two sets of characterized reference foods [14, 15] and human subjects with well-established plaque pH response profiles [1, 16, 17] encouraged us to perform a carefully controlled food comparison study.

Materials and Methods

The characteristics of the 5 human subjects used in this study have been described previously [16, 17]. They have an acidogenic plaque microflora, and their interproximal plaque pH consistently falls to approximately 4.0, when they are supplied with 10% sucrose rinses [1].

The method used to monitor changes in interproximal plaque pH with indwelling electrodes has been described [6, 16, 17]. The protocol involved the utilization of plaque which had accumulated on the electrodes for 3–7 days. The foods were tested individually by 4 of the subjects in early-morning sessions. 5-gram quantities of the solid foods were chewed for 60 s prior to swallowing, and 5 ml of each of the liquids was swished in the mouth for 60 s. Data were collected for 120 min and analyzed as described previously [18].

One set of reference foods [14] included potato chips, starch-lactalbumin-sucrose, milk chocolate A, and corn flakes and were obtained from the American Dental Association Health Foundation, Research Institute. Another set of foods [15] included skim milk powder, fruit beverage, caramel, snack cracker, sugar cookie, milk chocolate B, and wheat flake and were obtained from the Department of Food Science and Nutrition at Michigan State University. The aged Cheddar cheese was supplied by Dr. *Howard Morris*, University of Minnesota. The fruit beverage and skim milk powders were made up to 10% (w/v) with distilled water immediately prior to the test session.

Results

Analysis of the telemetry curves demonstrated that all of the foods caused a decrease in plaque pH. The minimum pH was obtained with the skim milk powder in approximately 13 min, while the snack cracker and wheat flake did not cause the pH to reach a minimum for 23 min. All of the other foods caused the pH to reach a minimum somewhere between these two times.

Figure 1 presents the minimum pH data obtained with the test foods. Except for the aged Cheddar cheese and skim milk solution the foods caused the pH to drop to close to 4.0. The results clearly demonstrate the marked acidogenic potential of 11 of the 13 foods, the comparability of the response between subjects, and indicate that minimum pH values are not useful for distinguishing between most of the foods.

However, if the area of the pH response curves below pH 5.7 is calculated for each food and the mean pH data plotted as in figure 2, the foods can be ordered from the least (aged Cheddar cheese) to the most (wheat flake) acidogenic. The basis for this ordering can be found

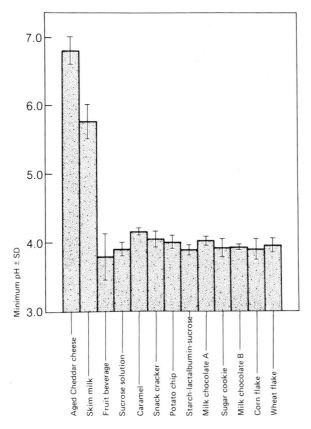

Fig. 1. Bar graph showing mean minimum pH and standard deviation obtained with the reference foods.

by looking at the telemetry curves presented in figure 3. Aged Cheddar cheese and the skim milk solution gave only a slight pH response, and there was a relatively rapid return to resting pH levels. The fruit drink caused a greater response with the minimum going to near 4.0 with a relatively rapid return towards the resting pH. The curves obtained with the remaining test foods are progressively more dramatic with the milk chocolate, sugar cookie, corn flake, and wheat flake showing virtually no return towards resting pH after 120 min. Thus, although most of the foods cause the pH to drop to approximately 4.0 they clearly cause the pH to remain at this level for different intervals.

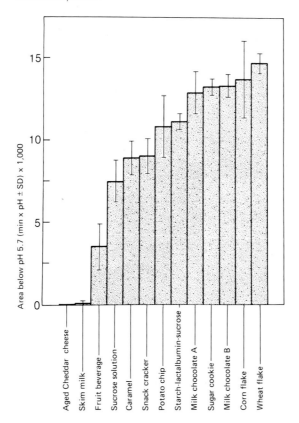

Fig. 2. Bar graph illustrating the mean area of the plaque pH curves under pH 5.7 with the standard deviation for each of the reference foods. Units are expressed as minutes multiplied by pH [17, 18].

Consequently, the area of the curves reflects the return of the pH curve towards preexposure levels.

From figure 2 it appears that the various foods might be placed into different groups based on the area of their curves below pH 5.7. If the foods are arbitrarily divided into five groups and the appropriate analyses performed, it can be demonstrated that the groups are statistically significantly different. The food groups, from least to most acidogenic, are: (1) aged Cheddar cheese; (2) nonfat dry milk solution; (3) 10% sucrose solution, fruit beverage; (4) caramel, snack cracker, potato chip, starch-lactalbumin-sucrose, and (5) milk chocolate (A and B), sugar cookie, corn flake, and wheat flake.

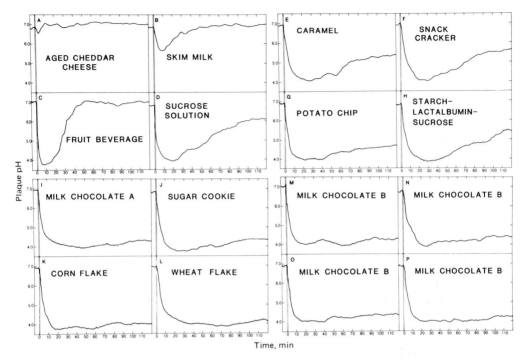

Fig. 3. Plaque pH telemetry curves obtained from 1 subject following ingestion of the various reference foods (A–L) and 4 subjects following ingestion of milk chocolate (M–P).

Discussion

The data presented in this communication supply an indirect, yet promising, answer to the question of whether foods can be ranked based on their cariogenic potential. It is envisioned that plaque pH data similar to that presented in figure 2 will eventually be integrated with results obtained from caries studies in rodent models and *in situ* demineralization investigations in humans. Although each of the models presents unique advantages and disadvantages, when taken as a whole, they should provide a good picture of the capacity of foods to contribute to dental caries, when the products are ingested by humans.

The results in figure 1 demonstrate that a wide variety of common foods containing fermentable carbohydrate drive the interproximal pH down to approximately 4.0, when they are ingested. This is not a surprising finding since, with the exception of the aged Cheddar, all of the food tested contained large quantities of fermentable carbohydrate [14, 15, 17]. Localization of the substrate at the interproximal site allowed the bacteria on the electrodes to metabolize the carbohydrate and produce large quantities of acid. Actually, the consistency of the minimum pH response with the foods may be considered a positive scientific finding as it presents a baseline for studies on the return of the pH towards resting levels.

As illustrated in figures 2 and 3 the reference foods can be separated by their response curves which differ primarily in the time and rate of their return towards resting pH. This latter parameter is important in that it might reflect a unique measure of oral clearance (i.e., the lowering of the acid concentration at interproximal sites). The concept of oral clearance as a factor in cariogenicity is not new, and, indeed, considerable data have been generated indicating that the time which a food or its breakdown products remain in the oral cavity can be related to disease [19–22]. We are confident that by carefully defining the study conditions, it is possible to rank foods with regard to their acidogenic potential at interproximal sites in the human dentition. The generation of this type of data base provides an important opportunity to begin evaluation of the relationship between acidogenic potential and disease.

Strong support for interproximal plaque pH as a means to assess cariogenic potential is obtained when the data in figure 2 are compared to results from caries studies in rats. Since the plaque pH data are obtained from a retentive site in the mouth, it is reasonable to look at the production of sulcal caries in the rat model. *Navia and Lopez* [23] have evaluated the reference caramel, sugar cookie, skim milk powder, snack cracker, and wheat flake using a carefully defined experimental procedure [9]. In agreement with the plaque pH data the skim milk powder was the least cariogenic food. The caramel was the next most cariogenic followed by the snack cracker, wheat flake, and sugar cookie. This ordering is almost identical to that obtained with plaque pH with 4 of the 5 foods being highly acidogenic and cariogenic.

Other rat caries studies with the remaining reference foods also provide supporting data [24] with high sulcal caries scores being obtained with starch-lactalbumin-sucrose, potato chips, milk chocolate, and corn flake. In general, the corn flake and starch-lactalbumin-sucrose gave the highest sulcal scores with the milk chocolate and potato chips showing slightly lower scores. The high acidogenic potential and cariogenicity of these reference foods and the variability of the rat data from the various laboratories make direct comparisons with the interproximal pH data difficult. The relatively high cariogenic potential of similar foods has been demonstrated in a separate study using a chocolate cookie with a soft filling, cereal with 8% sucrose, sugar-coated chocolate candy, potato chip, caramel, and chocolate bar [11].

The aged Cheddar cheese was included in the present study as an example of a food with little acidogenic potential. This and other cheeses have previously been shown by interproximal pH telemetry to be minimally acidogenic [25]. In addition, Cheddar cheese has been shown to have cariostatic effects in the rat model [12]. The aged Cheddar cheese results (fig. 2) clearly demonstrate the range of acidogenicity which can be found with commonly eaten foods.

The rat model is a useful tool for food evaluation, since it actually measures disease development. It is reasonable that there are components in various foods which will influence enamel dissolution, and such effects would not be detected by simply measuring plaque pH changes. Although the plaque pH and rat models are providing exciting results, future studies will need to be directed towards enamel demineralization [26–28]. Promising approachs would involve the use of ion-sensitive field effect transistors [1, 5] to monitor ions other than hydrogen at the interproximal site and placement of slabs of enamel at interproximal sites for demineralization studies with a controlled acid challenge from fermentable carbohydrate.

In conclusion, significant research progress is being made towards means to evaluate the cariogenic potential of foods. Reasonable test systems are being developed, and through collaborative studies it is likely that a scheme for testing foods will be developed. How such a scheme will be used to produce benefits for oral health should and will be the focus of considerable debate. Issues needing to be addressed will include: the effect of mixing of foods prior to and during ingestion; the sequence of eating different foods; the time of day when foods are eaten; the effect of changes in food form; variations in composition of a food, and, ultimately, the effect of foods with reduced cariogenic potential on disease development in humans. Until these and other issues are resolved, the most reasonable immediate goal in this area would be the global acceptance of the interproximal plaque pH test as a means to produce nonacidogenic products. The precedence for and success of this approach to reducing the cariogenic challenge to the teeth has been provided by our colleagues in Switzerland [29–33].

References

1   Schachtele, C.F.; Jensen, M.E.: Comparison of methods for monitoring changes in the pH of human dental plaque. J. dent. Res. *61:* 1117–1125 (1982).

2   Graf, H.; Mühlemann, H.R.: Telemetry of plaque pH from interdental areas. Helv. odont. Acta *10:* 94–101 (1966).

3   Clark, N.G.; Dowdell, L.R.: A radio-telemetric method for the study of pH and fluoride-ion concentrations in dental plaque and saliva. Med. biol. Eng. *11:* 159–163 (1973).

4   Newman, P.; MacFadyen, E.E.; Gillespie, F.C.; Stephen, K.W.: An indwelling electrode for in vivo measurement of the pH of dental plaque in man. Archs oral Biol. *24:* 501–507 (1979).

5   Yamada, T.; Igarashi, K.; Mitsudomi, M.: Evaluation of cariogenicity of glucosylsucrose by a new method to measure pH under human dental plaque in situ. J. dent. Res. *59:* 2157–2162 (1980).

6   Schachtele, C.F.; Jensen, M.E.: Human plaque pH studies: estimating the acidogenic potential of foods. Cereal Foods Wld *26:* 14–18 (1981).

7   Firestone, A.; Imfeld, T.; Schmid, R.; Mühlemann, H.R.: Cariogenicity of foods. J. Am. dent. Ass. dent. Cosmos *101:* 443–444 (1980).

8   Graf, H.: The glycolytic activity of plaque and its relation to hard tissue pathology. Recent findings from intraoral pH telemetry research. Int. dent. J. *20:* 426–435 (1970).

9   Navia, J.M.: Experimental and husbandry procedures in rat caries research; in Tanzer, Animal models in cariology, pp. 77–87 (Information Retrieval, Washington 1981).

10   Firestone, A.R.: Human interdental plaque pH data and rat caries tests: results with the same substance. J. dent. Res. *61:* 1130–1136 (1982).

11   Bowen, W.H.; Amsbaugh, S.M.; Monell-Torrens, S.; Brunelle, J.; Kuzmiak-Jones, H.; Cole, M.F.: A method to assess cariogenic potential of foodstuffs. J. Am. dent. Ass. dent. Cosmos *100:* 677–681 (1980).

12   Edgar, W.M.; Bowen, W.H.; Amsbaugh, S.; Monell-Torrens, E.; Brunelle, J.: Effects of different eating patterns on dental caries in rats. Caries Res. *16:* 384–389 (1982).

13   Jensen, M.E.; Schachtele, C.F.; Polansky, P.J.: Indwelling pH electrodes: analysis of human dental plaque responses at different sites; in Hefferren, Ayer, Koehler, Foods, nutrition and dental health, vol. 3, pp. 103–114 (Pathotox, Park Forest South 1981).

14   Li, B.W.: Chemical analysis of reference foods; in Hefferren, Ayer, McEnery, Foods, nutrition and dental health, vol. 4 (American Dental Association, Chicago, in press 1983).

15 Leveille, G.A.: Michigan State University reference foods; in Hefferren, Ayer, McEnery, Foods, nutrition and dental health, vol. 4 (American Dental Association, Chicago, in press 1983).

16 Schachtele, C.F.; Jensen, M.E.; Polansky, P.J.: Plaque models: monitoring pH changes following ingestion of test foods by human subjects; in Hefferren, Ayer, Koehler, Foods, nutrition and dental health, vol. 3, pp. 15–22 (Pathotox, Park Forest South 1981).

17 Jensen, M.E.; Aeppli, D.M.; Schachtele, C.F.: Evaluation of the acidogenic potential of reference foods by telemetry from interproximal sites in the human dentition; in Hefferren, McEnery, Foods, nutrition and dental health, vol. 5 (American Dental Association, Chicago, in press 1983).

18 Jensen, M.E.; Polansky, P.J.; Schachtele, C.F.: Plaque sampling and telemetry for monitoring acid production on human buccal tooth surfaces. Archs oral Biol. 27: 21–31 (1982).

19 Lundquist, C.: Oral sugar clearance: its influence on dental caries activity. Odont. Revy 3: 1–121 (1952).

20 Swenander Lanke, L.: Influence on salivary sugar of certain properties of foodstuffs and individual oral conditions. Acta odont. scand. 15: 1–156 (1957).

21 Caldwell, R.C.: A method for measuring the adhesion of foodstuffs to tooth surfaces. J. dent. Res. 38: 188–196 (1959).

22 MacGregor, A.B.: A new method for demonstrating the retention of foodstuffs in the mouth, with special reference to different forms of sweets. Proc. R. Soc. Med. 51: 41–44 (1958).

23 Navia, J.M.; Lopez, H.: Rat caries assay of reference foods and sugar containing snacks. J. dent. Res. (in press, 1983).

24 Navia, J.M.: Models for food cariogenicity testing: report of a collaborative study using animal models; in Hefferren, Ayer, Koehler, Foods, nutrition and dental health, vol. 3, pp. 1–12 (Pathotox, Park Forest South 1981).

25 Jensen, M.E.; Harlander, S.K.; Schachtele, C.F.; Halambeck, S.M.; Morris, H.A.: Evaluation of the acidogenic and antacid properties of cheeses by telemetric monitoring of human dental plaque pH; in Hefferren, Koehler, McEnery, Foods, nutrition and dental health, vol. 4 (American Dental Association, Chicago, in press 1983).

26 Bibby, B.G.; Mundorff, S.A.: Enamel demineralization by snack foods. J. dent. Res. 54: 461–470 (1975).

27 Bakhos, Y.; Brudevold, F.; Aasenden, R.: In vivo estimation of the permeability of surface human enamel. Archs oral Biol. 22: 599–603 (1977).

28 Koulourides, T.; Bodden, R.; Keller, S.; Manson-Hing, L.; Lastra, J.; Housch, T.: Cariogenicity of nine sugars tested with an intraoral device in man. Caries Res. 10: 427–441 (1976).

29 Imfeld, T.; Mühlemann, H.R.: Evaluation of sugar substitutes in preventive cariology. J. prev. Dent. 4: 8–14 (1977).

30 Imfeld, T.: Evaluation of the cariogenicity of confectionary by intra-oral wire-telemetry. Schweiz. Mschr. Zahnheilk. 87: 437–464 (1977).

31 Imfeld, T.; Hirsch, R.S.; Mühlemann, H.R.: Telemetric recordings of interdental plaque pH during different meal patterns. Br. dent. J. 144: 40–45 (1978).

32   Imfeld, T.; Mühlemann, H.R.: Cariogenicity and acidogenicity of food, confection-
     ary and beverages. Pharm. Therapeut. Dent. *3:* 53–68 (1978).
33   Mühlemann, H.R.: Sugar substitutes and plaque pH-telemetry in caries prevention.
     J. clin. Periodontol. *6:* suppl. 7, pp. 47–53 (1979).

Prof. C.F. Schachtele, School of Dentistry, 18–228 Health Sciences Unit A,
University of Minnesota, Minneapolis, MN 55455 (USA)

Cariology Today. Int. Congr., Zürich 1983, pp. 147–153 (Karger, Basel 1984)

Non-Acidogenic and Non-Cariogenic Sugar Substitutes and Sweeteners

T. Imfeld

Department of Cariology, Periodontology and Preventive Dentistry,
Dental Institute, University of Zurich, Switzerland

Available Possibilities

Sweetening agents proposed or used to replace acidogenic sugar as a means to reduce dental caries incidence can be divided into four categories: (1) intensive sweeteners; (2) sugar alcohols; (3) hypo-acidogenic sugars, and (4) the more recently developed hypo- or non-acidogenic derivatives of oligosaccharides, coupling sugars. The latter 3 groups are frequently termed sugar substitutes.

Intensive Sweeteners

There are two kinds of intensive sweeteners, the synthetic sweeteners such as cyclamate, saccharin, aspartame, etc. and the so-called sweeteners of natural origin such as dihydrochalcones, glycyr-rhizin, monellin, thaumatin, etc. They are of special interest in the production of low-calorie foods, beverages and confectionery products and for diabetics.

The vast literature concerning physiology, safety evaluations, legislation, food technology, etc. of intensive sweeteners has been reviewed and compiled elsewhere [1–3]. The calorie-free sweeteners saccharin and cyclamate and the low-calorie sweeteners aspartame, dihydrochalcones and glycyrrhizin are not metabolized by oral microorganisms. They are non-acidogenic in plaque-pH-telemetry [4] and have never been shown to be cariogenic in either animals or man. Saccharin [5], glycyrrhizin [6] and dihydrochalcones [7], have recently been reported to inhibit growth of *S. mutans* in vitro. Aspartame was reported effective in reducing plaque formation in vitro [8] and in reducing acid-induced enamel demineralization in the rat [9]. The actual or potential

Table I. Comparison of important characteristics of some polyols

Polyol	Commercial form	Price[1] sFr/kg	Relative sweetness (suc = 1)	Caloric yield	Suitable for diabetics	Food technological applications
Xylitol	crystalline	9.45	0.9–1.0	4 kcal/g	yes	candies, toffees, lozenges, chewing gum, chocolate, coatings, dragees, ice cream, jam, tinned fruits, medical syrups
Sorbitol	crystalline or syrup	3.90	0.5–0.6	4 kcal/g	yes	candies, toffees, lozenges, chewing gum, chocolate, coatings, dragees, medical syrups, humectant in toothpastes and pastry
Mannitol	crystalline	5.15	0.5–0.6	4 kcal/g	yes	same as sorbitol; special advantage: not hygroscopic, used for coatings and surface powdering
Maltitol (Malbit®)	crystalline or syrup	6.00[2]	0.9 0.6	approx. 2 kcal/g	yes	candies, toffees, jelly candies, pastry, tinned fruits, soft drinks, jam; disadvantage: highly hygroscopic
Lycasin® 8055	syrup	3.10[3]	0.75	4 kcal/g	no	candies, toffees, jelly cardies, plastifying phase of chewing gums, medical syrups; special advantage: crystallization inhibitor; advantage: not hygroscopic
Palatinit®	crystalline	5.10	0.45	approx. 2 kcal/g	yes	candies, toffees, drops, chewing gum, chocolate, marzipan products, ice cream, jam, pre-mixed doughs and cakes, icings, puddings, beverages; special advantage: not hygroscopic

[1] On industrial scale (> 5 tons), Switzerland, March 1981.
[2] Author's estimation.
[3] Per kilogram dry weight.

use of intensive sweeteners is, however, severely affected by regulatory actions. The sales volume of intensive sweeteners in the EEC is expected to increase by only 6% until 1985.

Sugar Alcohols

Polyols or polyalcohols are carbohydrates but not sugars in the strict sense because they have no reactive aldo group on carbon 1 or keto group on carbon 2. Each carbon of the skeleton has an alcohol group. They are generally produced by hydrogenation of sugars. Polyols are increasingly being used as substitutes for sugars, especially for sucrose, in confectionery products as a means of caries prevention.

The best known polyol compounds are xylitol (pentitol), sorbitol, mannitol (hexitols), maltitol, lactitol (12-carbon polyols), Lycasin® (hydrogenated starch hydrolysate), and Palatinit® (mixture of 12-carbon polyols). These sugar alcohols have proved to be non- or extremely low cariogenic in rat caries experimentation and some of them also in human clinical caries studies. They have equally been shown to be non- or hypo-acidogenic in plaque-pH-telemetry [for review, see 4]. With regard to the effect of sugar alcohols on oral bacterial colonization, *van Houte* [10] reported that their influence appeared to be similar to that of restriction of dietary carbohydrates, and *Havenaar* et al. [11] and *Carlsson* [12] concluded that there is a low risk of adaptation of the oral flora to polyols as main carbon and energy source in vivo.

The state of knowledge of sugar alcohols in animal and human nutrition is based on several hundred original publications that have successively been summarized [1, 2, 13–21]. The role of polyols in preventive dentistry has repeatedly been reviewed [4, 22–25]. Some important characteristics of the best known polyol sugar substitutes are given in table I.

Hypo-Acidogenic Sugars

Several sugars such as arabinose, ribose, xylose (pentoses), tagatose, sorbose (hexoses), melibiose, isomaltulose (Palatinose®) (12-carbon polys.), raffinose (18-carbon polys.) and Polydextrose are only slowly fermented by oral bacteria and proved hypo-acidogenic in plaque-pH-telemetry [4].

While most hypo-acidogenic sugars are not suitable because of toxicological and economic reasons, sorbose, xylose, Polydextrose and

Palatinose® have been considered as alternatives for sugar in confectionery products in order to render them less harmful to teeth. Recently *L*-sugars, especially *L*-fructose, have been proposed for use as non-calorific and non-cariogenic sweeteners [26]. Physiological evaluations and toxicity tests, however, remain to be accomplished.

Derivatives of Oligosaccharides

Japanese authors have reported the development of sugars of varying chemical structure designed for use as low-cariogenic sugar substitutes. *Okada* et al. [27], first reported that the incubation of starch, sucrose and cyclodextrin with glycosyltransferase from *Bacillus megaterium* yielded reaction products that are now termed *coupling sugars*. Coupling sugars, prepared as a white powder approximately half as sweet as sucrose, are composed of glucosylsucrose (G_2F), maltotriose (G_3), maltosylsucrose (G_3F), maltotetraose (G_4), G_4F, G_5, etc. as principle constituents but some also contain small amounts of glucose, fructose, sucrose and maltose. Their cariogenicity has been extensively assessed in several studies. They were reported to be a poor substrate for cellular aggregation, plaque formation, adherence of cells to glass surfaces and acid production when tested with *S. mutans*. Coupling sugars induced significantly less caries in gnotobiotic and normal rats than sucrose. They proved less acidogenic than sucrose in the Japanese plaque-pH-telemetry system [29] and less cariogenic than sucrose in the intraoral cariogenicity test (ICT) [for review, see 28].

A variety of confectioneries (candies, chocolate, cookies, jam, etc.) prepared with coupling sugars are currently marketed in Japan. Coupling sugar can be used as a food ingredient without specific labelling in that country [28]. Such candies, however, proved acidogenic in plaque-pH-telemetry in our laboratories. Patents for similar compounds, namely oligosaccharides of the type GF_2, GF_3, GF_4 and GF_5, claiming low cariogenicity have been submitted by a Japanese firm in different countries [30–32].

Restricted Realities

Non-acidogenic and non-cariogenic sweeteners and sugar substitutes have successfully been incorporated in confectionery products to reduce the cariogenic effect of frequently ingested snacks and sweets.

According to the legislation for the labelling of sweet confections with regard to dental caries introduced in 1969 by the Swiss Office of Health (Bundesamt für Gesundheitswesen), manufacturers are allowed to advertise those products as 'safe for teeth' in Switzerland that have proved in plaque-pH-telemetry not to depress the pH of interdental plaque below 5.7 by bacterial fermentation neither during consumption nor up to 30 min later. Up to now some 90 sweet confectionery products have been tested and approved safe for teeth in our laboratories. A comprehensive list of such products currently sold in Switzerland has recently been published [4]. In order to encourage consumer awareness and acceptance of products not harmful to teeth, a public relations campaign called 'Aktion Zahnfreundlich' has been inaugurated in Switzerland this year. Participants were drawn from the Swiss University Dental Institutes, from manufacturers of sweeteners and sugar substitutes and from producers of the final consumer products. Safe for teeth confections are now readily identified by the presence of a registered emblem. Sales figures of such alternatives to sugar-containing confectionery have been rising, especially for sugar-substituted chewing gums. The latter make up some 50% of the gum market in Switzerland.

On an international scale, however, the marketing of products sweetened by sugar alcohols and intensive sweeteners is severely affected by regulatory and economic constraints. Producers have to obtain premarketing clearance for food additives from the Health Authorities. In view of uncertain market prospects, the quantity and quality of data required for a food additive petition, especially with regard to safety, are often definitely prohibitive. Further, the legal status of polyols and sweeteners with regard to basic clearance, to restrictions for dosage, limitations of distribution and mandatory special labelling varies considerably between different countries. This lack of unanimity, even within organizations such as the EEC, inhibits free import and export of the consumer products thus diminishing economies of scale and discouraging industrial interest.

Similarly, there is no consensus as to the labelling of sugar-substituted confections with regard to dental health. Products sweetened by sugar alcohols are often described as 'sugar-free' or 'sugarless'. This term is of no value in preventive dentistry because its definition is not uniform everywhere and in many countries it only means 'without sucrose'. This does not exclude the presence of other sugars that may be fermented to yield organic acids in dental plaque.

The label 'safe for teeth' as used in the Swiss Food Ordinance is the only food regulation presently known that allows the consumers to exclude a caries risk when they select foods, snacks and beverages. Given that a numerical ranking of potential cariogenicity is not within the technological and methodological grasp of present-day dental science, the identification of non- or hypo-acidogenic foodstuffs by intraoral plaque-pH-telemetry seems the most valid contribution to dietary counselling in cariology available today.

As long as regulatory constraints remain as prohibitive as they are, already known but uncleared and possible new sugar substitutes exhibiting special food technological advantages favourable to consumer acceptance of the final product have no chance to be produced on an industrial scale. The public is thus deprived of a possible beneficial contribution to caries prevention. The dental profession should therefore influence the Health Authorities towards an international consensus on food additive regulations that could further preventive dentistry.

References

1   Shaw, J.H.; Roussos, G.G.: Sweeteners and dental caries. Spec. Suppl. Feeding, Weight and Obesity Abstracts (Information Retrieval Inc., Washington 1978).
2   Guggenheim, B.: Health and sugar substitutes. Proc. ERGOB Conf. (Karger, Basel 1978).
3   Shaw, J.H.: Sweeteners – an overview. I + II. Dent. Abstr. 26: 116, 172 (1981).
4   Imfeld, T.: Identification of low caries risk dietary components. Monogr. oral Sci., vol. 11 (Karger, Basel 1983).
5   Brown, A.T.; Breeding, L.C.; Grantham, W.C.: Interaction of saccharin and acesulfam with Streptococcus mutans. J. dent. Res. 61: suppl. A, p. 191 (1982).
6   Berry, C.W.; Henry, C.A.: Effect of glycyrrhizin on the growth and acid production of Streptococcus mutans. J. dent. Res. 61: suppl. A, p. 191 (1982).
7   Berry, C.W.; Henry, C.A.: Inhibition of growth and acid production of Streptococcus mutans by neohesperidin dihydrochalcone (Abstract). J. dent. Res. 62: 277 (1983).
8   Olson, B.: An in vitro study of the effect of artificial sweeteners on adherent plaque formation. J. dent. Res. 56: 1426 (1977).
9   Reussner, G.; Galimidi, A.; Coccodrilli, G.: Effects of aspartame and saccharin on tooth enamel demineralization. J. dent. Res. 61: suppl. A, p. 182 (1982).
10 Houte, J. van: Carbohydrates, sugar substitutes and oral bacterial colonization; in Guggenheim, Proc. ERGOB Conf., Health and Sugar Substitutes, pp. 109–204 (Karger, Basel 1978).

11   Havenaar, R.; Huis in't Veld, J.H.J.; Backer Dirks, O.; de Stoppelaar, J.D.: Some bacteriological aspects of sugar substitutes; in Guggenheim, Proc. ERGOB Conf., Health and Sugar Substitutes, pp. 192–198 (Karger, Basel 1978).

12   Carlsson, J.: Potentials of the oral microflora to utilize sugar substitutes as energy source; in Guggenheim, Proc. ERGOB Conf., Health and Sugar Substitutes, pp. 205–210 (Karger, Basel 1978).

13   Horecker, B.L.; Lang, K.; Takagi, Y.: Metabolism, physiology and clinical use of pentoses and pentitols (Springer, New York 1969).

14   Reported in Zuckersymposium Würzburg. Dt. zahnärztl. Z. *26:* 11 (1971).

15   Sipple, H.L.; McNutt, K.W.: Sugars in nutrition (Academic Press, New York 1974).

16   Zöllner, N.; Henckenkamp, I.-U.: Sugars and sugar substitutes. Nutr. Metab. *18:* suppl. 1 (1975).

17   Ritzel, G.; Brubacher, G.: Monosaccharides and polyalcohols in nutrition, therapy and dietetics. Suppl. Int. J. Vitam. Nutr. Res. (Huber, Bern 1976).

18   Schuberth, O.O.: Proceedings International Society of Parenteral Nutrition. Acta chir. scand., suppl. 466 (1976).

19   Reported in Zuckersymposium II Würzburg. Dt. zahnärztl. Z. *32:* suppl. 1 (1977).

20   Reported in Zuckerersatzstoffe – ihre Bedeutung in der heutigen Ernährung. Schriftenreihe der Schweiz. Vereinigung für Ernährung 40a (1979).

21   Koivistoinen, P.; Hyvönen, L.: Carbohydrate sweeteners in foods and nutrition (Academic Press, London 1980).

22   Frostell, G.; Edwardsson, S.; Birkhed, D.: Kariesgefahr bei Saccharose-Ersatz? Kariesprophylaxe *1:* 25 (1979).

23   Gehring, F.: Saccharose-Austauschstoffe und ihre Bedeutung für die Kariesprophylaxe, unter besonderer Berücksichtigung mikrobiologischer Aspekte. Kariesprophylaxe *1:* 77 (1979).

24   Scheinin, A.: Kohlenhydrate und Zahnkaries. Kariesprophylaxe *1:* 125 (1979).

25   Gehring, F.: Saccharose-Austauschstoffe in der Kariesprophylaxe. Kariesprophylaxe *3:* 1 (1981).

26   Reported in: A lefty eyes the sweetener game. Sci. News *119:* 276 (1981).

27   Okada, S.; Kitahata, S.: Preparation and some properties of sucrose-bound syrup. J. Jap. Food Ind. *22:* 6 (1975).

28   Ikeda, T.: Sugar substitutes: reasons and indications for their use. Int. dent. J. *32:* 33 (1982).

29   Igarashi, K.; Kamiyama, K.; Yamada, T.: Measurement of pH in human dental plaque in vivo with an ion-sensitive transistor electrode. Archs oral Biol. *26:* 203 (1981).

30   Meiji Seika Kaisha, Ltd.: Demande de Brevet d'Invention No. 8 106 308 (1981).

31   Meiji Seika Kaisha, Ltd.: Demande de Brevet d'Invention No. 8 115 868 (1981).

32   Meiji Seika Kaisha, Ltd.: Offenlegungsschrift DE 3 112 842 A1 (1982).

Dr. T. Imfeld, University Dental Institute,
Plattenstrasse 11, CH-8028 Zürich (Switzerland)

Cariology Today. Int. Congr., Zürich 1983, pp. 154–165 (Karger, Basel 1984)

The Value of Animal Models to Predict the Caries-Promoting Properties of Human Diet or Dietary Components[1]

Juan M. Navia

Schools of Public Health and Dentistry, University of Alabama in Birmingham, Birmingham, Ala., USA

Introduction

When the scientific method is used to solve a biomedical problem it involves the following steps: (a) recognizing and defining the problem; (b) gathering and organizing information about the problem; (c) formulating a question or hypothesis; (d) testing the hypothesis in a suitable model, and (e) drawing a conclusion from the results of the experiment. In testing the hypothesis it is essential that investigators understand and know the model to enable them to make appropriate inferences from the experiments performed. A number of animal models have been used in dental research [1] and specifically in caries research [2]. During the last 20 years great progress has been made in the improvement and understanding of animal models to study caries, and this has allowed major advances in the clarification and definition of mechanisms underlying oral diseases and in methods to prevent or control them. Animal models have been used to study the biology and pathology of oral tissues because: (a) there is a need to study biologic or disease processes under circumstances which are defined and standardized to decrease variability, and (b) a disease has to be induced or a toxic or even lethal procedure has to be imposed on the experimental subject.

[1] This paper is based on studies supported with grant NIH-NIDR DE-02670.

Ethical, legal and moral issues have been raised as a result of the use of experimental animals rather than human subjects in research. In the application of the scientific method to problem solving, an appropriate model has to be selected and a decision must be made to use humans, experimental animals or other alternative models. Three questions are usually asked at this time: (a) Is the answer to the research question specific for humans? (b) Are the proposed treatments safe for human subjects? (c) Would data derived from a study performed in animals contribute to the understanding of the research question? If the research question is for example: 'What is the cariostatic effectiveness of 1.5 ppm fluoride in the drinking water consumed by children aged 6–12 years?', then no measure of research with primates or rats would answer this question. If, however, the question asked is 'Will substance x be capable of inhibiting the implantation of microorganism M_1 when another microorganism M_2 is already established in the oral cavity?', then this question could be answered using data obtained with laboratory animals.

The research question being asked could also demand that testing be done under highly controlled and standardized conditions to facilitate evaluation of the effect. Use of highly inbred strains of laboratory animals which are genetically uniform, feeding chemically defined diets where all components are known and use of controlled environments which define the oral microbiota in gnotobiotes are some of the manipulations that can be easily performed in animals, but are impossible to achieve in humans. Results obtained under these conditions are also quite predictable. Precision is improved, tests can be repeated with a small margin for error, and the results obtained are useful in answering specific research questions. However, these are specific answers to the questions posed and do not necessarily imply that the same treatment will produce a similar response in humans. To understand the effect of a treatment for humans, other experiments should be set up using human subjects, assuming of course that toxicological studies have previously cleared the compound for human use. In general, a great deal of thought should be given to the formulation of research questions to experimental approaches and especially to the choice of experimental animals. Knowledge about the limitations and characteristics of the proposed model will enable the researcher to infer the right conclusion from his data and to determine the extent of extrapolation which can be done.

Dental Caries Assays

The assessment of the caries potential of foods or human diets presents special problems in that there is a need first to have a system that produces carious lesions that can be measured in a precise and accurate way, and secondly, the system should be reproducible and developed under healthy conditions to be sure that caries is the direct result of the oral cariogenic bacteria stimulated by dietary and oral substrates, acting on a susceptible tooth.

It is important to realize that dental caries has a complex multifactorial etiology where host, dietary and bacterial factors interact over a period of time to induce a characteristic demineralization in the carious lesion. The direct etiologic factors are specific acid-producing bacteria in dental plaque which use substrate coming from: (a) food debris held on oral tissues and in retentive tooth surfaces; (b) components from foods and liquids which come into direct contact with plaque when they are consumed, and (c) salivary and gingival fluid components. The combination of microbial and dietary factors is modulated by a series of host factors which includes among others: amount and composition of saliva, tooth morphology, structure and composition, immune competency of the host, positioning of the dentition, degree of occlusal erosion and abrasion and other factors which can modify profoundly the clinical expression of the disease. Because of these complex etiological interactions, the pathogenic process which leads to the formation of a carious lesion induced experimentally in a reproducible manner can be altered by interfering or enhancing one or more of the following six components of the cariogenic process: (a) implantation of the cariogenic bacteria; (b) colonization of the cariogenic bacteria to achieve a critical mass which can induce caries demineralization; (c) stimulation of growth of plaque bacteria which interact with the cariogenic bacteria to neutralize its cariogenic properties; (d) availability of substrate for the metabolic activity of the acid-producing cariogenic bacteria; (e) salivary flow or the composition of saliva coming in contact with plaque, and (f) remineralization reactions mediated by saliva and acquired pellicle on tooth enamel.

A variety of methods proposed to evaluate the caries-promoting potential of foods have been proposed and are listed in table I. Some of them involve human subjects, some are in vitro tests, others are conducted using laboratory animals. In general they can be grouped

Table I. Some methods to assess the caries-promoting properties of foods

---

Chemical assay of sugars and carbohydrate in foods
In vitro testing
    a   Acid production
    b   Enamel demineralization
Intraoral cariogenicity testing
Iodide permeability of enamel slabs exposed to a caries challenge intraorally
Human plaque pH
    a   Indwelling electrode
    b   Touch electrode
    c   Plaque collection
Rat plaque pH
Animal caries testing
    a   Programmed feeding
    b   Alternation procedure
    c   Ad lib conventional
Clinical and epidemiologic studies

---

into four categories: (a) those that measure plaque acid production; (b) others that evaluate changes in enamel slabs after a caries challenge; (c) still others that induce an experimental carious lesion in a laboratory animal, and (d) finally clinical or epidemiologic studies. The latter have been useful to detect the impact of some carbohydrates, such as sucrose [3] or xylitol [4], and some snacks such as chewing gum [5]. However, aside from the study done in Vipeholm [6], the use of humans to assess the caries-promoting properties of specific foods would be costly, difficult to interpret and subject to ethical, moral and legal challenges if the food to be tested were to be presumed to be highly caries conducive. For this reason major efforts have been directed to the use of in vitro or in vivo animal methods.

    Considering the six aspects of the carious process previously mentioned, it can be understood that these different methods do not necessarily have to agree. Plaque pH which measures the metabolic activity of plaque utilizing a carbohydrate substrate, does not respond to food effects directed to interfere with the implantation and colonization of bacteria, the immune reactions mediated through saliva or the remineralization reactions of enamel surfaces, all of which would affect also animal caries. Even within a method which uses laboratory animals, caries results could differ depending whether buccal or sulcal surfaces are considered, as these surfaces differ not only in flora [7], but also in accessibility to salivary components. Results using laboratory animals could also differ depending on background flora present and type of cariogenic bacteria used to superinfect the animals. A bacteria used to infect animals and which is highly sucrose dependent would show sucrose to be much more cariogenic than glucose, while another bacteria which is not so dependent on sucrose for implantation and colonization would show them to be equally cariogenic. Other organisms in plaque, such as Veillonella [8], may change the amount of acid available to attack the enamel, and still other organisms such as *Streptococcus faecalis* may change the capability of fermenting sugars and hydrolyzing starch in dental plaque, thus altering results of caries experiments depending on the biochemical properties of the plaque flora.

This understanding of the animal model to assess the effects of cariostatic or cariogenic agents has made it mandatory that in doing assays the following experimental conditions be carefully defined and controlled [9]: (a) species, strain and physical condition of animals; (b) environmental conditions: physical, chemical, microbiologic; (c) eruption time, morphology and composition of molars; (d) fluoride status; (e) salivary gland function and saliva composition; (f) diet composition (type, amount and texture) and dietary patterns (frequency of eating and drinking), and (g) background oral flora and degree of implantation and colonization of cariogenic strains of bacteria.

Each of these different factors can profoundly influence the caries result and their interactions confer a different degree of caries susceptibility in the animal model.

Assay of Food Cariogenicity

Foods fed to animals can stimulate or inhibit caries depending on their physical, biochemical or organoleptic properties in the following ways: (1) *physical:* particle size, impactation in fissures, disruption of plaque, adhesiveness, clearance or retention of diet in soft or hard tissues [10], and solubility (availability of nutrients); (2) *biochemical:* stimulation of bacterial colonization (plaque formation), stimulation of the metabolic activity of plaque [11], contribution to remineralization reactions, antibacterial activities, immune properties and systemic effects on oral tissue health [12]; (3) *organoleptic:* taste and smell which can affect the eating or drinking pattern of the animal [13].

Although all these physical, biochemical and organoleptic properties of foods can influence animal caries, they do not all enter into the determination of human caries, and, therefore, the animal caries assay should be designed in such a manner that all those aspects of the cariogenic process seen also in humans are included in the model. Tests of the caries-promoting properties of foods represent special cases of caries assay in that, if they are to be relevant to the human situation, they should be constructed in such a way that the caries effect is not due to artifactual factors such as particle size or organoleptic side effects (i.e. that may cause a change in the frequency of intake) rather than to the actual intrinsic properties of the food.

There is advantage in not using exclusively one animal model or one cariogenic microorganism with specific biochemical characteristics, because the results will be biased by the specific conditions used in the test. The caries effect in a human subject could be different because the food in this case is consumed in a different manner or frequency and the test food will exert its effect on a plaque flora which is hererogenous and endowed with different biochemical and metabolic capabilities. It is also important to use more than one type of carious lesion to evaluate the effect of foods, because different lesion sites will respond differently to the food that is being tested [14], depending on the accessibility of the tooth site to the food and the oral fluids, and the flora that colonizes that particular niche. Animal caries test will be more meaningful and relevant to humans, if they are performed in different animal models, with different types of conventional or gnotobiotic flora, evaluating different molar surfaces for carious lesions and controlling the feeding and eating pattern of the animal such as in a programmed feeding cage [15]. These recommendations are also in keeping with the requirements for a good experiment postulated by *Cox* [16], who emphasized the value of diversifying experimental conditions to increase the validity of results for extrapolation.

Animal Caries Models and Their Relevance to Human Caries

Several species of animals have been considered as possible models for caries research such as subhuman primates [17], rats [18], hamsters

Table II. Outline of a procedure to assay caries potential of foods using laboratory rats housed in a programmed feeder

Method	Remarks
1 Time pregnant rats (15 days pregnant) are purchased and shipped in filtered boxes using the most direct route; quarantined for 48 h	Assumes that young pups are not subjected to travel stress Filter cages protect rats from dust and vapors
2 Upon arrival, rats are caged in plastic cages conforming to DHEW recommendations [24] with beeding, stainless steel covers and filter covers; diet MIT 200 or 305 and distilled water offered	Cage and room environmental conditions are optimal for rats Diet provides all essential nutrients for growth and lactation Rat dams are swabbed to detect presence of *S. mutans* in the oral cavity
3 At day 2 after birth, rat pups are randomly distributed among dams and size of litter adjusted to 8 or 9 pups; body weights are recorded	Rats are not disturbed for 2 days after birth At 2 days, rat pups are randomized to avoid gestational differences between mothers Litters culled to 8–9 to ensure proper feeding and avoidance of runts
4 From day 3 to day 15, rat dams are rotated among litters; pups are identified by punching or tattooing the ears; they are weaned at 18 days, but left as a litter group	Rotation of dams eliminates the rat-dam effects due to differences in care, grooming and lactation Removal of the rat dam forces the pup to eat the diet exclusively at a time when 1st and 2nd molars are erupting
5 On days 18, 19 and 21 rat pups are orally infected using a minimum infecting dose (MID) consisting of 0.2 ml culture of a streptomycin-resistant *S. mutans* 6715 recently isolated from 'carrier rats'; either diet MIT 200 or 305 is fed to rats	An MID dose [25] is used to inoculate three times Concentration of cell culture (0.2 ml) is approximately 10^8 cells to ensure implantation [26–28]

6 At 22 days of age, the weanling rats are transferred to a programmed feeder apparatus (König-Hofer) with stainless steel cages	Rats usually are uniform in body weight (55–60 g) at this time; rats do not escape through the feeding tunnel and quickly learn the feeding routine
7 The test food is offered 10 times during the 12-hour night feeding period and the gel diet No. 456 is offered 5 times [29]; all food not consumed is collected and weighed; the programmed feeder assures that food is available a number of set times, but does not force the rat to eat; test food and gel diets should be controlled to provide slightly less (approximately 85%) of total calories required by the rats	Test food is cut into small discrete pieces and weighed daily and distributed among 10 trays The gel diet No. 456 has two functions: (a) provides the necessary nutrients for the rat to grow and develop normally, and (b) maintains a low level of sucrose in the oral cavity to facilitate the maintenance of the cariogenic flora and yet does not contribute essentially to the caries process
8 Experiments are usually terminated after 3 or 4 weeks in the programmed feeder; rats are weighed weekly and oral flora is monitored for presence of $S.\ mutans$; rats are euthanized using an excess dose of pentobarbitol (UTHOL) or a CO_2 chamber; heads are dissected with a guillotine	Moderate carious lesions develop on all molar surfaces of control rats Extension of the time beyond this number of days yields coalescence of lesions and makes caries scoring difficult Body weights are good indicators of health status and degree of acceptance of the feeding program
9 Heads are lightly autoclaved (5 psi for 5 min), soft tissue is removed, mandibles and maxillae are air dried and stained with murexide (ammonium purpurate); lingual surfaces are ground away and the mesiodistal section scored according to $Keyes$ [30] for buccal, sulcal and interproximal caries	No alterations of the carious lesions are produced by light steaming Murexide is a calcium chelator which readily discloses decayed areas of enamel and dentin, and does not stain intact, mature enamel Keyes procedure is useful and fast; morsal lesions are not recorded

[19], mice [20, 21], gerbils [22], cotton rats [23]. Selection of the most appropriate animal species for a caries research objective is usually made considering: (a) susceptibility to caries and time required to develop clinical lesions; (b) amount of background data and sources of information; (c) availability of the animal (determines group size); (d) health status (freedom from parasites, bacterial and viral infections); (e) genetic uniformity and mutant stocks; (f) low background oral flora (freedom from cariogenic bacteria); (g) adaptability to external manipulations; (h) requirements for housing and care (space and equipment), and (i) cost (animal purchase, board and personnel).

Considering these facts an appropriate selection can be made depending on the type of caries research study which is proposed. For the study of caries-promoting properties of foods the rat has been widely used, although as indicated previously subhuman primates, hamsters and mice have been also selected.

Using the laboratory rat as an animal model to assess the cariogenic properties of foods or diets a method has been proposed [14] which measures the intrinsic caries promoting properties of the food. The method and some remarks are included in table II.

In using this method, a control diet SSL consisting of a mixture of sucrose (20%), starch (65%) and lactalbumin (15%) is used as one of the test foods in an experimental run. This is useful because it allows expression of the caries potential of the test foods in terms of the SSL control diet, which is easily made and can be precisely reproduced in different laboratories. Using this procedure a number of foods have been studied. In general, this method of estimating the caries potential of snack foods does not distinguish minor differences, but it allows the use of either buccal or sulcal scores to assign foods to four major categories *high* (i.e. raisins), *moderate* (i.e. cookies, caramels), *low* (i.e. soda cracker, milk chocolate) and *very low* (i.e. skim milk, NGS No. 456 diet).

The methodology described is also useful in detecting the overall effect of combination of foods or beverages, thus it not only evaluates the caries effect of an isolated food, but the interaction between 2 or 3 foods fed in sequence or together. This animal caries procedure is a useful approach to evaluate caries-promoting properties of a food, but requires attention to detail and a high degree of standardization of all procedures and manipulations to maintain the necessary reproducibility of the method.

Conclusion

Animal models have been used widely in dental research, particularly, in caries investigations to test agents such as fluoride of known benefit to humans. The development of caries in the previously described rat caries assay for foods is based on the six components of the cariogenic process which occur both in humans and animals. The food to be tested contributes directly to the caries process, and the severity of lesions is, therefore, related to the intrinsic physical and biochemical properties of the snack food being tested. Foods, therefore, that are shown to have a low grade potential to promote caries in animals will have the same potential in humans and vice versa. However, it is important to recognize that the *actual* or real caries effect of these foods for humans can be very different. Results generally cannot be directly extrapolated from animals to humans, who could have a different caries response due to their characteristic dietary habits, the manner and frequency with which they consume snack foods and their individual oral health status. Regardless, results from animal caries assays represent an evaluation of actual caries potential of foods, which will be extremely valuable to consumers to guide their dietary habits, and also to food manufacturers who could use the information to direct their research and development efforts toward obtaining foods that will be safe for oral health.

References

1   Navia, J.M.: Animal models in dental research (University of Alabama Press, University 1977).
2   Tanzer, J.M.: Animal models in cariology, sp. suppl. Microbiology Abstracts (Information Retrieval Inc., Arlington 1981).
3   Newbrun, E.: Sugar and dental caries: a review of human studies. Science *217:* 418–423 (1982).
4   Mäkinen, K.K.: The use of xylitol in nutritional and medical research with special reference to dental caries; in Shaw, Roussos, Proc. Sweeteners and Dental Caries, sp. suppl. Feeding, Weight and Obesity Abstracts, pp. 193–220 (1978).
5   Finn, S.B.; Jamison, H.C.: The effect of dicalcium phosphate on caries incidence in children: 30-month results. J. Am. dent. Ass. *74:* 987–995 (1967).
6   Gustafsson, B.; Quensel, C.E.; Lanke, L.; Lundquist, C.; Grahnen, H.; Gonow, B.E.; Krasse, B.: The Vipeholm dental caries study: the effect of different levels of carbohydrate intake on caries activity in 436 individuals observed for five years. Acta odont. scand. *11:* 232–363 (1954).

7   Huxley, H.G.: The recovery of microorganisms from the fissures of rat molar teeth. Archs oral Biol. *17:* 1481–1485 (1972).
8   Mikx, F.H.M.; Hoeven, J.S. van der; König, K.G.; Plasschaert, A.J.M.; Guggenheim, B.: Establishment of defined microbial ecosystems in germ-free rats. I. Caries Res. *6:* 211–223 (1972).
9   Navia, J.M.: Experimental and husbandry procedures in rat caries research; in Tanzer, Proc. Symposium on Animal Models in Cariology, sp. suppl. Microbiology Abstracts, pp. 77–87 (1981).
10   Caldwell, R.C.: Adhesion of foods to teeth. J. dent. Res. *41:* 821–832 (1962).
11   Bowen, W.H.: Nature of plaque; in Melcher, Zarb, Preventive dentistry: nature, pathogenicity and clinical control of plaque. Oral Sci. Rev. *9:* 3–21 (1976).
12   Navia, J.M.: Perinatal nutritional influences on experimental rat caries; in Tanzer, Proc. Symposium on Animal Models in Cariology, sp. suppl. Microbiology Abstracts, pp. 319–328 (1981).
13   Mühlemann, H.R.; König, K.G.: The effect of addition of amylase, an amylase inhibitor and sodium chloride on the cariogenicity of a purified cornstarch in Osborne-Mendel rats. Helv. odont. Acta *11:* 152–156 (1967).
14   Navia, J.M.; Lopez, H.: Rat caries assay of reference foods on sugar containing snacks. J. dent. Res. *62:* 893–898 (1983).
15   König, K.G.; Schmid, P.; Schmid, R.: An apparatus for frequency controlled feeding of small rodents and its use in dental caries experiments. Archs oral Biol. *13:* 13–26 (1968).
16   Cox, D.R.: Planning of experiments (Wiley, New York 1958).
17   Bowen, W.H.: Dental caries in primates; in Tanzer, Proc. Symp. Animal Models in Cariology, sp. suppl. Microbiology Abstracts, pp. 131–135 (1981).
18   Guggenheim, B.; König, K.G.; Mühlemann, H.R.: Modifications of the oral bacterial flora and their influence on dental caries in the rat. Helv. odont. Acta *9:* 121–126 (1965).
19   Keyes, P.H.: Dental caries in the Syrian hamster. I. The character and distribution of lesions. J. dent. Res. *23:* 341–348 (1946).
20   Kamp, E.M.; Huis in't Veld, J.H.J.; Havenaar, R.; Backer Dirks, O.: Experimental dental caries in mice; in Proc. Symposium on Animal Models in Cariology, sp. suppl. Microbiology Abstracts, pp. 121–130 (1981).
21   Navia, J.M.; Hunt, C.E.: The PBB mouse: a new model for caries research (Abstract). Int. Ass. dent. Res. *807:* 249 (1972).
22   Fitzgerald, D.B.; Fitzgerald, R.J.: Induction of dental caries in gerbils. Archs oral Biol. *11:* 139–140 (1965).
23   Shaw, J.H.; Schweigert, B.S.; Elvehjem, C.A.; Phillips, P.H.: Dental caries in the cotton rat. II. Production and description of the carious lesions. J. dent. Res. *23:* 417–425 (1944).
24   Moreland, A.F.: Guide for the care and use of laboratory animals, DHEW Publ. No. (NIH) 78–23 (US Governmental Printing Office, Washington 1978).
25   Houte, J. van; Upeslacis, V.N.; Jordan, H.V.; Skobe, Z.; Green, D.B.: Role of sucrose in colonization of *Streptococcus mutans* in conventional Sprague-Dawley rats. J. dent. Res. *55:* 202–215 (1976).

26 Houte, J. van; Burgess, R.C.; Onose, H.: Oral implantation of human strains of *Streptococcus mutans* in rats fed sucrose or glucose diets. Archs oral Biol. *21:* 561–564 (1976).

27 Houte, J. van; Upeslacis, V.N.; Edelstein, S.: Decrease oral colonization of *Streptococcus mutans* during aging of Sprague-Dawley rats. Infect. Immunity *16:* 203–208 (1977).

28 Navia, J.M.; Lopez, H.: Sources of variability in rat caries studies: weaning age and diet fed during tooth eruption. J. dent. Res. *56:* 222–227 (1977).

29 Navia, J.M.: Models for food cariogenicity testing: Report of a collaborative study using animal models; in Hefferren, Ayer, Koehler, Fourth Annual Conference on Foods, Nutrition and Dental Health (Pathotox, Park Forest South 1981).

30 Keyes, P.H.: Dental caries in the molar teeth of rats. II. A method for diagnosing and scoring several types of lesions simultaneously. J. dent. Res. *37:* 1088–1099 (1958).

Prof. Juan M. Navia, PhD, Institute of Dental Research, Schools of Public Health and Dentistry, University of Alabama in Birmingham, University Station, Birmingham, AL 35294 (USA)

Cariology Today. Int. Congr., Zürich 1983, pp. 166–172 (Karger, Basel 1984)

Is the Ideal Diet for Preventing Dental Caries Physiologically Adequate?

James H. Shaw, Jelia C. Witschi

Harvard School of Dental Medicine and Harvard School of Public Health, Boston, Mass., USA

On the basis of present knowledge about the caries-producing potential of individual foods and eating patterns, no one should be so naive or brash as to attempt to describe an ideal diet which does not permit caries initiation and progression under every circumstance. In addition, individual food preferences and caloric needs differ widely. Even if an ideal non-cariogenic diet could be designed, it undoubtedly would be an experimental curiosity rather than eaten routinely.

A realistic approach is the application of current knowledge to develop guidelines for the selection of foods and eating habits which will result in little or no caries. From these guidelines, each individual can select meal patterns and snacking habits to fulfill caloric and other nutritional needs, utilizing preferred foods in that individual's social setting. Thus, the proposal is for a range of self-selected diets with the potential to approach the ideal: simultaneous low caries initiation and progression, and optimal nutrition.

Diet is discussed here in the context of a multi-faceted approach to caries prevention. It is assumed that an appropriate amount of systemic fluoride is provided during tooth development and maturation; that good oral hygiene is practiced with a fluoride dentifrice and, where appropriate, a fluoride rinse; and that dental care is available frequently.

Oral Considerations

Much information from varied sources has demonstrated a strong relationship between caries prevalence and the overall frequency of eating sweet foods. More specifically, caries prevalence is related to the length of time that readily fermentable carbohydrates and foods containing them are available to cariogenic microorganisms on susceptible tooth surfaces. Therefore, clear guidelines become available for menu planning and food consumption: reduce the total number of daily food contacts and reduce the caries potential of each contact by using foods with appropriate composition and low retentiveness, by short exposures in the mouth, and by appropriate sequencing of foods.

Nutritional Considerations

The best nutritional admonition is to eat a wide variety of foods. A common guideline for food selection to meet this goal is based on the daily use of an appropriate number of servings from each of the basic four food groups: (I) milk and its products; (II) meat, fish, poultry, eggs, cheese, dried legumes and nuts; (III) vegetables and fruit, and (IV) breads and cereals [1] (fig. 1). Basic nutritional needs can be obtained readily from the number of servings recommended for each food group. Caloric needs to maintain an appropriate body weight are fulfilled by adjusting the number of servings from each group according to individual preferences and by using food fats and other products not included in the above groups. Obviously, the various foods in each group plus combinations of foods from two or more groups in many recipes provide ample variety.

The nutritional quality of a diet can be estimated from the number of servings for each of the four food groups. However, in order to make valid comparisons with the Recommended Dietary Allowances (RDA) of the Food and Nutrition Board of the US National Research Council [2], quantitative calculations must be made for the amounts of nutrients consumed in these foods [3].

Nutritional Quality of Diets with Low Caries-Producing Potential

In order to respond to the question asked in the title, the nutritional quality of diets designed to have low caries-producing potentials is addressed as follows:

What will be the nutritional quality of diets where two-thirds of the kilocalories (kcal) are supplied by a normal food distribution from the basic four groups eaten at meals (major food contacts) and the remaining third are supplied by relatively noncariogenic (desirable) snacks between meals? To be as uncontroversial as possible, calculations for

A Guide to Good Eating

Use Daily:

Milk Group

3 or more glasses milk — Children
smaller glasses for some children under 8

4 or more glasses — Teen-agers

2 or more glasses — Adults

Cheese, ice cream and other milk-
made foods can supply part of the milk

Meat Group

2 or more servings

Meats, fish, poultry, eggs, or
cheese—with dry beans,
peas, nuts as alternates

Vegetables and Fruits

4 or more servings

Include dark green or
yellow vegetables;
citrus fruit or tomatoes

Breads and Cereals

4 or more servings

Enriched or whole grain
Added milk improves
nutritional values

This is the foundation for a good diet. Use
more of these and other foods as needed for
growth, for activity, and for desirable weight.

The nutritional statements made in this leaflet have been reviewed by the Council on
Foods and Nutrition of the American Medical Association and found consistent with
current authoritative medical opinion.

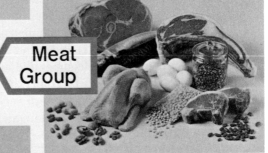

Fig. 1.

Table I. Composition of 2,100 kcal diet

Approximately 1,400 kcal will be provided in an appropriate distribution among the basic four food groups using the following amounts of food:

3 cups low fat milk, 2 oz lean ground beef, 2 oz light chicken meat without skin, 1 medium potato, 0.5 cup high calorie cooked vegetable, 1 cup tossed salad, 1 tbsp salad dressing, 1 serving fresh fruit, 3 slices bread, 1 cup corn or wheat flakes, 5 tsp soft margarine

Approximately 700 kcal will be provided from the following desirable snacks:

0.33 cup shelled, unsalted peanuts, 1 cup low fat milk, 2 servings fresh fruit, 1 oz natural or processed cheese, 1 cup unsweetened fruit juice

Approximately 700 kcal will be provided from the following less desirable snacks:
1 candy bar, 12 oz carbonated beverage, 2 doughnuts

Table II. Composition of 2,700 kcal diet

Approximately 1,800 kcal will be provided in an appropriate distribution among the basic four food groups using the following amounts of food:

4 cups low fat milk, 2 oz lean ground beef, 2 oz light chicken meat without skin, 1 medium potato, 1 cup high calorie cooked vegetable, 1 cup tossed salad, 2 tbsp salad dressing, 2 servings fresh fruit, 4 slices bread, 1 cup corn or wheat flakes, 6 tsp soft margarine

Approximately 900 kcal will be provided from the following desirable snacks:

0.5 shelled, unsalted peanuts, 1 cup low fat milk, 3 servings fresh fruit, 1 oz natural or processed cheese, 1 cup unsweetened fruit juice

Approximately 900 kcal will be provided from the following less desirable snacks:
2 candy bars, 12 oz carbonated beverages, 2 doughnuts

---

desirable snacks are based on fresh fruits, fruit juices, cheese and nuts which are not likely to be cariogenic. How will the nutritional quality be altered if the remaining third of the kcal were provided by less desirable snacks such as soft drinks, doughnuts and candy bars?

Calculations are presented for diets providing approximately 2,100 kcal per day, which is the mean recommended daily energy intake for females in both the 15- to 18- and 19- to 22-year-old groups. Calculations are also given for diets providing 2,700 kcal which is the mean value recommended for 11- to 14-year-old boys and 23- to 50-year-old men. Sedentary individuals need appreciably less and very active individuals considerably more. The standards for nutritional quality used for the 2,100 kcal diet are the RDA for 15- to 18-year-old girls and for the 2,700 kcal diet, 11- to 14-year-old boys [2].

Table III. Comparison of total daily food intake with use of desirable (low caries-potential) snacks or less desirable (high caries-potential) snacks

	15- to 18-year-old girls			11- to 14-year-old boys		
	RDA	actual with desirable snacks	actual with less desirable snacks	RDA	actual with desirable snacks	actual with less desirable snacks
Calories	2,100	2,130	2,170	2,700	2,710	2,740
Protein, g	46	110	89	45	132	107
Fat, g	–	85	82	–	114	107
CHO., g	–	245	279	–	312	349
Chol., mg	–	190	180	–	212	202
Sodium, mg	–	1,990	2,030	–	2,470	2,570
Calcium, mg	1,200	1,860	1,270	1,200	2,300	1,700
Iron, mg	18	11.3	9.6	18	14.7	12.2
Vitamin A, IU	4,000	5,450	3,930	5,000	6,600	4,840
Thiamin, mg	1.1	1.7	1.3	1.4	2.1	1.6
Riboflavin, mg	1.3	3.3	2.6	1.6	4.0	3.3
Niacin, mg	14	28	18	18	34	20
Ascorbic acid, mg	60	256	84	50	318	122

RDA = Recommended dietary allowances, 9th revised edition, National Academy of Sciences, Washington 1980.

In these comparisons two problems arise. The first concerns selecting appropriate values for nutrient intake where no generally accepted standard is available. Fat is the best example of a major food component without an established value. The average calorie contribution from fat in the United States is in excess of 40%. A recent guideline proposed that 30–35% would be more desirable [4].

The second problem concerns the variation in nutrient contributions that different acceptable foods make within each basic four-food group. The accompanying data are conservative values based on typical distribution of foods consumed in American households [5]. Thus, for a diet providing 2,100 kcal/day (table I), the data are expressed for nutrients provided from the two sources: the contributions provided with 1,400 kcal eaten in meals; and the contributions provided with 700 kcal eaten as between-meal snacks. The same procedure is followed for the 2,700 kcal diet with 1,800 kcal from meals and 900 kcal from snacks (table II).

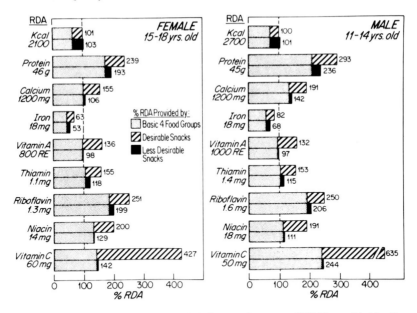

Fig. 2. Comparison of % recommended dietary allowances (RDA) provided by the basic four food groups at meals plus either desirable or less desirable snacks. The comparison is made for diets providing either 2,100 or 2,700 kcal daily.

Results

The data in table III and fig. 2 compare the total nutrient intakes of meals plus desirable snacks with the intakes from meals plus less desirable snacks. Using calcium in a 2,100 kcal diet as an example, the food consumed at meals contributed 1,210 mg of calcium (101% RDA); desirable snacks contained 650 mg for a total of 1,860 mg or 156% RDA. In contrast, less desirable snacks contributed only 60 mg of calcium. Except for iron, the remaining nutrients are all supplied generously by the meals plus desirable snacks in both the 2,100 and 2,700 kcal diets. As with calcium, lesser amounts of each were contributed by less desirable snacks.

Since only about 6 mg of iron are obtainable per 1,000 kcal, the RDA is virtually impossible to fulfill by consumption of a normal distribution of foods. The use of desirable snacks with meals is clearly advantageous for iron in that 63% RDA is obtained in contrast to 53% when less desirable snacks were used.

Fat concentrations as a percentage of calories and cholesterol levels were within desirable ranges for both diets with either desirable or less desirable snacks. The caloric contributions from fats were 36.1 and 33.8% for the 2,100 kcal diet with desirable and less desirable snacks, and 37.7 and 35.3% for the 2,700 kcal diets. Cholesterol levels were well below the usual recommendation of less than 300 mg/day. Sodium concentrations in all diets were kept low by the use of unsalted peanuts as a desirable snack and by omission of salt as a condiment. Replacement of some or all cheese by fresh vegetables would further reduce sodium, fat, and cholesterol intake.

Conclusion

The above calculations indicate that various diets with low caries-producing potentials are adequate nutritionally and physiologically. Desirable snacks contribute somewhat larger amounts of nutrients than less desirable snacks.

References

1   Hill, M.M.: Food to satisfy; in Stefferud, Consumers all, the yearbook of agriculture 1965, pp. 393–397 (US Department of Agriculture, Superintendent of Documents, US Government Printing Office, Washington 1965).
2   Committee on Dietary Allowances: Recommended dietary allowances; 9th revised ed. (Office of Publications, National Research Council, Washington 1980).
3   Witschi, J.; Kowaloff, H.; Bloom, S.; Slack, W.: Analysis of dietary data. An interactive computer method for storage and retrieval. J. Am. diet. Ass. *78:* 609–613 (1981).
4   Anon: Nutrition and your health: dietary guidelines for Americans. US Department of Agriculture, and US Department of Health and Human Services, Home and Garden Bulletin No. 232 (Superintendent of Documents, US Government Printing Office, Washington 1980).
5   Mitchell, H.; Rynbergen, H.; Anderson, L.; Dibble, M.: Nutrition in health and disease; 16th ed., table 10-2. Evaluation of a pattern dietary for its nutritive content, p. 162 (Lippincott, Philadelphia 1968).

James H. Shaw, PhD, Department of Nutrition, Harvard School of
Dental Medicine, 188 Longwood Avenue, Boston, MA 02115 (USA)

Plaque

Moderator: R.J. Gibbons, Boston, Mass., USA

Cariology Today. Int. Congr., Zürich 1983, pp. 173–181 (Karger, Basel 1984)

Streptococcus mutans and Caries: State of the Art 1983

G.H. Bowden[a], A.R. Milnes[b], R. Boyar[c]

Departments of [a]Oral Biology, [b]Preventive Dental Science and [c]Stomatology, Faculty of Dentistry, University of Manitoba, Winnipeg, Manitoba, Canada

Introduction

At this time there is ample evidence that *Streptococcus mutans* has a close association with dental caries in man [1–4]. This fact, coupled to the results of an array of animal studies [5], indicates the potential pathogenicity of this species or group of species [6]. The basis for many of the studies on the biology of *S. mutans* is the objective of devising strategies to control this bacterial component of the caries process in man. Many aspects of *S. mutans* are covered in an extensive review by *Hamada and Slade* [7] and discussion of these would be superfluous in this short paper. The object of this paper will be to view caries as a disease resulting from changes in the ecology of bacterial communities in the mouth.

Caries is a disease with fascinating aspects for the microbiologist. Faced in most cases with definite pathogens in infectious disease, the microbiologist must recognize that carious lesions develop as a result of a change in the ecosystem at the tooth surface [8]. One of the results of changes in the ecosystem is that shifts in the microbial community occur to accommodate to the changed environment. This adaptation is a recognized response of any bacterial community and is not limited to the mouth [9]. If the changes in the environment lead to destruction of tissue we recognize a disease state, however, many changes must occur which are regarded as normal.

Is there then evidence that ecological 'imbalances' in the bacterial communities on tooth surfaces predispose or predict a carious lesion [10]? Ecological imbalance should be viewed in a wide sense, that is, between individual populations in the community, and the community and the host. One of the known features of the adaptation of bacterial communities to a changing environment is the elimination of, or the sudden increase in a bacterial population, stimulated in an attempt by the community to adapt [9]. Examples of such changes in the environment of dental plaque which introduce bacterial changes are high carbohydrate intake [11] and xerostomia [12]. Dramatic shifts in the populations within the microbial community may lead to one species becoming dominant [9].

A Role for S. mutans in the Formation of Carious Lesions

Most the evidence for the relationships of *S. mutans* to caries in man depends on associating the effect of a change in a bacterial community, i.e. an increase in the population to dominance, with the development of a carious lesion. Several studies, both cross-sectional and longitudinal, have addressed the question, 'Do increased levels of *S. mutans* in localized areas of dental plaque correlate with the presence or development of carious lesions?' Almost all studies have been able to answer this question and detect such correlations [2–4, 13, 14]. However, the studies have revealed more than an association of high levels of *S. mutans* with caries lesions [2–4] and have encouraged interest in plaque ecology. In considering caries as a disease arising from changes in the environment, one could expect that the results might not be absolutely clear-cut, as the ecosystem combines all features of the environment including those which are the result of disease activity. The levels of *S. mutans* in plaque are only one facet of a multifactorial disease. Consequently, other community interactions could be involved in the final outcome of the balance between the environment, the plaque microflora and the integrity of the tooth enamel. Although *S. mutans* in high (dominant) levels is associated with many carious lesions, other pertinent questions can be asked if our anticaries strategies are to be based on *S. mutans* as the sole pathogen. These questions would be: (1) Is *S. mutans* obligatory for the production of a carious lesion in man? (2) Are other bacteria involved to a significant extent in the production of carious lesions? (3) Can sites which do not develop caries harbour high levels of *S. mutans*? (4) What environmental stresses applied to the plaque community stimulate changes to a pathogenic plaque? (5) Can the environment be modified to reduce caries?

The first question is the most difficult to answer. It is unlikely that *S. mutans* could be totally excluded from the human oral cavity without alteration in some other parameters. Given the problem of accurate sampling of approximal and occlusal sites [4, 15], negative findings could always be attributed to sampling inaccuracies. Very few examples of caries occurring in the apparent absence of *S. mutans* have been recorded [4], although lesions have developed with very low levels of *S. mutans* [2]. In those instances where *S. mutans* was absent or present in low numbers the lesion has been associated with lactobacilli [2–4]. It is not inconceivable that in these lesions *S. mutans* has been eliminated from the community by the more aciduric lactobacilli [24]. Thus, the plaque samples for assay may have been taken at too late a stage in the carious process. There is, therefore, little data to show that a lesion can occur in the complete absence of *S. mutans*. However, relatively few observations would be necessary to disprove an absolute requirement for these species. Moreover, the cariogenic capacity of other oral micro-organisms has been demonstrated in some animal models [16].

The observations on lactobacilli stated above lead to question 2. The association of *Lactobacillus* sp. with caries has been known for over 50 years. In almost all studies on caries, lactobacilli have been shown to have a strong correlation with the lesions. Moreover, as lactobacilli are present in low levels on smooth tooth surfaces their association with caries would indicate an even more precise ecological selection than that of *S. mutans*. One might consider bacterial succession in the development of caries, with *S. mutans* as a major initiator of the lesion and *Lactobacillus* as a later colonizer. In order to demonstrate such successions, microbial analyzes must be carried out on a longitudinal basis and recent studies (table I) [*Milnes and Bowden*, unpublished data] have suggested succession. Recent studies [17, 18] on incipient approximal lesions in children living in an area with water fluoridation indicate a relationship between lactobacilli and the risk of lesion progression to a point needing restoration (table II). One lesion has progressed without lactobacilli. Such bacterial relationships to caries cannot be ignored if control of caries is sought at the microbial level.

Question 3 is very easily answered, in many studies dominant levels of *S. mutans* have been detected in the absence of caries [2–4] (table I).

Table I. The levels of S. mutans and Lactobacillus sp. associated with the developing lesions of nursing caries and intact tooth surfaces in 2 Canadian Indian children

Site[a]	Subject		Sample time (1-month intervals)							
			1	2	3	4	5	6	7	8
		Caries state	0	0	0	0	WS	WS	L1	2
1	C.H.	S. mutans	–	–	–	0	29[b]	–	40	20
		Lactobacillus	–	–	–	0	0	–	3	12
1	K.T.	S. mutans	0	0	0	0	39	20	NT	NT
		Lactobacillus	0	0	0	0	0	0.002	NT	NT
		Caries state	0	0	0	0	0	0	0	0
2	C.H.	S. mutans	–	–	–	0	52	–	3	12
		Lactobacillus	–	–	–	0	0	–	0	0.2
2	K.T.	S. mutans	0	0	0	0	41	56	NT	NT
		Lactobacillus	0	0	0	0	0	0	NT	NT

WS = White spot; L = cavitation; – = not sampled; NT = not yet sampled.
[a] Site 1 = labial max. prim. incisor; site 2 = palatal max. prim. incisor.
[b] % of total cultivable flora.

These data indicate that colonization and successful competition in the community on an enamel surface need not be associated with decalcification and re-emphasize the multifactorial nature of the caries process.

One of the major problems in making an accurate assessment of the types of microbiological data mentioned above is when caries is diagnosed in tooth surfaces which cannot be seen by the clinician. Diagnosis of initiation and progression is based on X-ray and clinical examination and this may not provide an accurate assessment of the state of the enamel [19, 20]. One form of caries does produce lesions in full view of the clinician; this is nursing bottle caries where lesions occur on the incisors [21]. A recent study on this disease in Canadian Indian children [22] has produced interesting data on the microbiology of lesions, examples of which are shown in table I. Lesions develop rapidly (3 months) and are easily visible to the clinician. Thus, intact enamel, white spots and initial cavitation can be sampled sequentially and precisely. The early results show the following microbiological features of lesion development: (1) Dominance by S. mutans on the tooth surface precedes the formation of a white spot lesion in some

Table II. The presence of *S. mutans* and *Lactobacillus* sp. associated with the progression of incipient lesions in the teeth of children living in an area with water fluoridation

Subject	Organisms	Sample period (total 12–18 months)										Caries state
		1	2	3	4	5	6	7	8	9	10	
R.T.	*S. mutans*	8[a]	5	9	12R	3	–	–	–	–	–	progression
	Lactobacillus	6	–	–	0.9	–	–	–	–	–	–	
M.I.	*S. mutans*	15	–	–	12	16	14	18	21R	8	3	
	Lactobacillus	–	–	–	–	–	–	0.3	9	–	–	
B.R.	*S. mutans*	7	9	7	7R	4	–	–	–			
	Lactobacillus	0.02	0.01	0.06	0.1	–						
B.B.	*S. mutans*	4	7	3	5	6	8	8	7			no progression
	Lactobacillus	–	–	–	–	–	–	–	–			
M.V.	*S. mutans*	10	9	15	18	17	18	16	14			
	Lactobacillus	–	–	–	–	–	–	–	–			
S.B.	*S. mutans*	3	–	–	2	7	–	5	5			
	Lactobacillus	–	–	–	–	–	–	–	–			
Mean for 6 subjects	*S. mutans*	6	6	6	6	11[b]	10[b]	7[b]				control intact surface
	Lactobacillus	–	–	–	–	–	–	–				

– = Not detected; R = restored.
[a] % cultivable flora.
[b] Mean of 4 subjects.

surfaces. (2) Susceptible surfaces in the same child can show equivalent dominance of the community by *S. mutans* populations, yet the surfaces do not decalcify. (3) White spot lesions are colonized by lactobacilli prior to cavitation. (4) As the white spot develops, the complexity of the bacterial community is reduced. The data from this study reaffirm those from previous studies and avoid the criticism of accuracy of diagnosis and sampling. There can be no doubt of the significance of *S. mutans* as a potential pathogen in caries in man. However, acceptance of this significant pathogenic role must not blind us to the other factors involved, as the production of a lesion does not necessarily follow dominance of the community by *S. mutans*.

Are there any data suggesting which of the changes in the environment allows *S. mutans* to colonize and dominate a bacterial community (question 4)? Characteristics which could be regarded as bestowing virulence on *S. mutans* have been extensively studied [7, 23] and include environment [24], aciduricity [25], acid production [26] and adherence (27, 28]. These characteristics can relate to high carbohydrate intake and the loss of buffer in xerostomia, all of which can lead to high levels of *S. mutans* on the tooth surface.

As *S. mutans* is responsive to changes in the environment which provide advantages in the oral cavity, it could also be adversely influenced by other environmental changes. Dietary control has been used as one component of a preventive programme which resulted in a reduction in the levels of *S. mutans* [29]. Perhaps the major environmental change which influences caries is the intake of fluoride [30]. As water fluoridation reduces caries, does it at the same time produce a dramatic difference in the levels of *S. mutans,* or is *S. mutans* eliminated? Most detailed studies indicate that fluoride intake even to relatively high levels does not introduce major shifts in the oral flora [31, 32]. However, very high levels of fluoride can control the populations of aciduric bacteria in xerostomia [12]. While it is recognized that fluoride influences enamel remineralization, it does seem likely that it affects the metabolism of the bacterial population in dental plaque [32–34]. If this influence reduces the ability of *S. mutans* to dominate a community in the presence of carbohydrate [12, 33], it could affect caries experience. The data for fluoride direct attention to the fact that environmental controls can reduce caries in the presence of *S. mutans*.

In this short discussion of *S. mutans* and its role in caries, emphasis has been placed on the ecology of the disease, recognizing the other parameters involved. Perhaps the data on nursing caries, albeit rather little, could serve as a model: (1) The ability of *S. mutans* to colonize a habitat and achieve dominance in a bacterial community is directly related to the environment. In the case of nursing caries the prime factor is high carbohydrate intake. (2) Dominance alone is not of itself sufficient for the underlying enamel to be decalcified, the local environment is important. (3) Lactobacilli play a significant role in extension of the lesion to a point of cavitation and possibly compete with *S. mutans* in that habitat.

Given the above statements, would the elimination of *S. mutans* eliminate caries by preventing initial enamel decalcification? In order to give a definite yes to this question one would have to be absolutely certain that no other combination of oral bacteria could decalcify enamel and this does not seem likely [24]. Consideration should be given to the condition where *S. mutans* would be eliminated but the caries challenge remains high, e.g. high carbohydrate intake. This situation could easily arise if the public were 'protected' from caries by the elimination of *S. mutans,* when the need for diet control might seem less pressing. In this context *Lactobacillus* sp. could still be present in the oral cavity and available to colonize any sufficiently decalcified area. Moreover, lactobacilli are relatively resistant to fluoride [18, 35] and could prove less responsive to its anticaries effect.

In summary, *S. mutans* is a major pathogen in caries in man. However: (1) Its pathogenic potential can be modified by changes in the environment even on similar tooth surfaces in the same mouth. (2) *Lactobacillus* plays a major role in the development of a lesion, this may be particularly true in the presence of fluoride. (3) Control of the environment can lead to the control of caries without the elimination of *S. mutans*. (4) Elimination of *S. mutans* will reduce caries in man, however, *Lactobacillus* sp. could pose a problem in subjects with a high carbohydrate intake. We may reduce caries significantly by eliminating *S. mutans,* however, *Lactobacillus* might be 'waiting in the wings' to take over the spotlight that it enjoyed over 50 years ago.

References

1   Gibbons, R.J.; Van Houte, J.: Dental caries. A. Rev. Med. *26:* 121–136 (1975).
2   Bowden, G.H.; Hardie, J.M.; McKee, A.S.; Marsh, P.D.; Fillery, E.D.; Slack, G.L.: The microflora associated with developing carious lesions on the distal

surfaces on the upper first premolars in 13–14-year-old children; in Stiles, Loesche, O'Brien, Microbial aspects of dental caries, vol. 1. Microbiol. Abstr. Spec. Suppl., pp. 223–241 (Information Retrieval, Washington 1976).

3   Hardie, J.M.; Thompson, P.L.; South, R.J.; Marsh, P.D.; Bowden, G.H.; McKee, A.S.; Fillery, E.D.; Slack, G.L.: A longitudinal epidemiological study on dental plaque and the development of dental caries. J. dent. Res. *56:* suppl., pp. 90–98 (1977).

4   Loesche, W.J.; Straffon, L.H.: Longitudinal investigation of the role of *Streptococcus mutans* in human tissue decay. Infect. Immunity *26:* 498–507 (1979).

5   Tanzer, J.M.: Symposium on animal models in cariology. Microbiol. Abstr. Spec. Suppl. (Information Retrieval, Washington 1981).

6   Coykendall, A.L.: Proposal to elevate the subspecies of *Streptococcus mutans* to species status, based on their molecular composition. Int. J. Syst. Bacteriol. *27:* 26–30 (1977).

7   Hamada, S.; Slade, H.: Biology, immunology, and cariogenicity of *Streptococcus mutans*. Microbiol. Rev. *44:* 331–384 (1980).

8   Bowden, G.H.W.; Ellwood, D.C.; Hamilton, I.R.: Microbial ecology of the oral cavity; in Alexander, Advances in microbial ecology, vol. 3, pp. 157–160 (Plenum Press, New York 1979).

9   Alexander, M.: Microbial ecology, pp. 57–58, 165–223 (Wiley & Sons, New York 1971).

10 Bowden, G.H.; Hardie, J.M.; Fillery, E.D.; Marsh, P.D.; Slack, G.L.: Microbial analyses related to caries susceptibility; in Bibby, Shern, Methods of caries prediction. Microbiol. Abstr. Spec. Suppl., pp. 83–97 (Information Retrieval, Washington 1978).

11 Krasse, B.: Effect of dietaries on oral microbiology; in Harris, Art and science of dental caries research, pp. 111–120 (Academic Press, New York 1968).

12 Brown, L.R.; Dreizen, S.; Handler, S.: Effects of selected caries preventive regimens on microbial changes following irradiation induced xerostomia in cancer patients; in Stiles, Loesche, O'Brien, Microbial aspects of dental caries, vol. 1. Microbiol. Abstr. Spec. Suppl., pp. 275–290 (Information Retrieval, Washington 1976).

13 Ikeda, T.; Sandham, H.J.; Bradley, E.L.: Changes in *Streptococcus mutans* and lactobacilli in relation to the initiation of dental caries in Negro children. Archs oral Biol. *18:* 555–566 (1973).

14 Loesche, W.J.; Rowan, J.; Straffon, L.H.; Loos, P.J.: Association of *Streptococcus mutans* with human dental decay. Infect. Immunity *11:* 1252–1260 (1975).

15 Bowden, G.H.; Hardie, J.M.; Slack, G.L.; Microbial variations in approximal dental plaque. Caries Res. *9:* 253–277 (1975).

16 Mikx, F.H.M.: Multiple association of experimental animals with oral microorganisms; in Tanzer, Symposium on animal models in cariology. Microbiol. Abstr. Spec. Suppl., pp. 271–279 (Information Retrieval, Washington 1981).

17 Boyar, R.; Bowden, G.: Longitudinal observation of the microflora associated with incipient approximal lesions. Annu. Sess. AADR. J. dent. Res. *61:* 252 (1982).

18 Boyar, R.; Bowden, G.H.: The association of lactobacillus with progressing incipient carious lesions in children from a water fluoridated area. Annu. Sess. AADR. J. dent. Res. *62:* 176 (1983).

19 Growndahl, H.G.: Radiographic caries diagnosis and treatment decisions. Swed. dent. J. *3:* 109–117 (1979).

20 Ruiken, H.M.; Ruiken, H.M.; Irvin, G.J.; Konig, K.C.: Feasibility of radiographic diagnosis in 8-year-old school children with low caries activity. Caries Res. *16:* 398–403 (1982).

21 Ripa, L.W.: Nursing habits and dental decay in infants: nursing bottle caries, J. Dent. Child. *45:* 274–275 (1978).

22 Milnes, A.R.; Bowden, G.H.: A longitudinal microbiological investigation of nursing caries in Canadian Indian children. Annu. Sess. AADR. J. dent. Res. *62:* 270 (1983).

23 Freedman, M.L.; Tanzer, J.M.; Coykendall, A.L.: The use of genetic variants in the study of dental caries; in Tanzer, Symposium on animal models in cariology. Microbiol Abstr. Spec. Suppl., pp. 247–269 (Information Retrieval, Washington 1981).

24 Minah, G.E.; Lovekin, G.B.; Finney, J.P.: Sucrose induced ecological response of experimental dental plaques from caries-free and caries-susceptible human volunteers. Infect. Immunity *34:* 662–675 (1981).

25 Svanberg, M.: *Streptococcus mutans* in plaque after mouthrinsing with buffers at varying pH values. Scad. J. dent. Res. *88:* 76–78 (1980).

26 Hoeven, J.S. van der; Franken, H.C.M.: Production of acids in rat dental plaque with or without *Streptococcus mutans.* Caries Res. *16:* 375–383 (1982).

27 Gibbons, R.J.; Houte, J. van: Bacterial adherence in oral microbial ecology. A. Rev. Microbiol. *29:* 19–33 (1975).

28 Hoeven, J.S. van der; Rogers, A.H.: Initial adherence and minimum infective dose for rats of *Streptococcus mutans* T2 grown under differing conditions. Caries Res. *17:* 62–80 (1983).

29 Klock, B.; Krasse, B.: Effect of caries-preventive measures in children with high numbers of *S. mutans* and lactobacilli. Scand. J. dent. Res. *86:* 221–230 (1978).

30 Ericsson, S.Y.: Cariostatic mechanisms of fluorides: clinical observations. Caries Res. *11:* suppl. 1, pp. 2–41 (1977).

31 Kilian, M.; Thylstrup, A.; Fejerskov, O.: Predominant plaque flora of Tanzanian children exposed to high and low water fluoride concentrations. Caries Res. *13:* 330–343 (1979).

32 Bowden, G.H.W.; Odlum, O.; Nolette, N.; Hamilton, I.R.: Microbial populations growing in the presence of fluoride at low pH isolated from dental plaque of children living in an area with fluoridated water. Infect. Immunity *36:* 247–254 (1982).

33 Hamilton, I.R.; Bowden, G.H.: Response of freshly isolated strains of *Streptococcus mutans* and *Streptococcus mitior* to change in pH in the presence and absence of fluoride during growth in continuous culture. Infect. Immunity *36:* 255–262 (1982).

34 Okuda, K.; Frostell, G.: The effect of fluoride on the acid production of *Streptococcus mutans* and other oral streptococci. Swed. dent. J. *6:* 29–36 (1982).

35 Maltz, M.; Ericson, C.G.: Susceptibility of oral bacteria to various fluoride salts; Diss. Faculty of Odontology, University of Goteborg (1981).

G.H. Bowden, PhD, Department of Oral Biology, Faculty of Dentistry,
University of Manitoba, Winnipeg, Manitoba R3E OW3 (Canada)

Cariology Today. Int. Congr., Zürich 1983, pp. 182–190 (Karger, Basel 1984)

Are the Concepts Proposed for Dental Plaque Formation Valid?

J. van Houte

Department of Oral Microbiology, Forsyth Dental Center, Boston, Mass., USA

Introduction

Our understanding of dental plaque formation has increased enormously during the past two decades. This must be attributed mainly to the recognition and subsequent intensive study of aspects related to bacterial adhesion. Much information is still needed, however. Below an attempt will be made, within the allotted space, to identify some areas which require further clarification. An outline of plaque development, reflecting current thinking, will be used as a basis for discussion. For acquaintance with most literature the reader is referred to pertinent reviews [1, 3, 7, 8, 10, 11].

Nature of Dental Plaque and Plaque Development

Dental plaque can be defined as an adherent mass of bacteria covering tooth surfaces [3, 7, 11]. Coronal plaques, indispensable for caries formation on the crowns of teeth and to which our discussion will be confined, are present in fissures or on buccal, lingual, or approximal tooth surface areas. Coronal plaques are generally separated from the tooth enamel by the acquired pellicle. This thin layer (0.05 to about 0.5 μm) is thought to be formed by the rapid, selective adsorption of different salivary glycoproteins such as high molecular weight mucinous glycoproteins; immunoglobulins (IgA, IgG, IgM), extracellular bacterial polysaccharides, and enzymes (e.g., lysozyme, amylase) may also be present [3, 11]. There is evidence that pellicle material can be gradually altered or degraded by enzymatic and other processes leading to changes in its solubility, perm-selective properties as well as bacterial adherence [4].

Cultural studies indicate that the predominant bacterial groups in coronal plaque consist of streptococci *(S. sanguis, S. mitior, S. milleri, S. mutans)*, actinomycetes *(A. viscosus, A. naeslundii, A. odontolyticus, A. israelii)*, veillonellae; staphylococci, enterococci, *Streptococcus salivarius*, neisseriae, lactobacilli, and most other gram-positive or gram-negative rod-like species generally comprise less than 1% of all cultivable bacteria [10].

Plaque bacteria are generally surrounded by an interbacterial plaque matrix. Bacterial extracellular polymers, e.g., glucans synthesized from sucrose by *S. mutans,* or host-derived products, e.g., salivary glycoproteins, appear to be matrix constituents. The plaque matrix is responsible for interbacterial adhesion and, thereby, the structural integrity of plaque [7].

Considerable information exists with respect to plaque morphogenesis on smooth tooth surfaces [8]. Such surfaces, when devoid of pellicle and exposed to the oral environment, will first be covered by pellicle material. Subsequent bacterial colonization on top of this pellicle appears to start by the adherence of predominantly single cells, doublets, or sometimes very small cell aggregates rather than of larger cell aggregates; the latter appear to adhere less well than the former. Adhering cells are initially well isolated; in relatively retentive areas near the gingiva about 10^3-10^4 cells/mm^2 may be found within 2 h after oral exposure which represents coverage of about 0.1–1% of the total available surface area. Within 1 or 2 days a continuous bacterial layer can be formed by further adherence and lateral in situ bacterial growth. The rate of bacterial colonization varies greatly between fissures and smoother, less retentive tooth surface areas, and some areas may remain practically free of bacteria. Although less well studied, plaque morphogenesis in fissures is probably quite comparable to that on smooth surfaces.

Plaque accumulation, commencing after a continuous bacterial layer is formed, entails further bacterial attachment as well as outward and lateral growth of attached bacteria. This may lead to plaques with a thickness of up to 500 μm or more depending on the locally prevailing oral cleansing forces, oral hygiene, and other factors.

Bacterial Colonization of the Acquired Pellicle

Abundant evidence indicates that bacterial adhesion to the tooth surface is a prerequisite for plaque formation; only bacteria with a sufficient adherence ability can resist the powerful oral cleansing forces [3, 11]. This appears to apply even to the retentive fissures, although the role of entrapment, for example, via food, needs further evaluation.

Initially, the numbers of a given type of organism on the pellicle is determined by its innate affinity and its numbers available for attachment. The former depends on the number of adhesins (binding sites) on the bacterial cell surface and the strength of the bond between the adhesins and the receptors on the pellicle surface.

As may be expected from the heterogeneous and varied nature of bacterial and oral surfaces, bacterial adhesion to the pellicle appears to be highly specific [3, 11]. Different bacteria appear to possess different adhesins which interact with different receptors on the pellicle surface. Recent evidence also indicates that one particular organism can possess different adhesins [6]. Some investigations have suggested nonspecific bacterial adherence. However, pitfalls such as the use of only high cell concentrations in the assays rather than a range of cell concentrations causing 'masking' of highly specific binding sites only demonstrable with low cell concentrations may be responsible [6]. Analysis of bacterial adhesion to saliva-coated hydroxyapatite according to the Langmuir model or other comparable models, although initially controversial, allows differentiation between the number of adhesins and the strength of their bond with pellicle receptors and may provide valuable data about the nature of bacterial adhesion [3, 11].

Variation in the composition of the cell surface among bacteria appears also responsible for their selective attachment to the acquired pellicle or to different oral epithelial surfaces and adequately explains their variable preference for these oral surfaces [3, 11]. In vitro and in vivo studies provide some basis for a provisional ranking of oral bacteria with respect to their adherence ability to the pellicle. Generally, organisms such as S. sanguis, S. mitior, A. viscosus or A. naeslundii may rank high when compared to S. mutans, S. salivarius, different Lactobacillus species or Veillonella, Neisseria, or Actinobacillus species.

Some evidence implicates high molecular weight, mucinous, blood group reactive glycoproteins in bacterial adherence to the pellicle. Recent work also suggests that secretory immunoglobulins may increase the adherence of some but decrease that of other bacteria [3, 11]. Clearly, further information is needed about (1) the nature of pellicle components and (2) the role of such components which are known to include different types of salivary glycoproteins, enzymes, and bacterial polysaccharides as receptors for bacterial adherence.

Salivary components such as high molecular weight mucinous glycoproteins or immunoglobulins are known to be present on the surface of bacteria in vivo [3, 11]. Such components can induce bacterial aggregation in vitro and are undoubtedly also responsible for the formation of bacterial aggregates in vivo. As mentioned earlier, this may reduce bacterial attachment to oral surfaces and thus promote oral bacterial clearance. Salivary components, when bound to bacterial cells, may also decrease their attachment to the pellicle by 'masking' cell surface adhesins.

From the above it appears that salivary components, including immunoglobulins, play a dual role in bacterial adhesion. When present in the pellicle or plaque matrix, they can enhance bacterial attachment to the tooth surface or the structural integrity of the plaque mass. However, when present on attaching organisms they may diminish their adherence to the pellicle or other oral surfaces.

Salivary components which aggregate some oral organisms also appear to be similar to those which mediate their attachment to the pellicle. This suggests that in vivo the binding of some bacteria to the pellicle surface is mediated at least in part by adhesins unoccupied by salivary components. Further work is needed to (1) identify salivary components which can bind to different oral bacteria; (2) determine which of those components is present in the pellicle; (3) determine the validity of the concept of binding of bacteria to pellicle via receptors unoccupied by salivary components and the prevalence of this process; (4) determine the role in bacterial adhesion to the pellicle of salivary components which can bind to bacteria, but are absent in the pellicle, and (5) since different salivary glycoproteins can also interact with each other, it would be of interest to know whether the apparently weaker interactions between the pellicle and cell-bound salivary components could indeed contribute to bacterial adhesion under some conditions.

Extracellular polymers synthesized by plaque bacteria include glucans (dextran, mutan), fructans (levan, inulin), various heteropolysaccharides, and glycogen-like polymers [3, 11]. Some polymers, e.g., glucans, have been detected in the pellicle and, according to some evidence, can enhance the attachment of *S. mutans* strains. On the other hand, cell-bound glucans may not favor the adherence of *S. mutans* to pellicle; an extracellular heteropolysaccharide produced by *A. viscosus* appears to greatly inhibit the adherence of *A. viscosus* to pellicle by 'masking' adhesins on surface appendages (fimbriae) involved in attachment [3, 11]. It seems possible that some extracellular polymers, which are present in the pellicle and on the bacterial cell surface, may play the same dual role in cell adhesion as has been proposed for salivary components. Further clarification of the role of different bacterial extracellular polymers will necessitate (1) analysis of pellicle material for their presence; (2) evaluation of their effect on bacterial binding when present in pellicle or on the bacterial cell surface, and (3) determination of their relative resistance to enzymatic degradation.

Plaque Accumulation

Bacterial interactions during plaque accumulation would appear even more complex than those associated with the colonization of the acquired pellicle, because they comprise in addition interactions with plaque matrix components, bacterial coaggregations, i.e., adhesion via direct contact between the cell surfaces of different organisms [1], as well as effects on bacterial growth rate.

Formation of the plaque matrix via adhesion between bacteria and matrix components such as bacterial extracellular polymers or salivary components appears a very attractive hypothesis. Other processes considered in the past, such as mucin precipitation via locally produced bacterial acids or via enzymatic alteration of mucin molecules [7], appear to have been largely discredited, but may merit reevaluation as supplementary mechanisms. Matrix formation may involve in situ bacterial polymer synthesis or adhesion of salivary components to organisms in the plaque periphery as well as incorporation of such components associated with bacteria adhering to the plaque periphery.

Extracellular glucan synthesis appears to promote the accumulation of *S. mutans* on human teeth, but not that of another glucan-synthesizing species, i.e., *S. sanguis*. Generally, it is unclear to what extent differences among a variety of glucan-producing plaque bacteria with respect to the effect of glucan on their colonization are due to lack of glucan-binding sites on the cell surface, inability of the cells to bind glucosyltransferase(s) involved in the conversion of sucrose to glucan, or differences in the nature of the glucans synthesized. Bacterial glucosyltransferases in plaque probably diffuse away to some extent from the producing cells. In vitro studies suggest that this could affect accumulation by other organisms because (1) some plaque organisms which are unable to produce glucosyltransferase, e.g., Veillonella species, can bind these enzymes and, as a result, synthesize glucan which only then enables them to form plaque, and (2) glucans synthesized by cell-free enzymes may promote accumulation of other, nearby located, organisms by glucan-mediated adhesion or, possibly, entrapment [3, 11].

Further study is required to determine the nature, conditions for synthesis, and resistance to degradation of extracellular polymers synthesized by plaque bacteria as well as their role as plaque matrix components or as substrates for bacterial degradation and energy production. It may be suspected that bacterium-polymer interactions other than those between S. mutans and glucan may play a role in plaque accumulation, also, because of the probably wide range of the strength of the adhesive interactions sufficient for effective cell-to-cell binding under varying plaque conditions.

Salivary components undoubtedly contribute to the plaque matrix, but more work is needed to identify such components in plaque as well to clarify their role [3, 11]. Most attention so far has been paid only to high molecular weight mucinous glycoproteins. Such glycoproteins also appear capable of mediating attachment between similar as well dissimilar organisms and may thus function as potentially very versatile plaque matrix components.

Nature of Bacterial Attachment

Considerable attention is focused at present upon the mechanisms of bacterial attachment occurring during plaque formation. Long-range forces (van der Waals' and electrostatic forces) as well as different short-range forces are potential determinants of adhesion. Potential modes of attachment may include:

(1) Simple electrostatic, relatively nonspecific forces which mediate an initial, relatively weak association between bacteria and the acquired pellicle or other organisms; this is followed by stronger binding involving short-range forces. Such a biphasic process, entailing initially reversible and subsequent 'irreversible' attachment, has been proposed,

for example, in the case of the attachment of marine bacteria [3, 11]. During reversible attachment a gap between organism and attachment surface exists which reflects the balance between the attractive van der Waals and the repulsive electrostatic forces; this gap may be bridged via bacterial polymer synthesis leading to much stronger binding. The attachment of some *S. mutans* strains to the pellicle or the accumulation of *S. mutans* cells in plaque via in situ glucan synthesis (polymeric bridging) may proceed analogously.

(2) Direct, strong binding may occur via fimbriae possessed by many oral bacteria [3, 11]. Fimbriae, by extending from the cell surface, may make the long-range forces ineffective.

(3) Effective bacterial adhesion occurring solely via electrostatic forces has also been considered. This has been postulated to explain bacterial binding to the acquired pellicle with bridging via calcium ions as essential component or the alleged glucan-mediated enhanced attachment of *S. mutans* cells via glucan-entrapped lipoteichoic acid causing an increase in the net negative cell surface charge; lipoteichoic acid may possibly also mediate hydrophobic bonding [3, 11].

Strong binding via a short-range lectin-receptor type interaction has been implicated in many host-parasite adhesive interactions. It has also been implicated in bacterial attachment to the pellicle, in coaggregations, in saliva-induced bacterial aggregation, as well as in the binding of extracellular bacterial polymers to the bacterial cell surface [3, 11]. Recent evidence has in addition suggested the importance of hydrophobic interactions in the case of some organisms [2, 5, 9]. Both types of interactions have been associated with fimbriae.

Elucidation of the mechanisms of bacterial attachment is obviously a complex task. It is also of potential significance for prevention of dental diseases. Whatever the mechanisms that are proposed, they should account for the evidently high degree of specificity characteristic of the attachment of different bacteria to various oral surfaces. Consequently, a trend of oral research is emerging which is primarily concerned with short-range, highly specific forces and stereochemical detail.

Shifts in Plaque Flora

Extreme changes in saliva production or exposure of teeth to dietary carbohydrate resulting from xerostomia, feeding by gastric intubation, hereditary fructose intolerance, 'nursing bottle' syndrome, etc. generally lead to pronounced changes in plaque flora [10]. The observed shifts with respect to *S. mutans* and lactobacilli may be related in part to the effect of sucrose-induced glucan synthesis on *S. mutans* accumulation; fluctuations in plaque acidity caused by changes in carbohydrate intake or salivary flow may also be responsible because acidic conditions selectively favor both groups of organisms [10].

Aging of a 'normally' developing plaque also appears to be often accompanied by a shift from coccal to rod-like organisms. Microscopic studies of smooth surface plaque also suggest a preponderance of mainly coccal organisms in plaque a few days to about 1 week of age but more variation in bacterial composition in peripheral areas of older plaques [8]. Also, in young plaques columns of apparently similar organisms can be found frequently to extend from the pellicle surface towards the plaque periphery; in older plaques organisms in the peripheral area are often less oriented. These observations suggest first of all that early plaque may contain many distinct communities each consisting of microcolonies of one type of organism. Secondly, it suggests that the total mass of early plaque is determined by bacterial growth. On the other hand, selective bacterial adherence is probably largely responsible for its bacterial composition.

It is possible that the range of organisms possessing effective binding mechanisms for the peripheral plaque surface, composed of salivary and bacterial extracellular and cellsurface components, is wider, or different, than that for the acquired pellicle; differences in the types of salivary components contributing to the pellicle and to the plaque periphery (plaque matrix) may also exist. Such differences could be responsible for the different composition of peripheral areas in older plaques. Bacterial coaggregation may play a special role here as strongly suggested by studies indicating a dependence of *Bacteroides melaninogenicus* or Veillonella species on the prior presence of gram-positive organisms for their tooth surface colonization [3, 11].

The role of differences in growth rate among plaque bacteria, as also influenced by potentially toxic products such as bacteriocins, in shifts of the plaque flora is unclear. Equally unclear is the relative contribution of the factors bacterial adhesion and growth to the bacterial composition and the total mass of older developing plaque.

Aging of plaque is also accompanied by an increase in bacterial density which is generally more pronounced in the inner part of plaque.

Degradation of pellicle or plaque matrix components and reorganization of microbial structure appears to occur progressively and causes undoubtedly changes in the interbacterial binding responsible for the plaque's structural integrity. It is possible that coaggregations assume more significance during aging of the plaque.

References

1 Cisar, J.O.: Coaggregation reactions between oral bacteria: studies of specific cell-to-cell adherence mediated by microbial lectins; in Genco, Mergenhagen, Host-parasite interactions in periodontal diseases, pp. 121–131 (American Society for Microbiology, Washington 1982).
2 Etherden, I.; Gibbons, R.J.: Comparative hydrophobicities of selected oral bacteria (Abstract No. 965). J. dent. Res. *62:* 276 (1983).
3 Gibbons, R.J.: Adhesion of bacteria to the surfaces of the mouth; in Berkeley, Lynch, Melling, Rutter, Vincent, Microbial adhesion to surfaces, pp. 351–388 (Ellis Horwood, Chichester 1980).
4 Gibbons, R.J.; Etherden, I.: Enzymatic modification of bacterial receptors on saliva-treated hydroxyapatite surfaces. Infect Immunity *36:* 52–58 (1982).
5 Gibbons, R.J.; Moreno, E.C.; Etherden, I.: The nature of pellicle binding sites for *Streptococcus sanguis* C5 (Abstract No. 790). J. dent. Res. *62:* 257 (1983).
6 Gibbons, R.J.; Moreno, E.C.; Etherden, I.: Concentration-dependent multiple binding sites on saliva-treated hydroxyapatite for *Streptococcus sanguis* Infect Immunity *39:* 280–289 (1983).
7 Gibbons, R.J.; Houte, J. van: On the formation of dental plaques. J. Periodont. *44:* 347–360 (1973).
8 Guggenheim, B.: Ultrastructure and some biochemical aspects of dental plaque: a review. Microbiol. Abstr., suppl. 1, pp. 89–107 (1976).
9 Nesbitt, W.E.; Doyle, R.S.; Taylor, K.G.: Hydrophobic interactions and the adherence of *Streptococcus sanguis* to hydroxyapatite. Infect. Immunity *38:* 637–644 (1982).
10 Houte, J. van: Bacterial specificity in the etiology of dental caries. Int. dent. J. *30:* 305–326 (1980).
11 Houte, J. van: Bacterial adherence and dental plaque formation. Infection *10:* 252–260 (1982).

Dr. J. van Houte, Department of Oral Microbiology, Forsyth Dental Center, Boston, MA 02115 (USA)

Cariology Today. Int. Congr., Zürich 1983, pp. 191–198 (Karger, Basel 1984)

A Brief Survey of Recent in vitro Work on Diffusion of Small Ions and Molecules in Dental Plaque

G.H. Dibdin

Medical Research Council Dental Unit, Bristol, England

Introduction

Diffusion through plaque has frequently been proposed as an important factor in initiation and progress of dental caries. Thus, caries is favoured if sugars can diffuse easily into the plaque or if clearance of acids produced near the tooth surface is restricted. On the other hand, factors preventing mineral breakdown products at the tooth surface from diffusing away are cariostatic. Both perm selectivity and absolute permeability of the plaque are, therefore, important, and there has been a growing interest in obtaining quantitative data on them [1, 2, 4, 8–12, 14, 15, 17–21]. Extracellular polysaccharide is a particular component of plaque which it has been suggested may have diffusion-restricting properties [5, 7].

Survey of Methods

The study of diffusion in reactive heterogeneous systems like dental plaque is complicated [6, 13], and there is no uniform nomenclature for the various diffusion coefficients [1]. Furthermore, the coefficients obtained may depend on the experimental procedures used [1, 13] and can differ in their relevance to the caries process. The 4 groups who have recently studied diffusion in plaque have used different methods, although 2 are related.

Melsen et al. [14, 15] packed plaque into 2-mm plastic tubes (fig. 1a), with 10 μl of diffusate solution on top. After a few minutes diffusion, the tubes were frozen in liquid N_2 and analyzed. Results were expressed in terms of penetration depth, and no attempt was made to calculate diffusion coefficients.

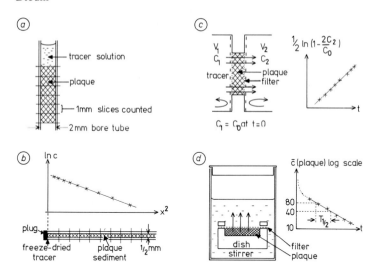

Fig. 1. Methods used by various authors for studying diffusion. *a Melsen* et al. [14, 15]. *b Tatevossian* [18–20] and *Tatevossian and Newbrun* [21]. *c Dibdin* [1] and *Dibdin* et al. [2]. *d McNee* [8] and *McNee* et al. [9–12].

The technique of *Tatevossian* [19] was similar (fig. 1b) except that he used 0.5-mm bore plastic tubes packed with plaque sediment by centrifugation. The tracer was freeze-dried onto a small stainless steel plug which was pressed into one end of each tube. After several hours the tubes were frozen, sliced, and analyzed for diffusate. Diffusion coefficients were calculated from tracer distribution along these tubes using the method of *Redwood* et al. [16].

Dibdin [1] and *Dibdin* et al. [2] used a diaphragm diffusion cell (fig. 1c) with the plaque membrane separating two chambers, identical except that one contained labelled and the other unlabelled diffusate. Diffusion coefficients were obtained from the diffusion resistance of the plaque after subtracting the resistance of the enclosing filters [1].

Geddes [4], *McNee* [8], and *McNee* et al. [10–12] used a desorption method (fig. 1d). Plaque contained in a small disc-shaped depression in a metal plate and covered by a bacteriological filter was equilibrated with diffusate. Clearance of diffusate into another solution was then monitored for about 15 min. The concentration left in the plaque was also measured, and a curve of ln C (sample) versus time was constructed. After an initial adjustment this gave a linear negative slope, from which a diffusion coefficient was calculated [8, 10]. Clearance of ^{133}Xe from plaque [9] was also measured by directly monitoring γ-rays from the samples.

An obvious disadvantage of these in vitro methods is that the samples were scraped from teeth, so that some large-scale structure was lost. However, this is a general problem in plaque studies, and it is difficult to see how diffusion could properly be studied in vivo.

The diffusion coefficients obtained are not all equivalent. The measurements of *Dibdin* [1] and *Dibdin* et al. [2] give an apparent diffusion coefficient (D_a) from the steady state flux condition. On the other hand, the other methods, in which the driving force for diffusion is taken as the gradient of total diffusate concentration within the plaque, give a different coefficient (D_e). The total diffusate concentration consists of (a) mobile diffusate and (b) reversibly bound (sorbed) diffusate in equilibrium with (a). Irreversibly bound or changed molecules, being no longer in equilibrium with the original diffusate, have effectively been removed from the system and should, strictly, be ignored. The relationship between the two coefficients is given [1] by

$$D_a = {_m}\lambda_s \cdot D_e \qquad (1)$$

where ${_m}\lambda_s$ is the partition coefficient between plaque membrane and bathing solution.

Dibdin [1] *and Dibdin* et al. [2] prevented metabolism in many experiments by heating the plaque to 60 °C for 30 min before measurement. More recently *Tatevossian* [20] too has adopted this technique when studying sugar diffusion in plaque. *McNee* [8] and *McNee* et al. [11, 12] fixed plaques with glutaraldehyde to avoid metabolism. Neither procedure necessarily deals with all the problems of irreversible binding, except in the diaphragm method, where concentration effects due to irreversible *and* reversible binding are excluded. This exclusion of all concentration effects of binding, which is inherent in measurements of D_a, has been criticized by *Tatevossion and Newbrun* [21].

Tatevossian's procedure has been criticized by *McNee* et al. [9, 11] and *Dibdin* [1] for its inclusion of irreversibly bound label in the concentration gradient. A common way of avoiding this is to equilibrate samples with unlabelled diffusate, adding tracer in small enough quantities to avoid upsetting the established equilibrium. This was the procedure adopted by *Flim and Arends* [3] for analogous studies of diffusion in enamel.

The method of *McNee* [8] and *McNee* et al. [10, 11] relies on a knowledge of the concentration (C_p) of diffusate left in the sample and, depending on how this is estimated, may or may not include irreversible binding. If C_p is estimated from the amount diffused out after an extended clearance time, then it does not. However, if, as seems the case [8, 10], C_p was estimated from the amount diffused out plus the *total* remaining in the plaque, then it too may have included irreversibly bound diffusate.

As an example of error of interpretation which such binding could cause in extreme cases, consider a hypothetical experiment in which clearance of ^{45}Ca from the crystals of a highly mineralized system is being monitored. Here the rate-controlling step is likely to be dissolution of the mineral phase and quite unconnected with any bulk diffusion processes.

A quite different point, made by *Tatevossian and Newbrun* [21] was that equilibrating with simple buffers before [8, 10] or during [1, 2] a diffusion study could cause plaque fluid constitutents to be lost and thus lead to errors. This point is important if the results of *Tatevossian* [19] and *Tatevossian and Newbrun* [21] for plaque fluid are accepted. It has been answered to some extent, in the case of NaF diffusion, by the use [8, 10] of saliva supernatant for equilibration. Furthermore, a brief study [*Dibdin*, unpublished], which used plaque fluid, saliva supernatant, or simple buffer as bathing solutions in a microdiffusion cell, suggests that the choice of fluid has little effect on the diffusivity ratio: $D(^{14}C\text{-lactate})/D(^3H_2O)$.

Table I. Comparison of diffusion coefficients ($cm^2 \cdot s^{-1} \times 10^6$) and diffusivity ratios (D/D_{aq}) in plaque or plaque residue, measured by different authors in vitro

Diffusing species	*Tatevossian* [19] and *Tatevossian and Newbrun* [21] plaque residue		*McNee* et al. [9–11] plaque		*Dibdin* [1] plaque	
	Dp	Dp/D$_{Aq}$	Dp	Dp/D$_{Aq}$	Dp	Dp/D$_{Aq}$
^3H_2O	–		–		10.9	0.34
Xenon	–		7.2[a]	0.46	–	
Acetate	1.29[a,e]	0.12	5.0[c,e]	0.31	{3.88[b] / 4.06[a]	0.26
Propionate	–		–		{3.23[b] / 2.98[a]	0.25
Lactate	1.42[a,e]	0.14	4.8[c,e]	0.31	{3.25[b] / 3.93[b,d]	0.24 / 0.29
n.butyrate	0.96[a,e]		–		–	
NaF	–		{4.2[a] / 4.7[c]	0.22 / 0.25	–	
Na^{36}Cl	9.0[a]	0.41	–		–	
^{45}Ca Cl$_2$	0.44[a]	0.025	–		–	
NaH$_2$ ^{32}PO$_4$	1.99[a]		–		–	
Na$_2$H ^{32}PO$_4$	1.52[a]	0.076	–		–	
Na$_2$ ^{35}SO$_4$	1.15[a]		–		–	
NaH ^{14}CO$_3$	0.97[a]	0.08	–		–	
Glucose	–		–		2.51[b]	0.27
Fructose	–		–		2.59[b]	0.27
Xylitol	–		{2.3[a] / 2.8[c]		–	
Sucrose	0.92[a]	0.125	3.0[c]	0.43	1.64[b]	0.23

[a] Live plaque.
[b] Plaque killed by heating to 60 °C for 30 min.
[c] Plaque killed by fixation with glutaraldehyde.
[d] pH = 3.
[e] Sodium salt.

Diffusion of Small Molecules and Ions in Plaque

Table I shows diffusion coefficients measured in plaque residue by *Tatevossian* [19] and *Tatevossian and Newbrun* [21] and in pooled plaque by *McNee* et al. [9, 10, 12] and *Dibdin* [1]. The figures of *Dibdin* [13] are based on his 20-mg samples. Perm selectivity is conveniently shown by differences between the diffusivity ratios of diffusates [D(plaque)/ D(aqueous solution)]. Only the results of *Tatevossian* [19] and *Tatevossian and Newbrun* [21] suggest much perm selectivity, and his diffusion coefficients are generally lower than found by *McNee* et al. [9–11] or by *Dibdin* [1] whose results did nevertheless show a small increase in D (lactate) at pH 3 (table I). To some extent it is possible to relate the penetration figures of *Melsen* et al. [14, 15] with the diffusivities found by other authors. For example, *Melsen* et al. [14] found that $CaCl_2$ penetrated plaque very much more than did glucose, the opposite finding of *Tatevossian* [19] and *Tatevossian and Newbrun* [21]. These authors showed a dependence of diffusion coefficient on packing density of the plaque residue, produced by increasing the centrifuge speed from 5,000 up to 74,000 *g*.

Diffusion in Plaque Fluid, Saliva, and Water

For most of the diffusates shown in column 1 of table I *Tatevossian* [19] and *Tatevossian and Newbrun* [21] have also obtained diffusion coefficients in plaque fluid and in water [19], and some also in saliva [21]. Except for $Na^{36}Cl$ and sucrose their results suggest considerable reductions of D compared with water. Therefore, these authors believe that the diffusion behaviour of whole plaque is markedly affected by the plaque fluid. *Dibdin* [1] and *McNee* et al. [11] have criticized these results on other grounds, pointing out that values obtained for diffusion of sucrose in water and in plaque fluid [18, 19] are unchanged between 5 and 37 °C, whereas accurate aqueous values in the literature show D (37 °C) to be about 2.5 times D (5 °C), in close agreement with theory. In addition *McNee* et al. [12] have criticized the large coefficients of variation (up to 114%).

Effect of Extracellular Polysaccharide (EPS) on Diffusion in Plaque and in Bacterial Sediments

Geddes [4], *McNee* [8], and *McNee* et al. [12] found a rise in diffusion of NaF with the carbohydrate content (and presumably, therefore, EPS content) of *Streptococcus sanguis* sediments which had been cultured with 5% sucrose. In glutaraldehyde-fixed sediments D (NaF) showed a similar correlation, but that for D (sucrose) was much less marked. In plaque samples they found a barely significant correlation of D (NaF) with carbohydrate content.

Dibdin et al. [2] compared fasted plaque with plaque cultured for up to 90 h using different sucrose concentrations in the membrane assembly of their apparatus (fig. 1c). ^3H_2O diffusion was compared with ^{14}C-sucrose diffusion in one group and with ^{14}C-sorbitol diffusion in the other. Samples were analyzed for protein, EPS, and dry weight. Partial correlation analyses showed a strong positive correlation with dry weight, but no correlation between either D (acetate) or sugar/acetate diffusivity ratio and the polysaccharide-to-protein ratio. *McNee* [8] and *McNee* et al. [12] found a small increase in D (NaF) after culturing three plaque samples in the diffusion well of their apparatus (fig. 1d). *Tatevossian* [20] has also studied the effect of polysaccharide on diffusion in plaque and has come to the conclusion that its presence causes a slight reduction in D.

Concluding Remarks

Neglecting, in the first instance, possible errors in obtaining the diffusion coefficients of table I, it is useful to consider their practical implications in caries. D_a and D_e are related by $_m\lambda_s$ (>1 if binding predominates, <1 if excluded volume predominates, see equation 1). D_a is a measure of the diffusate flux for a given activity gradient and D_e the rate at which a front moves through the sample [1]. Thus, if one is interested in the degree to which the effect of changes at one point in the plaque are felt at another point, then D_e is appropriate. On the other hand, D_a gives an indication of the rate of supply or removal of some moiety for a given concentration at the source. For example, once binding sites are in equilibrium, the rate at which calcium ions may be removed from the tooth surface will depend on D_a (calcium) for plaque and on the calcium activity gradient between tooth surface and saliva. However, if the binding sites are undersaturated, then the initial loss of calcium from the tooth will be faster, even though D_e may be low – possibly only a fraction of D_a. On the other hand the effects of cyclic changes in calcium levels will penetrate slowly, in line with the low value of D_e.

Turning to a comparison of results, there now seems to be some agreement that extracellular glucan does not form a major barrier to diffusion in plaque, but that dry weight or packing density is important. It is probable also that the observation [10] that NaF diffuses easily through plaque will also find general acceptance. See also *Melsen* et al. [15]. The differences between the three sets of figures in table I can be seen to be quite large, even though not many diffusates are common to all three, but the reasons for the differences are not altogether clear. The samples of *Tatevossian and Newbrun* [21] were centrifuged at 5,000 *g* causing 70% of the plaque fluid to be removed in the process, suggesting that increased packing density could be the reason. However, all three groups consider their samples to have about the same water content (80–85%). Perhaps centrifugation changes the balance between cellular and extracellular content without much change in water content; certainly packing density and, therefore, tortuosity of the diffusion pathways seem [1, 2, 19, 21] to be one of the main factors controlling rates of diffusion. This cannot, however, account for the very high values of *Tatevossian and Newbrun* [21] for D (NaCl) (see table I). The figures of *Dibdin* [1], being for D_a, can only be compared with the others by measuring $_m\lambda_s$, but those of *McNee* et al. [11] and *Tatevossian and Newbrun* [21] should coincide. One useful comparison experiment would be to study plaque sediment using the methods of *Dibdin* [1] and *McNee* et al. [10]. The effect on D of possible loss of plaque fluid constituents [19, 21] should also be further investigated, as mentioned earlier. On the other side of the argument, the effects of irreversible binding need further study.

In this very brief survey I have tried to give some indication of the problems and current progress in understanding diffusion in plaque. I hope that it may provide a starting point for fruitful discussions on this subject at 'Cariology 83', when we meet to honour Prof. *Mühlemann*.

References

1   Dibdin, G.H.: Diffusion of sugars and carboxylic acids through human dental plaque in vitro. Archs oral Biol. *26:* 515–523 (1981).
2   Dibdin, G.H.; Wilson, C.M.; Shellis, R.P.: Effect of packing density and polysaccharide to protein ratio of plaque samples cultured in vitro upon their permeability. Caries Res. *17:* 52–58 (1983).

3   Flim, G.J.; Arends, J.: Diffusion of ^{45}Ca in bovine enamel. Calcif. Tissue Res. *24:* 59–64 (1977).

4   Geddes, D.A.M.: Studies on metabolism of dental plaque: diffusion and acid production in human dental plaque. Front. oral Physiol, vol. 3, pp. 78–87 (Karger, Basel 1981).

5   Hojo, S.; Higuchi, M.; Araya, S.: Glucan inhibition of diffusion in dental plaque. J. dent. Res. *55:* 169 (1976).

6   Jost, W.: Diffusion in solids (Academic Press, New York 1960).

7   Kleinberg, I.: Formation and accumulation of acid on the tooth surface. J. dent. Res. *49:* 1300–1316 (1970).

8   McNee, S.G.: Diffusion properties of dental plaque in relation to dental caries; thesis Glasgow (1981).

9   McNee, S.G.; Geddes, D.A.M.; Main, C.; Gillespie, F.C.: Measurement of the rate of diffusion of radioactive xenon in human dental plaque in vitro. Archs oral Biol. *24:* 359–362 (1979).

10 McNee, S.G.; Geddes, D.A.M.; Main, C.; Gillespie, F.C.: Measurement of the diffusion coefficient of NaF in human dental plaque in vitro. Archs oral Biol. *25:* 819–823 (1980).

11 McNee, S.G.; Geddes, D.A.M.; Wheetman, D.A.: Diffusion of sugars and acids in human dental plaque in vitro. Archs oral Biol. *27:* 975–979 (1982).

12 McNee, S.G.; Geddes, D.A.M.; Wheetman, D.A.; Sweeney, D.; Beeley, J.A.: Effect of extracellular polysaccharides on diffusion of NaF and ^{14}C-sucrose in human dental plaque and in sediments of the bacterium *Streptococcus sanguis* 804 (NCTC 10904). Archs oral Biol. *27:* 981–986 (1982).

13 Meares, P.: Transport in ion-exchange polymers; in Crank, Diffusion in polymers, pp. 373–428 (Academic Press, London 1968).

14 Melsen, B.; Kaae, O.; Rolla, G.; Fejerskov, O.; Karring, T.: Penetration of ions in human dental plaque. Archs oral Biol. *24:* 75–81 (1979).

15 Melsen, B.; Kaae, O.; Rolla, G.: Penetration of fluoride and chlorhexidine in human dental plaque in vitro. Caries Res. *17:* 113–117 (1983).

16 Redwood, W.R.; Rall, E.; Perl, W: Red cell membrane permeability deduced from bulk diffusion coefficients. J. gen. Physiol. *64:* 706–729 (1974).

17 Shellis, R.P.; Wilson, C.M.; Dibdin, G.H.: Metabolic artifacts in measurement of diffusion rates in dental plaque. J. dent. Res. *61:* 250 (1982).

18 Tatevossian, A.: Salivary exchange of sucrose and lactate with dental plaque; in Kleinberg, Saliva and dental caries. Microbiol. Abstracts; suppl., pp. 333–342 (1979).

19 Tatevossian, A.: Diffusion of radiotracers in human dental plaque. Caries Res. *13:* 154–162 (1979).

20 Tatevossian, A.: Some factors affecting the diffusion of sucrose in dental plaque in vitro. J. dent. Res. *60:* 1165 (1981).

21 Tatevossian, A.; Newbrun, E.: Diffusion of small ionic species in human saliva, plaque fluid and plaque residue in vitro. Archs oral Biol. *28:* 109–115 (1983).

G.H. Dibdin, PhD, Medical Research Council Dental Unit,
Lower Maudlin Street, Bristol BS1 2LY (England)

Cariology Today. Int. Congr., Zürich 1983, pp. 199–204 (Karger, Basel 1984)

Current View of Plaque Acidogenicity

D.A.M. Geddes

Glasgow Dental Hospital and School, University of Glasgow,
Glasgow, Scotland

Introduction

Advances in the knowledge of plaque acidogenicity have largely resulted from improvements in the sensitivity of the analytical methods available. Traditionally, acidogenicity of dental plaque has been assessed either by measurement of pH or by qualitative and quantitative analysis of carboxylic acid anions. Some studies have combined both methods. There are three methods, employing a range of types of electrode systems, for measuring plaque pH following fermentation of carbohydrate in situ. The probing method [21] permits direct reading from plaque on individual tooth sites using antimony or glass electrodes. The indwelling method pioneered in Zurich by *Graf and Mühlemann* [15] permits continuous measurement from glass and more recently semi-conductor electrode systems housed in a denture assembly. The oldest technique [1] still in use employs an external pH electrode system (the 'one drop') to measure small samples of plaque removed from the teeth after fermentation in situ. This method has the advantage that it can readily be used in conjunction with anion estimation [6]. Numerous workers using one or more of these methods have confirmed and extended *Stephan's* [21] observation that where plaque on the tooth surface is exposed to carbohydrate, which can readily be metabolised by the bacteria in plaque, the pH rapidly decreases then subsequently rises, more slowly, to approach neutrality (the 'Stephan Curve').

Early studies measuring pH values and lactate concentrations [18] showed a significant negative correlation between pH and lactate concentration; however, volatile acid anions were not estimated. Volatile acid anions were subsequently identified from in vitro fermentations [7, 9, 14, 19, 20]. Quantitative anion analysis after fermentation in situ became possible with refinement of the gas-liquid chromatography (GLC) technique [6, 13]. This somewhat exacting procedure has now been superseded by isotachophoresis [3, 11] and liquid chromatography (HPLC) [2, 23]. Both new techniques provide quantitative analysis of the range of volatile and non-volatile acids in submilligram amounts of plaque with the minimum of sample preparation. This short paper is confined to the consideration of the data available from recent studies of acid anions and corresponding pH measurement from plaque before and after fermentation in situ.

Review of Acid Anion Profiles and pH

Some general conclusions about acid anion profiles and pH in dental plaque in situ may be drawn from these [2, 3, 6, 11, 13, 23] and other recent studies [8, 12, 24]. In 'starved' plaques (samples after overnight fasting) and 'resting' plaques (samples not less than 2 h after the last consumption of food or drink containing carbohydrate capable of fermentation by plaque bacteria) acetate is the major anion present and lactate concentration is minimal. This general finding holds true for samples of 'young' plaques (24-hour accumulation from subjects with healthy mouths) and 'old' plaques (from subjects with poor oral hygiene and dental disease), for samples from adults and from comparable samples from deciduous teeth in children (unpublished data), and for plaques from caries-resistant as well as from caries-susceptible subjects [2, 24]. Typical values for acetate concentration are 40–50 nmol mg^{-1} wet weight of plaque and for the acetate:lactate ratio 10:1. Propionate, succinate, formate, butyrate and pyruvate are commonly present as minor constituents in 'starved' and 'resting' plaques.

After exposure in situ to sucrose or glucose, the pH of plaque falls rapidly, reaching its minimum value usually within 20 min. However, the most rapid pH decrease occurs early and a significant ($p < 0.01$) increase in lactate has been observed within 1 min [12]. This is consistent with the findings of our [17] and other recent studies on the diffusion of sugars and acids in human dental plaque which are reviewed elsewhere in the symposium [*Dibdin, this volume*]. Lactate concentrations are highest around the time of the pH minimum (fig. 1) [12]. Lactate analysis by GLC, HPLC or by isotachophoresis does not differentiate between the $L(+)$ and $D(-)$ isomers of lactic acid but in an earlier study lactate was quantified enzymically and the presence of both isomers established [7]. In 'resting' plaque, the $D(-)$ form predominated. After fermentation, the ratio of $D(-):L(+)$ was reversed. It was concluded that although the volatiles are the dominant acid anions around neutral ('resting') pH, the rapid pH decrease typical of the Stephan Curve, depends upon the release of $L(+)$ and to a lesser extent $D(-)$ lactate. The amount and rate of lactate production was found to be higher in plaques of caries-susceptible compared with caries-resistant subjects in one study [24] but not in another [2].

Although formate was tentatively identified by *Muntz* [19] in 1943 and *Ranke* et al. [20] in 1964, it has until recently not been quantified

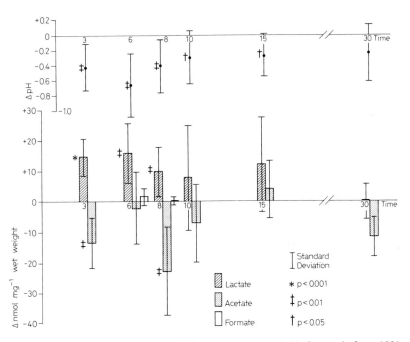

Fig. 1. Changes in acid anions and pH from plaques sampled before and after a 10% sucrose rinse. 24-hour plaques were sampled individually, from 9 healthy subjects. The anions were estimated by isotachophoresis and pH using the 'one-drop' electrode. Statistical analysis was by Student's t test [12].

from plaque fermentation in situ because of technical difficulties. The available data [2, 3, 12, 13, 24] allow the tentative suggestion that the occurrence and concentration of formate increases with plaque age. The highest concentrations reported are from '7-day', interstitial plaque [13] and the lowest from '24-h' samples [12].

The general conclusions that may be drawn about the anion profiles during the 'recovery phase' (pH minimum to 'resting' pH) of the Stephan Curve are that lactate decreases and volatile acid anions increase, but that the anion concentrations take longer than pH to return to the 'resting' values.

Discussion

Lactic acid, and in 'old' plaques perhaps also formic acid, are the major plaque metabolites responsible for the rapid fall to acid pH after exogenous carbohydrate fermentation. However, the metabolic pathways leading to, and the consequences of, the high acetate levels found in 'resting' or 'starved' plaques around neutral pH are less clearly understood. It is likely that acetate accumulation is the result of a number of metabolic processes within the complex, dynamic plaque eco-system [10]. Lactate may be considered as an intermediate metabolite in plaque, providing substrate for obligate lactate utilizing bacteria and resulting in acetate formation. Acetate can also arise from the breakdown of intracellular and extracellular carbohydrate storage compounds and from heterofermentation pathways. The regulation of sugar metabolism in plaque is reviewed elsewhere in the symposium [*Carlsson,* this volume]. It has also been suggested [8, 24] that another source of substrate for acetate production could be amino acid catabolism from the proteins and peptides in saliva and crevicular fluid. Nitrogen metabolism in plaque is reviewed elsewhere in the symposium [*Curtis,* this volume].

At pH values around neutrality, the acids found in plaque are almost completely dissociated, therefore differences between high pK (butyric, propionic, acetic) and low pK (lactic, formic, pyruvic) are unimportant with respect to base consumption in 'resting' and 'starved' plaque. *Vratsanos* [23] argues that, as pH falls, the weak, high-pK acids develop a potential acidity (undissociated form) contributing to the buffer capacity of plaque, thus controlling the level of the pH minimum and he further postulates that this buffering capacity gives a protective role for the high pK acids [24]. However, *Gray* [16], studying the kinetics of 'white spot' formation within the enamel, concluded that not only pH but also the types of anions present affected acid dissolution. He postulated that increased buffer capacity and buffer strength would increase caries activity, so that the anion profiles would be an important factor in caries development.

The loss of acetate frequently observed around the pH minimum of the Stephan Curve [3, 6, 12] has been attributed to the dilution and washing effects of saliva [5]. However, *Featherstone and Rodgers* [4] suggest that rapid diffusion into enamel of the high pK acids in their undissociated form could also contribute to the observed loss of acetate in vivo. Acetate has been identified as an anion from organic acid residues in human enamel 'white spot' lesions [22]. Recent evidence on diffusion and enamel caries development [discussed elsewhere in the symposium; *Featherstone*, this volume] supports the hypothesis that acid diffuses into enamel in its undissociated form and that the rate of lesion progress is a function of unionized acid concentration and pK. Thus acetic acid (and other high-pK acids) may make a major contribution to lesion formation with mixtures of acetic and lactic acids having additive demineralizing properties [4].

References

1   Campaigne, E.E.; Fosdick, L.D.: Production and characteristics of synthetic mucin plaques. Bull. N.West. Univ. dent. Sch. *38:* 14–17 (1938).

2   Distler, W.; Kröncke, A.: In vivo acid formation by human dental plaque. Zahn-, Mund- u. Kieferheilk. Vortr. *69:* 743 (1981).

3   Edgar, W.M.: Isotachophoretic analysis of major acids in human plaque fluid before and after sugar consumption. Zahn-, Mund- u. Kieferheilk. Vortr. *69:* 744 (1981).

4   Featherstone, J.D.B.; Rodgers, B.E.: Effect of acetic, lactic and other organic acids on the formation of artificial carious lesions. Caries Res. *15:* 377–385 (1981).

5   Geddes, D.A.M.: Studies on acid production in human dental plaque in relation to dental caries; PhD thesis Newcastle upon Tyne (1974).

6   Geddes, D.A.M.: Acids produced by human dental plaque metabolism in situ. Caries Res. *9:* 98–109 (1975).

7   Geddes, D.A.M.: The production of $L(+)$ and $D(-)$ lactic acid and volatile acids by human dental plaque and the effect of plaque buffering and acidic strength on pH. Archs oral Biol. *17:* 537–545 (1972).

8 Geddes, D.A.M.: Diffusion and acid production in human dental plaque; in Kawamura, Front. oral Physiol., vol. 3, edited by D.B. Ferguson, pp. 78–87 (Karger, Basel 1981).

9 Geddes, D.A.M.; Gilmour, M.N.: The reproducibility of acid production by human, unhomogenized, dental plaques. J. dent. Res. *48:* 1106 (1969).

10 Geddes, D.A.M.; Jenkins, G.N.: Intrinsic and extrinsic factors influencing the flora of the mouth; in Skinner, Sykes, The normal microbial flora of man. SAB Symp. No. 3 (Academic Press, London 1974).

11 Geddes, D.A.M.; Weetman, D.A.: Estimation of organic acids in human dental plaque by isotachophoresis. Zahn-, Mund- u. Kieferheilk. Vortr. *69:* 744 (1981).

12 Geddes, D.A.M.; Weetman, D.A.: Acid anion profiles in dental plaque (Abstract No. 47). Caries Res. *17:* 173 (1983).

13 Gilmour, M.N.; Greene, G.C.; Zahn, L.M.; Sparmann, C.D.; Pearlman, J.: C1–C4 monocarboxylic and lactic acids in dental plaques before and after exposure to sucrose in vivo; in Stiles, Loesche, O'Brien, Microbial aspects of dental caries. Microb. Abstr., suppl. 2, pp. 539–556 (1976).

14 Gilmour, N.; Poole, A.E.: The fermentation capabilities of dental plaque. Caries Res. *1:* 247–260 (1967).

15 Graf, H.; Mühlemann, H.R.: Telemetry of plaque pH from interdental area. Helv. odont. Acta *10:* 94–101 (1966).

16 Gray, J.A.: Kinetics of enamel dissolution during formation of incipient caries-like lesions. Archs oral Biol. *11:* 397–421 (1966).

17 McNee, S.G.; Geddes, D.A.M.; Weetman, D.A.: Diffusion of sugars and acids in human dental plaque. Archs oral Biol. *27:* 987–991 (1982).

18 Moore, B.W.; Carter, W.J.; Dunn, J.K.; Fosdick, L.S.: The formation of lactic acid in dental plaques in caries-active individuals. J. dent. Res. *35:* 778–785 (1956).

19 Muntz, J.A.: Production of acids from glucose by dental plaque material. J. biol. Chem. *148:* 225–236 (1943).

20 Ranke, B.; Bramstedt, F.; Naujoks, R.: Untersuchungen mit markierten Verbindungen über den Kohlenhydratabbau in den plaques. Adv. Fluorine Res. dent. Caries Prev. *2:* 189–193 (1964).

21 Stephan, R.M.: Changes in the hydrogen ion concentration on tooth surfaces and in carious lesions. J. Am. dent. Ass. *27:* 718–723 (1940).

22 Tyler, J.E.: Quantitative estimation of volatile fatty acids in carious enamel by gas chromatography of their methyl esters. J. dent. Res. *50:* 1189 (1971).

23 Vratsanos, S.M.: Chromatographic micro analysis of organic acids in plaque, related to food cariogenicity; in Foods, nutrition and dental Health (Pathotox 1981), Park Forest South 1981, vol. 3.

24 Vratsanos, S.M.; Mandel, I.D.: Comparative plaque acidogenesis of caries-resitant vs. caries-susceptible adults. J. dent. Res. *61:* 465–468 (1982).

D.A.M. Geddes, MD, Glasgow Dental Hospital and School,
University of Glasgow, Glasgow (Scotland)

Cariology Today. Int. Congr., Zürich 1983, pp. 205–211 (Karger, Basel 1984)

Regulation of Sugar Metabolism in Relation to the Feast-and-Famine Existence of Plaque

Jan Carlsson

Department of Oral Microbiology, University of Umeå, Sweden

A natural microbiota usually develops in its habitat, until it has exploited the nutritional resources, and become inhibited by shortage of nutrients. In many natural habitats, however, there could from time to time be unannounced and irregular periods of food in excess. To survive under such conditions the organisms of the microbiota do not only have to be able to grow under chronic starvation, they also have to respond quickly to the windfalls of food [18]. This ability is important, since it has been demonstrated in the laboratory that starving microorganisms might be killed by nutrients in excess [9].

The main source of nutrients to the oral microbiota are the salivary secretions [7]. The concentration of glucose in these secretions is, however, only 5–40 μM [17]. The sugar level in the oral fluids may, however, increase 1,000-fold upon food intake, and there is an obvious risk that the starving microorganisms are killed by this sugar ('sugar killing'). To survive under these conditions the microorganisms have defense mechanisms. In recent years, we have gained some insight into how a predominant group of dental microorganisms, the streptococci, regulate their sugar metabolism in order to adapt to their feast-and-famine existence on the teeth.

The sugar metabolism is regulated at three levels, i.e. the transport of the sugar, the glycolytic pathway, and the conversion of pyruvate into metabolic end-products. The transport of sugar from the external environment through the cell membrane into the cytoplasm requires specific proteins (carriers) in the cell membrane. There is usually a specific transport system for each sugar, and for a given sugar there may be more than one system. For the efficient use of the nutritional resources and for the defense against 'sugar killing' these transport systems have to be regulated. The synthesis of the transport proteins can thus be induced and repressed, and the activity of the transport systems can be modulated by cellular metabolites [10].

Streptococci have often two transport systems for each sugar, a phosphoenolpyruvate: sugar phosphotransferase system and a proton-linked active sugar transport. The phosphotransferase system usually has high affinity for the sugar and is induced, when the sugar is present at low concentration, whereas the proton-linked system is used at higher sugar levels and at low pH. The phosphoenolpyruvate:glucose phosphotransferase system (fig. 1a, A) of *Streptococcus mutans* works with half-maximum rate already at a glucose concentration of less then 10 μM and is obviously well-suited for taking care of the glucose in the salivary secretions. The proton-linked active glucose transport (fig. 1b, B) works with half-maximum rate at 100–200 μM of glucose [15]. For sucrose there are three transport systems in *S. mutans* [11, 21].

After the sugar has entered the cell, it is degraded by the glycolytic enzymes. In most organisms, the Embden-Meyerhof pathway is the main route (from G6P to PYR in fig. 1), but also the hexose mono-phosphate pathway (not shown) is used in order to provide cellular precursors and reducing power (NADPH) for biosynthetic reactions. *S. mutans* and *Streptococcus salivarius* do not have the oxidative por-tion of the hexose monophosphate pathway [5, 26]. To get NADPH, these streptococci have a specific NADPH-dependent glyceraldehyde 3-phosphate dehydrogenase (fig. 1, C) [8]. This enzyme oxidizes gly-ceraldehyde 3-phosphate into 3-phosphoglycerate instead of 1,3-bisphosphoglycerate as the ordinary NAD-dependent enzyme (fig. 1, D) of the Embden-Meyerhof pathway. To get the cellular precursors of the hexose monophosphate pathway *S. mutans* and *S. salivarius* have, however, the nonoxidative portion of this pathway [4].

Pyruvate kinase (fig. 1, E) is the main regulatory site of the Embden-Meyerhof pathway in streptococci [16, 28]. When sugars limit the growth, this enzyme is inhibited by the intracellular level of inorgan-ic phosphate [2]. By this inhibition a pool of phosphoenolpyruvate is created for an efficient transport of the sugar into the cell by the phosphotransferase system (fig. 1a, A). Phosphoenolpyruvate may also activate (fig. 1a, F) glycogen phosphorylase (fig. 1a, R) and this initiates the use of intracellular polysaccharides as energy reserve [22]. The end-product of the Embden-Meyerhof pathway, pyruvate, is subsequently converted by the inducible pyruvate formatelyase (fig. 1, G) into for-mate and acetyl-CoA [29]. The further fate of acetyl-CoA is determined by the oxidation-reduction balance of the cell. The degradation of one molecule of glucose by the Embden-Meyerhof pathway gives two molecules of pyruvate and two molecules of NADH. To preserve the oxidation-reduction balance, the NADH has to be reoxidized. By converting acetyl-CoA (fig. 1a, H) first into acetaldehyde and after that (fig. 1a, I) into ethanol, the two NADH are oxidized. The other acetyl-CoA from pyruvate is converted (fig. 1a, J) into acetylphosphate. The energy of acetylphosphate is conserved in ATP (fig. 1a, K) and acetate is formed [1, 23]. Each molecule of glucose will thus give two molecules of formate and one each of ethanol and acetate [6].

When starving microorganisms are exposed to an excess of sugars, glycolytic intermediates might be built up in the cell to such high levels that they become toxic. There are several regulatory mechanisms, which may keep the glycolytic intermediates at nontoxic levels. Against high concentrations of sucrose some streptococci have a unique first line of defense in the form of extracellular enzymes, which convert the glucose or the fructose moiety of sucrose into polymers outside the cell wall. In this way, the net sugar load on the organism is halved. The formation of these polymers may also be favorable to the dental microorganisms in other ways. They may serve as an energy reserve and as a protection against dehydration. They may also help in retaining the microorganisms at the tooth surface [12, 14].

To keep the glycolytic intermediates at nontoxic levels, the activity of the glycolytic enzymes may be modulated by the intracellular level of specific glycolytic intermediates, or by the concerted action of several glycolytic intermediates and ATP, ADP, AMP or inorganic phosphate. Two important regulators are glucose 6-phosphate and fructose 1,6-bisphosphate. In S. mutans and S. salivarius, glucose 6-phosphate abolishes (fig. 1b, L) the phosphate inhibition of pyruvate kinase (fig. 1, E) and increases the rate of glycolysis [2, 28]. In Streptococcus sanguis and Streptococcus mitis, fructose 1,6-bisphosphate plays the same role [3] in draining the cell of glycolytic intermediates. Fructose 1,6-bisphosphate may also be of significance in keeping the glycolytic intermediates at nontoxic levels by activating (fig. 1b, M) ADP-glucose phosphorylase (fig. 1b, S), and initiating the synthesis of intracellular polysaccharides, 'glycogen' [19].

The most important defense against 'sugar killing' is, however, the 'lactate gate'. Lactate dehydrogenase (fig. 1b, N) is a constitutive enzyme that is always present in high amounts in streptococci [1, 27].

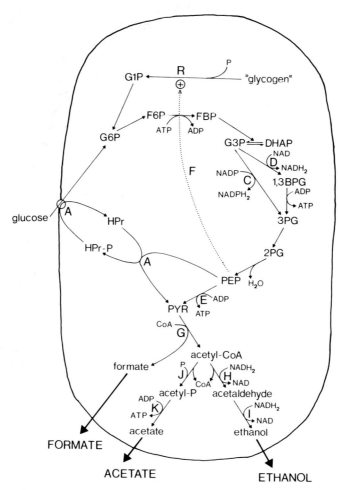

Fig. 1. Regulation of sugar metabolism. *a* Limited supply of glucose. Lactate gate closed. *b* Excess of glucose. Lactate gate open (N). Further explanations are given in the text.

This enzyme is absolutely dependent on fructose 1,6-bisphosphate for activity, and under conditions of sugar limitation the intracellular pool of fructose 1,6-bisphosphate is too low to activate the enzyme. The lactate gate is closed. When the level of fructose 1,6-bisphosphate increases upon exposure of the cell to sugar, lactate dehydrogenase (fig. 1, N) is activated (fig. 1, O). The lactate gate opens and the glycolytic intermediates are rapidly drained off the cell. A large amount of lactate is excreted. Also acetate, formate and ethanol are formed although the

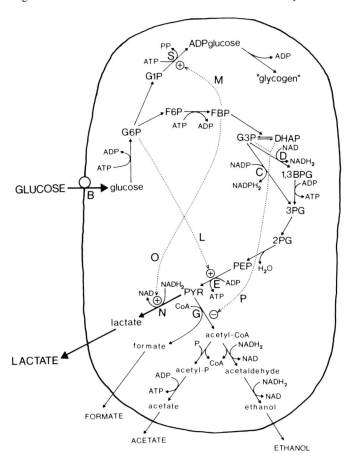

b

activity of pyruvate formate-lyase (fig. 1, G) is inhibited (fig. 1b, P) by glyceraldehyde 3-phosphate and dihydroxyacetone phosphate [1, 23, 29]. The lactate gate may be more common among oral bacteria than has been appreciated. So far, lactate dehydrogenases with an absolute requirement for fructose 1,6-bisphosphate have been found in strepto-cocci, lactobacilli [24], and bifidobacteria [25].

There may, in some cases, be no defense against sugar killing. A well-known example is xylitol, which in some organisms is transported into the cell by a phosphoenolpyruvate:fructose phosphotransferase system, and xylitol 5-phosphate is formed. The organism is unable to degrade this intermediate. It accumulates in the cell and kills the organism [20].

Upon exposure of dental plaque to high sugar levels there is a very rapid drop of pH and an increase in the concentration of lactate [13]. The concentration of acids in the plaque may be so high that the tooth minerals are solubilized. Against this background, the lactate gate stands out as a crucial microbial characteristic in the initiation of dental caries. We have in the previous discussion considered the lactate gate as a requisite for the survival of microorganisms during their feast-and-famine existence on the teeth. We may now conclude that the microorganisms escape from sugar killing by sacrificing the integrity of the tooth surface to which they adhere.

References

1   Abbe, K.; Takahashi, S.; Yamada, T.: Involvement of oxygen-sensitive pyruvate formate-lyase in mixed-acid fermentation by *Streptococcus mutans* under strictly anaerobic conditions. J. Bact. *152:* 175–182 (1982).

2   Abbe, K.; Yamada, T.: Purification and properties of pyruvate kinase from *Streptococcus mutans*. J. Bact. *149:* 299–305 (1982).

3   Abbe, K.; Takahashi, S.; Yamada, T.: Purification and properties of pyruvate kinase from *Streptococcus sanguis,* and activator specificity of pyruvate kinase from oral streptococci. Infect. Immunity *39/3* (1983).

4   Bridges, R.B.: Ribose biosynthesis in *Streptococcus mutans*. Archs oral Biol. *22:* 139–145 (1977).

5   Brown, A.T.; Wittenberger, C.L.: The occurrence of multiple glyceraldehyde-3-phosphate dehydrogenases in cariogenic streptococci. Biochem. biophys. Res. Commun. *43:* 217–224 (1971).

6   Carlsson, J.; Griffith, C.J.: Fermentation products and bacterial yields in glucose-limited and nitrogen-limited cultures of streptococci. Archs oral Biol. *19:* 1105–1109 (1974).

7   Carlsson, J.; Johansson, T.: Sugar and the production of bacteria in the human mouth. Caries Res. *7:* 273–282 (1973).

8   Crow, V.L.; Wittenberger, C.L.: Separation and properties of NAD- and NADP-dependent glyceraldehyde-3-phosphate dehydrogenases from *Streptococcus mutans*. J. biol. Chem. *254:* 1134–1142 (1979).

9   Dawes, E.A.: Endogenous metabolism and the survival of starved prokaryotes; in Gray, Postgate, 26th Symp. Soc. Gen. Microbiol. The survival of vegetative microbes, pp. 19–53 (Cambridge University Press, Cambridge 1976)

10 Dills, S.S.; Apperson, A.; Schmidt, M.R.; Saier, M.H.R., Jr.: Carbohydrate transport in bacteria. Microbiol. Rev. *44:* 385–418 (1980)

11 Ellwood, D.C.; Hamilton, I.R.: Properties of *Streptococcus mutans* Ingbritt growing on limiting sucrose in a chemostat: repression of the phosphoenolpyruvate phosphotransferase transport system. Infect. Immunity *36:* 576–581 (1982).

12 Gibbons, R.J.; van Houte, J.: Bacterial adherence in oral microbial ecology. A. Rev. Microbiol. *29:* 19–44 (1975).

13 Geddes, D.A.M.: Acids produced by human dental plaque metabolism in situ. Caries Res. *9:* 98–109 (1975).

14 Guggenheim, B.: Extracellular polysaccharides and microbial plaque. Int. dent. J., Lond. *20:* 657–678 (1970).

15 Hamilton, I.R.; St. Martin, E.J.: Evidence for the involvement of proton motive force in the transport of glucose by a mutant of *Streptococcus mutans* strain DR0001 defective in glucose-phosphoenolpyruvate phosphotransferase activity. Infect. Immunity *36:* 567–575 (1982).

16 Iwami, Y.; Yamada, T.: Rate-limiting steps of the glycolytic pathway in the oral bacteria *Streptococcus mutans* and *Streptococcus sanguis* and the influence of acidic pH on the glucose metabolism. Archs oral Biol. *25:* 163–169 (1980).

17 Kelsay, J.L.; McCague, K.E.; Holden, J.M.: Variations in flow rate, metabolites and enzyme activities of fasting human parotid saliva. Archs oral Biol. *17:* 439–445 (1972).

18 Koch, A.L.: The adaptive responses of *Escherichia coli* to a feast and famine existence. Adv. Microbiol. Physiol. *6:* 147–217 (1971).

19 Mattingly, S.J.; Daneo-Moore, L.; Shockman, G.D.: Factors regulating cell wall thickening and intracellular iodophilic polysaccharide storage in *Streptococcus mutans.* Infect. Immunity *16:* 967–973 (1977).

20 Reiner, A.M.: Xylitol and *d*-arabitol toxicities due to derepressed fructose, galactitol, and sorbitol phosphotransferases of *Escherichia coli.* J. Bact. *132:* 166–173 (1977).

21 Slee, A.M.; Tanzer, J.M.: Sucrose transport by *Streptococcus mutans.* Evidence for multiple transport systems. Biochim. biophys. Acta *692:* 415–424 (1982).

22 Spearman, T.N.; Khandelwal, R.L.; Hamilton, I.R.: Some regulatory properties of glycogen phosphorylase from *Streptococcus salivarius.* Archs Biochem. Biophys. *154:* 306–313 (1973).

23 Takahashi, S.; Abbe, K.; Yamada, T.: Purification of pyruvate formate-lyase from *Streptococcus mutans* and its regulatory properties. J. Bact. *149:* 1034–1040 (1982).

24 de Vries, W.; Kapteijn, W.M.C.; Van Der Beek, E.G.; Stouthamer, A.H.: Molar growth yields and fermentation balances of *Lactobacillus casei* L3 in batch cultures and in continuous cultures. J. gen. Microbiol. *63:* 333–345 (1970).

25 de Vries, W.; Stouthamer, A.H.: Fermentation of glucose, lactose, galactose, mannitol, and xylose by bifidobacteria. J. Bact. *96:* 472–478 (1968).

26 Yamada, T.; Carlsson, J.: Phosphoenolpyruvate carboxylase and ammonium metabolism in oral streptococci, Archs oral Biol. *18:* 799–812 (1973).

27 Yamada, T.; Carlsson, J.: Regulation of lactate dehydrogenase and change of fermentation products in streptococci. J. Bact. *124:* 55–61 (1975).

28 Yamada, T.; Carlsson, J.: Glucose-6-phosphate-dependent pyruvate kinase in *Streptococcus mutans.* J. Bact. *124:* 562–563 (1975).

29 Yamada, T.; Carlsson. J.: The role of pyruvate formate-lyase in glucose metabolism of *Streptococcus mutans;* in Stiles, Loesche, O'Brien, Microbial aspects of dental caries. Microbiol. Abstr., suppl. 2, pp. 809–819 (1976).

Jan Carlsson, MD, Oral Microbiology, University of Umeå,
S-901 87 Umeå (Sweden)

Cariology Today. Int. Congr., Zürich 1983, pp. 212–222 (Karger, Basel 1984)

Nitrogen Metabolism in Dental Plaque

M.A. Curtis, C.W. Kemp[1]

National Caries Program, National Institute of Dental Research,
National Institutes of Health, Bethesda, Md., USA

Introduction

In the same way that analysis of the end-products of carbohydrate metabolism in the extracellular phase of dental plaque has provided much information regarding the extent and diversity of the fermentation activities of the oral microbiota [1–4], examination of the free amino acid, amine and ammonia levels in plaque may give some insight into the metabolism of nitrogen at the tooth surface.

The ammonium concentration of plaque fluid has been reported to be 18 mM in humans [5] and 50 mM in experimental monkeys [6]. Both values were determined in resting plaque. The source of this abundant ion may be assumed to be predominantly from the catabolism of amino acids and urea. The latter is secreted continuously in saliva and elevation of its normal level in patients with renal disorders has been implicated in the low caries incidence of these subjects [7]. The precise mechanism of breakdown of urea in plaque is not fully established, though the lack of stoichiometric release of NH_3 and CO_2 suggests a reaction other than that catalyzed by the enzyme urease [8]. The general elevation of the total concentration of free amino acids at the tooth surface to approximately tenfold that in whole saliva [6, 9] probably reflects the extensive proteolytic activity associated with plaque [10–12]

[1] We thank Drs. *M.F. Cole* and *D.B. Mirth* for their critical review of this manuscript.

directed towards both salivary and possibly dietary substrates. The high concentration of glutamic acid, however, accounting for approximately 25% of the total free amino acid pool, is more likely a result of the anabolic activities of the plaque microbiota. Glutamate is present at a very high intracellular concentration in gram-positive bacteria [13]; the formation of glutamic acid through the action of NADPH-linked glutamate dehydrogenase is thought to be the principal mechanism of ammonia assimilation by the oral streptococci [14].

Despite these elevated levels of free amino acids it is suggested that their concentrations will still be insufficient, when used as substrates for decarboxylation reactions [15] to have any significant neutralization effect upon the large amounts of acid which accumulate at the tooth surface following the dietary carbohydrate challenge [16, 17]. The low levels of amines in plaque [18], although thus far only determined in 'starved' plaque samples, support this view.

A more consistent feature of amino acid metabolism, which may have a bearing on the overal pH balance of plaque, is their deamination during fermentation. With the notable exception of arginine [19, 20] few data are available on the fermentation of amino acids in plaque. Degradation of arginine in plaque is thought to proceed via the widespread arginine deiminase pathway [20]. The repression of this pathway in streptococci, however, by low extracellular glucose levels [21, 22] suggests that base formation from arginine may only occur during periods of carbohydrate limitation in plaque. The extremely low concentration of free arginine in resting plaque samples [9] perhaps signifies this utilization.

Fermentation of other amino acids in plaque has not been widely investigated despite the potential for ammonia formation. For example, during the fermentation of aspartic acid by washed cells of *Bacteroides melaninogenicus* over 95% of the substrate is deaminated [23]. The effect of base generated through the activities of amino acid fermentors including the bacteroides, fusobacteria, peptococci and peptostreptococci in plaque is largely unknown. However, since many of the substrates for these reactions are unlikely to be limiting, given the protein-rich nature of the oral secretions, it is perhaps worthy of further investigation.

During the course of free amino acid analyses of plaque fluid we observed a high concentration of a ninhydrin-positive component previously unreported in the oral environment [24]. On the basis of its retention time and subsequent GC/MS analysis [manuscript in preparation], it was identified as δ-NH$_2$ valeric acid. Though this compound comprised 20–25% of the total extracellular free amino acid pool, it was absent from the ductal salivary secretions and its presence in the mouth was, therefore, assumed to be a product of microbial action [6]. The production of δ-NH$_2$ valeric acid is classically associated with the genus *Clostridium* utilizing the Stickland reaction [25–27]. Essentially, this reaction involves the oxidation of one amino acid to a fatty acid, CO$_2$ and ammonia, while two molecules of another amino acid act as hydrogen acceptors and are thereby reduced. In the case of noncyclic amino acids, reduction leads to the release of ammonia whereas reduction of proline leads to ring cleavage and the formation of δ-NH$_2$ valeric acid. Keto acids may participate in the reaction provided they are structurally related to an amino acid. In addition, it is suggested that molecular hydrogen may replace the oxidizable amino acid in the reaction providing a hydrogenase system is present [28].

Given the importance of ammonia generation in plaque and the high concentration of proline in the salivary secretions [29], we have conducted experiments to examine the source of the reducing power for the formation of δ-NH$_2$ valeric acid in plaque and the organisms involved. This paper presents the results of some preliminary investigations.

Materials and Methods

Growth Characteristics of a Proline-Reducing Microorganism from Human Saliva.
The utilization of amino acids during the growth of a human salivary isolate (KC11) with proline reductase activity was examined. KC11 was originally isolated on blood agar in close association with a second colony type. The dependency of KC11 on the other organism was evident in that optimal growth of KC11 could only be achieved in the filtrate of the spent medium following growth of the mixture of organisms. The nature of this dependency has not been established, though it did not appear to be related to a deficiency in the medium of amino acids, organic acids or vitamins.

The mixture of organisms from which KC11 was isolated was inoculated into brain-heart infusion medium and incubated anaerobically at 37 °C. After cessation of growth, the medium was filter-sterilized, enriched with proline to a concentration of 22 mM, reinoculated with a pure culture of KC11 and incubated at 37 °C under 95% N$_2$/5% CO$_2$ in a tube fermentor. At 15-min intervals during the course of growht, aliquots were aseptically removed and the optical density at 600 nm determined. Filter-sterilized samples were then frozen prior to analysis.

Amino Acid Analysis. Alterations in the amino acid and ammonia profile of the medium were examined with a Beckmann 121MB automatic analyzer using modified citrate buffers for elution [30] and Trione (Pickering Labs, Calif.) for detection. The samples were initially rendered free of high molecular weight proteins using sulfosalicylic acid (4%) precipitation followed by centrifugation at 10,000 g for 30 min.

HPLC Analysis. The carboxylic acids produced during growth of KC11 and *Peptostreptococcus anaerobius* (ATCC 27337) in peptone yeast extract medium supplemented with glucose (0.2%), Tween and proline (20 mM) (PYGTP) were examined using HPLC [31]. Analyses were performed on a Waters HPLC system equipped with a Bio Rad HPX87H column using 10.8% (v/v) acetonitrile in 0.007 N H_2SO_4 as the mobile phase at a flow rate of 0.5 ml/min. Absorbance was monitored at 210 nm. A standard solution containing the volatile acids C_1–C_6, a-ketoglutaric, malonic, methyl malonic, pyruvic, succinic, lactic, fumaric, phenylacetic, OH-phenylacetic, phenylpropionic and OH-phenylpropionic acids was used for calibration.

Plaque Fluid Analysis. The organic acid profile of plaque fluid was examined by GLC and by the HPLC technique described earlier. In order to obtain sufficient material for the HPLC analyses, whole-mouth plaque was pooled from 4 monkeys *(Macaca fascicularis)* maintained on a high sucrose cariogenic diet [32]. Plaque samples were collected after overnight fasting, centrifuged at 18,000 g at 4 °C for 1 h and stored on ice prior to analysis.

Gas Chromatography. Volatile fatty acids were determined using a Hewlett-Packard 5840 chromatograph equipped with a 25-meter capillary Carbowax column and flame ionization detector (FID). Conditions were as follows: injection port temperature, 250 °C; oven temperature, 105 °C; FID temperature, 300 °C; carrier gas, helium, 1.5 kg/cm²; make-up gas nitrogen, 30 ml/min. A split ratio of 1:100 was used.

Plaque Incubation. Whole-mouth plaque from monkeys (*M. fascicularis*) was pooled and stored on ice for no longer than 2 h prior to use. It was then homogenized in preduced saline and aliquots incubated with the appropriate substrates at 37 °C in capped microcentrifuge tubes. In a preliminary series of experiments the suspensions were incubated in phosphate-buffered saline, pH 7.0, in the presence of proline (20 mM) and one of a variety of the possible oxidizable substrates commonly found in dental plaque. After incubation for 4 h the homogenates were centrifuged at 10,000 g for 15 min at 4 °C and the supernatants removed. Analysis of δ-NH_2 valeric acid was performed directly on the supernatants by gas chromatography using the conditions described previously except that the injection port temperature was raised to 270 °C. The rates of proline reduction by alanine, glucose and lactic acid were examined in a series of timed plaque incubations. Equal volumes (50 μl) of the plaque homogenate (150 mg/ml saline) were incubated in phosphate-buffered saline, pH 7.0 and pH 5.5, with proline alone, proline and alanine, lithium-L-lactate or glucose. All final concentrations were 20 mM except glucose, 10 mM. The final volume in all cases was 350 μl. At intervals up to 24 h, one tube from each series was chilled on crushed ice, centrifuged as described earlier and the supernatant removed. Analysis of the δ-NH_2 valeric acid content was performed on a Beckman 121 MB automatic analyser as described earlier.

Results

Characterization of KC11

Oral-isolate KC11 was a gram-positive coccus growing in chains. The staining, cellular morphology and anaerobic nature of the organism categorized it as a member of the genus *Peptostreptococcus* and the diversity of its end products as *Peptostreptococcus anaerobius* [33]. However, the failure of the organism to produce isocaproic and phenyl propionic acids differentiates it from other *P. anaerobius* strains [31, 34, 35]. In addition, no immunological cross-reactivity was found between KC11 and stock *P. anaerobius* strain ATCC 27337. However, all stock and clinical isolates of *P. anaerobius* thus far examined contain proline reductase activity.

Metabolism of KC11

Growth of KC11 resulted in an almost complete exhaustion of free proline from the medium (falling in concentration by approximately 19 mM.) The disappearance of proline yielded an approximately stoichiometric increase in the concentration of δ-NH$_2$ valeric acid–slope 0.93 (fig. 1). The reduction of proline was linear with respect to growth as measured by increase in optical density. Amino acids other than proline which suffered a substantial fall in concentration during growth were threonine, serine, valine, methionine, isoleucine, leucine, tyrosine and phenylalanine. With the exception of methionine and threonine, these amino acids have been demonstrated to act as hydrogen donators

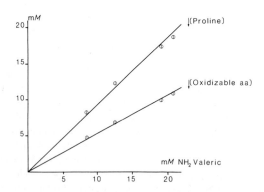

Fig. 1. The utilization of proline and oxidizable amino acids and production of δ-NH$_2$ valeric acid during growth of oral isolate KC11.

in coupled oxidation-reduction reactions in *Clostridium sporogones* [25, 26]. A plot of the disappearance of these oxidizable amino acids versus proline reduction gave a slope of 0.54 (fig. 1). An accurate quantitation of ammonia in the medium was not possible by amino acid analysis because of high blank values from the buffer system. An increase in the ammonia concentration of approximately 6 mM was estimated, however.

Plaque Fluid Composition

The results of the HPCL and GLC analyses of plaque fluid are shown in table I. The individual concentrations of phenyl acetic and 3-OH phenylpropionic acid could not be established because of coelution of these two compounds from the Aminex column. The disparity between the level of isocaproic acid as determined by the two methods is also indicative of coelution with an unknown component during the HPLC analysis.

Plaque Incubations

The amino acids alanine, tyrosine and arginine, the organic pyruvic and lactic acids, and glucose all stimulated the reduction of proline. Plaque incubations containing proline alone showed a low level of δ-NH$_2$ valeric acid production, presumably as a result of the oxidation

Table I. Organic acid composition of plaque fluid from pooled starved monkey plaque samples

Acid	Concentration mM	Acid	Concentration mM
Acetic	39.8 (30.9)	Pyruvic	0.7
Butyric	13.2 (8.8)	Isobutyric	0.6 (0.6)
Lactic	8.9	Isovaleric	(0.6)
δ-NH$_2$ Valeric	8.2[1]	Isocaproic	7.9 (0.5)
Propionic	8.2	3-Phenylpropionic	0.4
Succinic	4.8	3-OH Phenylpropionic	0.2
Formic	3.2	Phenylacetic	
α-Ketoglutaric	0.8	Valeric	(0.1)
		Fumaric	0.01

Figures in parentheses determined via GLC.
[1] n = 24; data from ref. [9].

of substrates within the plaque sample. At pH 7.0, glucose (10 mM) and lactate 20 mM) gave identical initial rates of proline reduction (27.3 μmol proline reduced/g wet weight plaque/h). The initial rate of proline reduction by alanine was somewhat lower at 17.1 μmol proline reduced/g wet weight plaque/h. At pH 5.5, the rates of proline reduction by lactate and alanine were 88 and 77% of the rates at pH 7.0, respectively. Glucose was ineffective at pH 5.5.

Discussion

The highly anaerobic nature of dental plaque demands a resourcefulness on the part of the microbial community for means to eliminate the reducing power generated by the oxidation of their substrates for growth. The reduction of amino acids is an example of one such mechanism utilized by anaerobic microorganisms [25, 26]. The abundance of proline in the salivary secretions [29] and its relatively high free concentration at the tooth surface [9] make this imino acid a major candidate for utilization as an electron sink in plaque and this probably accounts for the high levels of δ-NH$_2$ valeric acid in plaque fluid.

The oral isolate KC11, presumptively identified as *P. anaerobius* utilized amino acids during the course of exponential growth in approximate accordance with the stoichiometry expected for the Stickland reaction: a ratio of 0.54 was observed for the millimolar fall in concentration of free oxidizable amino acids versus the rise in concentration of δ-NH$_2$ valeric acid. A theoretical value of 0.5 would be expected. However, the observed value may have been influenced not only by the fermentation of bound amino acids, which were not determined, but also by the assimilation of medium amino acid into cellular proteins.

In terms of the acid-base balance of plaque, the most obvious beneficial effect of amino acid utilization via Stickland reactions is the production of ammonia. Since one can assume that these processes are not normally subject to substrate limitation given the protein-rich nature of the salivary secretions, the metabolism of the amino-acid-fermenting anaerobes is probably a consistent feature of the overall biochemistry of the oral microbiota. The high concentration of δ-NH$_2$ valeric acid and perhaps also of ammonia [5, 6, 9] testify to this continuity. The use of amino acids other than proline as oxidants in coupled oxidation-reduction reactions would lead to a higher ammonia yield. Though proline may be considered to be the foremost hydrogen acceptor in these reactions given its high concentration in the oral environment, it is possible that other equally abundant amino acids in plaque may function in a similar capacity. However, the contribution of amino acids such as glycine and aspartic acid is difficult to assess simply by examination of the fermentation products of plaque fluid since the reductive deamination products of these substrates, acetic and succinic acids, respectively, are also end-products of microbial glucose metabolism.

Proline reduction was stimulated by both glucose and lactic acid in plaque incubations. The utilization of leucine as a hydrogen acceptor in *P. anaerobius* has been demonstrated during the anaerobic fermentation of glucose and pyruvate [36]. Such activity may account for the proline reduction in plaque incubations in the presence of glucose at pH 7.0 in the present investigation. Alternatively, lactic acid produced by the glucose fermentation of other members of the plaque microbiota may be responsible. A similar confusion surrounds the role of lactic acid in proline reduction in plaque. In the mixed microbiota of dental plaque certain bacteria, notably veillonella, are capable of the oxidation of lactate to acetate, propionate and hydrogen. The molecular hydrogen evolved during such a reaction could be responsible for the proline reduction in the lactate incubations seen in this study. Another and more intriguing possibility, however, is that lactate may be oxidized directly in a Stickland reaction with proline. Though organisms of the genera *Clostridium* [37] and *Peptostreptococcus* [35, 38] are known to contain lactate dehydrogenase activity, the use of amino acids as hydrogen acceptors during the oxidation of lactate have thus far not been reported. Whether lactate is used directly in the Stickland reaction or whether the molecular hydrogen from lactate oxidation by the veillonella is responsible for the reduction of proline, the formation of δ-NH_2 valeric acid from proline will lead to a decreased lactate concentration at the tooth surface. This will occur either by a direct action on the lactate or by the removal of hydrogen causing a shift in the equilibrium of the lactate oxidation. Some of the possible sources of hydrogen for the reduction of proline in plaque are summarized in figure 2.

Data concerning the nitrogenous composition of plaque used throughout this paper have, per force, referred only to resting plaque

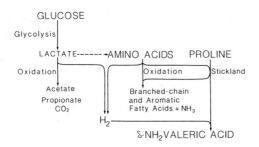

Fig. 2. Possible sources of reduction of proline in dental plaque.

concentrations. However, nitrogen metabolism at the tooth surface cannot be regarded as a static process and will be subject to the same environmental alterations which so dramatically affect the end-products of carbohydrate metabolism. Information pertaining to these alterations would therefore, be of value in determining which aspects of the nitrogen metabolism of the oral microbiota are of most importance in helping to achieve both the pH homeostasis of resting plaque and the return of plaque pH to neutrality following carbohydrate ingestion.

References

1   Geddes, D.: The production of $L(+)$ and $D(-)$ lactic acid and volatile acids by human dental plaque and the effect of plaque buffering and acidic strength on pH. Archs oral Biol. *17:* 537–545 (1972).
2   Geddes, D.: Acids produced by human dental plaque *in situ.* Caries Res. *9:* 98–109 (1975).
3   Gilmour, M.; Green, G.; Zahn, L.; Sparmann, C.; Pearlman, J.: The C_1–C_4 mono-carboxylic and lactic acids in dental plaques before and after exposure to sucrose in vivo; in Stiles, Loesche, O'Brien, Microbial aspects of dental caries. Microbiol. Abstr., suppl. 2, pp. 539–556 (1976).
4   Cole, M.; Bowden, G.; Korts, D.; Bowen, W.: The effect of pyridoxine, phytate and invert sugar on production of plaque acids in situ in the monkey *(M. fascicularis).* Caries Res. *12:* 190–201 (1978).
5   Tatevossian, A.; Gould, C.: The composition of the aqueous phase in human dental plaque. Archs oral Biol. *21:* 319–323 (1976).
6   Curtis, M.: Studies in the chemical composition and nitrogen metabolism of dental plaque from the monkey *Macaca fascicularis;* PhD thesis London (1980).
7   Stoppelaar, J. de: Urea and ammonia in saliva of caries inactive children with renal disease (Abstract No. 424). J. dent. Res. *61:* 225 (1982).

8   Biswas, S.; Kleinberg, I.: Effect of urea concentration on its utilisation, on the pH and the formation of ammonia and carbon dioxide in a human salivary sediment system. Archs oral Biol. *16:* 759–780 (1971).

9   Curtis, M.; Eastoe, J.: Comparison of free amino acid pools in dental plaque fluid from monkeys *(Macaca fascicularis)* fed on high and low sugar diets. Archs oral Biol. *23:* 989–992 (1978).

10 Soder, P.-O.; Frostell, G.: Proteolytic activity of dental plaque material. I. Action of dental plaque material on azocoll, casein and gelatin. Acta odont. scand. *24:* 501–516 (1966).

11 Soder, P.-O.: Proteolytic activity in the oral cavity: proteolytic enzymes from human saliva and dental plaque material. J. dent. Res. *51:* 389–393 (1972).

12 Tatevossian, A.; Newbrun, E.: Enzymic activities in the aqueous phase of human dental plaque. Archs oral Biol. *24:* 657–662 (1979).

13 Tempest, D.; Meers, J.; Brown, C.: The influence of environment on the content and composition of microbial free amino acid pools. J. gen. Microbiol. *64:* 171–185 (1970).

14 Griffith, C.; Carlsson, J.: Mechanism of ammonia assimilation in streptococci. J. gen. Microbiol. *82:* 253–260 (1974).

15 Gale, E.: The bacterial amino acid decarboxylases. Adv. Enzymol. *6:* 1–32 (1946).

16 Hayes, M.; Hyatt, A.: The decarboxylation of amino acids by bacteria derived from human dental plaque. Archs oral Biol. *19:* 361–369 (1974).

17 Cole, M.; Curtis, M.; Bowen, W.: Ornithine decarboxylase activity in tooth surface plaque from monkeys *(Macaca fascicularis)* fed pyridoxine, phytate and invert sugar. Archs oral Biol. *22:* 503–506 (1977).

18 Hyatt, A.; Hayes, M.: Free amino acids and amines in human dental plaque. Archs oral Biol. *20:* 203–209 (1975).

19 Kleinberg, I.; Kanapka, J.; Craw, D.: The effect of saliva and salivary factors on the metabolism of the mixed oral flora; in Stiles, Loesche, O'Brien, Microbial aspects of dental caries. Microbiol. Abstr., suppl. 2, pp. 433–464 (1976).

20 Kleinberg, I.; Kanapka, J.; Chatterjee, R.; Craw, D.; D'Angelo, N.; Sandham, H.: Metabolism of nitrogen by the oral mixed bacteria; in Kleinberg, Ellison, Mandel, Saliva and dental caries. Microbiol. Abstr., suppl., pp. 357–377 (1979).

21 Crow, V.; Thomas, T.: Arginine metabolism in lactic streptococci. J. Bact. *150:* 1024–1032 (1982).

22 Ferro, K.; Bender, G.R.; Marquis, R.E.: Repressible arginine deiminase system in *Streptococcus sanguis* NCTC 10904 (Abstract No. 557). J. dent. Res. *62:* 231 (1983).

23 Wong, J.; Dyer, J.; Tribble, J.: Fermentation of *L*-aspartate by a saccharolytic strain of *Bacteroides melaninogenicus.* Appl. environ. Microbiol. *33:* 69–73 (1977).

24 Curtis, M.; Eastoe, J.: A preliminary investigation into the identity of a major ninhydrin-positive compenent of dental plaque fluid from the monkey *Macaca fascicularis.* Archs oral Biol. *23:* 421–423 (1978).

25 Stickland, L.: The chemical reactions by which *C. sporogenes* obtains its energy. Biochem. J. *28:* 1746–1759 (1934).

26 Stickland, L.: The oxidation of alanine by *C. sporogenes.* Biochem. J. *29:* 889–896 (1935).

27 Nisman, B.: The Stickland reaction. Bact. Rev. *18:* 16–42 (1954).

28 Hoogerheide, J.; Kochalty, W.: Metabolism of the strict anaerobes (genus: Clo-
    stridium). II. Reduction of amino acids with gaseous hydrogen by suspensions of
    Cl. sporogones. Biochem. J. *32:* 949–957 (1938).
29 Levine, M.; Ellison, S.: Immunoelectrophoretic and chemical analyses of human
    parotid saliva. Archs oral Biol. *18:* 839–853 (1973).
30 Barbarash, G.; Quarles, R.: Single column amino acid analysis with o-phthal-
    aldehyde: An evaluation of two commercial buffer systems. Analyt. Biochem. *119:*
    177–184 (1982).
31 Guerrant, G.; Lambert, M.; Moss, C.: Analysis of short chain acids from anaerobic
    bacteria by high-performance liquid chromatography. J. clin. Microbiol. *16:*
    355–360 (1982).
32 Bowen, W.: The induction of rampant caries in monkeys *(Macaca irus)*. Caries Res.
    3: 227–237 (1969).
33 Holdemann, L.; Cato, E.; Moore, E.: Anaerobe laboratory manual; 4th ed. (Vir-
    ginia Polytechnic Institute and State University, Blacksburg 1977).
34 Babcock, J.: Tyrosine degradation in presumptive identification of *Peptostreptococ-
    cus anaerobius*. J. clin. Microbiol. *9:* 358–361 (1979).
35 Lambert, M.; Moss, C.: Production of *p*-hydroxyhydrocinnamic acid from tyrosine
    by *Peptostreptococcus anaerobius*. J. clin. Microbiol. *12:* 291–293 (1980).
36 Hoshino, E.; Frolander, F.; Carlsson, J.: Oxygen and the metabolism of *Pepto-
    streptococcus anaerobius* VPI 4330-1. J. gen. Microbiol. *107:* 235–248 (1978).
37 Bard, R.; Gunsalus, I.: Glucose metabolism of *Clostridium perfringens:* existence of
    a metallaldolase. J. Bact. *59:* 387–400 (1950).
38 Somerville, H.: Enzymic studies of the biosynthesis of amino acids from lactate by
    Peptostreptococcus elsdenii. Biochem. J. *108:* 107–119 (1968).

M.A. Curtis, National Caries Program, National Institute of Dental
Research, National Institutes of Health, Bethesda, MD 20205 (USA)

Fluoride and Enamel

Moderator: O. Fejerskov, Aarhus, Denmark

Cariology Today. Int. Congr., Zürich 1983, pp. 223–230 (Karger, Basel 1984)

The Concept of Enamel Resistance –
A Critical Review

J.A. Weatherell, C. Robinson, A.S. Hallsworth

Department of Oral Biology, School of Dentistry, University of Leeds, Leeds, UK

There would seem to be no such thing as absolute resistance to caries. Enamel consists of calcium phosphate and, given a sufficiently severe challenge by the bacterially produced acid, a carious lesion will probably develop. Its capacity to resist such lesion formation is, however, variable. It is curious that the FDI Committee included the word 'relative' in their definition of susceptibility and yet omitted it from their concept of caries resistance [1].

Inorganic Composition of Enamel and Caries Resistance

Enamel consists almost entirely of mineral and, carious attack being associated with acid dissolution, it is not surprising that caries resistance has often been considered to reflect the reaction of the enamel mineral towards an acidic environment. Some clinically effective anticaries substances can certainly reduce the mineral's solubility in acid. The best documented example is fluoride. Whether supplied in the drinking water, or by topical application or via some other vehicle, the caries prevalence of the population decreases. In vitro, its incorporation into enamel has been shown to reduce its acid solubility [2, 3] and there is almost certainly a relationship between this effect, explicable in purely crystallographic [4, 5] and thermodynamic [6] terms, and the inhibition of caries attack.

Unfortunately, it cannot be simply or solely a question of increased resistance to acid. Materials which reduce the rate of acid dissolution might have no effect on resistance to caries [7, 8]. In the previous Zürich Symposium, *Bibby* [9] suggested that such materials might reduce solubility by producing a protective patina on the tooth surface but that this is worn off when subjected to the rigours of the oral environment.

Fluoride can affect the mineral's solubility in a much more fundamental way, however. Incorporated into the crystal lattice, it can influence the nature and quality of the mineral. Crystallites become more stable, more crystalline [10] and consequently intrinsically more resistant to acid dissolution. Other substances known from clinical or experimental observations to change the resistance of enamel to carious attack probably also act by bringing about a more than superficial change in the nature of the enamel. The alleged deleterious effect of carbonate on caries resistance, for instance [11], could be linked to the adverse effect the ion is known to have on apatite formation and its crystalline structure [12–15]. The mechanism by which strontium achieves the reported reduction in caries incidence [16, 17] is perhaps also linked to its incorporation in the crystal lattice [18]. It is difficult to imagine how its presence could increase the stability of the lattice directly but the ion could act synergistically by influencing the incorporation of other ions into the lattice, enhancing the concentration of fluoride [17] or decreasing the concentration of carbonate [20]. As *Hegsted* [19] pointed out, practically everything in a closely integrated system affects everything else.

The composition and structure of the enamel surface does not remain constant. Carbonate and magnesium at the surface of the enamel are probably leached out slowly and fluoride tends to accumulate by ion exchange. Should the pH at the enamel surface fall, such changes will be accelerated. Thus, during incipient carious attack, carbonate and magnesium are removed preferentially [21–23] and fluoride uptake increases [24–26]. The resistance of the enamel will correspondingly change. *Nikiforuk* [27] put both observations together, proposing that the CO_2/F ratio might serve as an index of caries susceptibility.

Crystallite size alone could influence resistance to carious attack. The larger they are, the smaller is their specific surface area and the less easily they dissolve. Crystallites at the surface of the enamel increase in size after eruption [28], probably a manifestation of the tendency for crystallites to grow when in contact with the supersaturated oral fluids. Enamel consequently becomes more caries resistant.

The disposition and orientation of the crystallites may also affect resistance by governing accessibility of their surface to acid. It has been suggested that the alignment of hydroxyapatite crystallites varied from one individual to another, being perhaps nutritionally or genetically determined. In the outer layer of enamel, thought to act as a tooth-protecting barrier, the alignment of the hydroxyapatite microcrystals was reported to be superior in caries-resistant than in caries-susceptible teeth [29].

Tooth Structure and Caries Resistance

Such crystallographic and ultrastructural considerations are obviously of great importance when attempting to evaluate the innate resistance of dental enamel but the nature of the mineral should not be taken as the sole criterion. In the mouth, there is never a bare mineral surface and penetration to the enamel is first of all restricted by the organic pellicle on the tooth surface. Once in the enamel, which is a complex biological structure, further migration takes place by diffusion along striae of Retzius, prismatic boundaries, lamellae, cracks and other biological interfaces [30, 31]. Some workers regard the process of diffusion as a critical determinant in lesion development, which could therefore be influenced or even controlled by activity in the pulpal cavity [32–34], by the genetic dysfunction of odontoblasts [35], by temperature gradients [36] or any other factors which influence fluid flow in the enamel [37].

On the other hand, obvious increases in the size of diffusion pathways in enamel are not always or obviously associated with decreased caries resistance. Cracks or lamellae extending from the enamel surface to the underlying dentine, relatively porous regions with massive tracts of tuft protein, or the porous enamel of fluorotic teeth do not stand out as caries-susceptible features [31, 38–40].

One possible explanation is that protein and other organic materials instantly acquired from the oral fluids will render such areas less permeable and the enamel mineral less acid soluble [41] because it is no longer so accessible to acid from the overlying plaque. Alternatively, the higher levels of fluoride, preferentially acquired by such areas, will have an effect.

Another possible explanation is that, since enamel is bathed for most of the time in fluid which is supersaturated with respect to the tooth mineral, crystallites will generally tend to grow rather than to dissolve. Only when the degree of saturation falls, due e.g. to a reduction in pH, will mineral ions dissolve and diffuse out of the tooth. Soon, a condition of supersaturation will be re-established. If, however, the escaping ions meanwhile precipitate in the plaque, migrate away or are swept away from the tooth surface, space will be left in the enamel and porosity will develop. The surface of enamel, being most of the time in contact with these supersaturated oral fluids, will tend to remain intact. Any porosity which develops will therefore tend to do so below the enamel surface.

In some recent experiments, lesions similar to natural caries were produced by placing teeth in the vapour of volatile acids. Conditions were very different from those of natural caries. The pH at the tooth surface, which did not fluctuate, was about 2.4. There was no organic pellicle or dental plaque. No weak acid anions were present other than those of the enamel mineral itself. What the situation probably had in common with the oral environment, however, was a degree of supersaturation at the tooth surface. On this basis, the rapid formation of caries-like lesions at relatively low pH, could be explained [42].

This view of lesion development places more emphasis on the degree of environmental saturation than on a tendency for acid to attack enamel directly and moves the emphasis of the discussion away from a consideration of the enamel itself towards the changing relationship between the enamel and the fluids which form its external environment. Factors which increased the degree of saturation and encouraged crystallite growth would reduce the tendency for caries formation. Changes which decreased saturation would encourage the formation of a carious lesion. Agents which reduce the acid solubility of enamel without affecting either the degree of saturation of the environment or growth of enamel crystallites would, on this hypothesis, have little effect on resistance to carious attack. This is an alternative solution to *Bibby's* [9] conundrum about solubility and caries resistance.

The Oral Environment and Caries Resistance

The hypothesis, correct or not, at least serves to make the point that caries resistance is a function of two inseparable and mutually dependent variables: (a) the nature of the enamel itself and (b) the nature of its external environment. One of the main difficulties in studying the caries resistance of enamel is to establish that a tooth *is* genuinely caries resistant. Tooth survival, which the phrase implies, is not in itself a sufficient criterion. Teeth which remain caries-free when the caries prevalence of the population has achieved a plateau value cannot be called resistant without knowing something about the severity of cariogenic challenge to which they have been subjected. Caries-free dentitions in a population of immigrants, previously accustomed to unrefined foodstuffs, can become carious when challenged by a more severely cariogenic diet. A smooth enamel surface will not readily decay until a stagnation area forms by occlusion with a neighbouring tooth [43]. The removal of such a tooth would decrease the chance that the adjacent surface will decay, without implying any change in the innate caries resistance of its enamel.

Interdependence between the Nature of Enamel and Its Environment

These two broad areas (a) the enamel, which may be more or less caries resistant and (b) the environment, which may be more or less cariogenic are, however, to some extent interdependent. The size of a tooth and the form and texture of its surface together with the anatomy of the mouth largely determine the degree of stagnation in the environment. It has even been suggested that fluoride could influence the size and shape of molar crowns [44, 45]. Hypoplastic roughness of the enamel surface resulting from vitamin D deficiency was thought to account for high caries prevalence [46, 47].

Conversely, as already described, the enamel can become increasingly resistant as a result of compositional and structural changes brought about by the environment. Finally, ions could inhibit carious attack by altering the degree of supersaturation in the environment at the enamel surface.

Unfortunately, those who search for the single overriding factor or who claim that one or another feature of enamel or its environment crucially dictates caries resistance are likely to be disappointed. None of the above points are mutually exclusive.

References

1   Baume, L.J.: FDI special commission on oral and dental statistics. Standardization of dental caries statistics. Int. dent. J., Lond. *12:* 65–75 (1962).
2   Volker, J.F.: Effect of fluorine on solubility of enamel and dentin. Proc. Soc. exp. Biol. Med. *42:* 725–727 (1939).

3 Mühlemann, H.R.; Schmid, H.; König, K.G.: Enamel solubility reduction studies with inorganic and organic fluorides. Helv. odont. Acta *1:* 23–33 (1957).

4 Kay, M.I.; Young, R.A.; Posner, A.S.: Crystal structure of hydroxyapatite. Nature, Lond. *204:* 1050–1052 (1964).

5 Elliott, J.C.: Recent progress in the chemistry, crystal chemistry and structure of the apatites. Calcif. Tissue Res. *3:* 293–307 (1969).

6 Brown, W.E.; Gregory, T.M.; Chow, L.C.: Effects of fluoride on enamel solubility and cariostasis. Caries Res. *11:* suppl. 1, pp. 118–141 (1977).

7 Bibby, B.G.: Passive changes in the enamel surface and dental caries. Dent. J. Austr. *26:* 127–131 (1954).

8 König, K.G.; Mühlemann, H.R.: Caries inhibiting effect of amine fluoride containing dentifrices tested in an animal experiment and in a clinical study; in Mühlemann, König, Caries Symp., Zürich 1961, pp. 126–132 (Huber, Berne 1961).

9 Bibby, B.G.: Fluoride-phosphate interrelationships; in Mühlemann, König, Caries Symp., Zürich 1961, pp. 146–153 (Huber, Berne 1961).

10 Zipkin, I.; Posner, A.S.; Eanes, E.D.: The effect of fluoride on the X-ray diffraction pattern of the apatite of human bone. Biochim. biophys. Acta *59:* 255–258 (1962).

11 Sobel, A.E.; Hanok, A.: Calcification. XVI. Composition of bones and teeth in relation to blood and diet in the cotton rat. J. dent. Res. *37:* 631–637 (1958).

12 Trautz, O.R.; Zapanta, R.R.: Experiments with calcium carbonate phosphates and the effect of topical application of sodium fluoride. Archs oral Biol. *4:* 122–133 (1961).

13 Bachra, B.N.; Trautz, O.R.: Carbonic anhydrase and the precipitation of apatite. Science *137:* 337–338 (1962).

14 Ingram, G.S.: The role of carbonate in dental mineral. Caries Res. *7:* 217–230 (1973).

15 Blumenthal, N.C.; Betts, F.; Posner, A.S.: Effect of carbonate and biological macromolecules on formation and properties of hydroxyapatite. Calcif. Tissue Res. *18:* 81–90 (1975).

16 Curzon, M.E.J.; Losee, F.L.: Strontium content of enamel and dental caries. Caries Res. *11:* 321–326 (1977).

17 Spector, P.C.; Curzon, M.E.J.: Surface enamel fluoride and strontium in relation to caries prevalence in man. Caries Res. *13:* 227–230 (1979).

18 Johnson, A.R.; Armstrong, W.D.; Singer, L.: The solubility of the mineral phase in the rat of powdered bone and dentine laden with strontium. Archs oral Biol. *15:* 401–409 (1970).

19 Hegsted, D.M.: Closing remarks; in Conference on Micronutrients Interactions. Vitamins, minerals and hazardous elements. Ann. N.Y. Acad. Sci. *335:* 366–370 (1980).

20 Legeros, R.Z.; Miravite, M.A.; Quirolgico, G.B.; Curzon, M.E.J.: The effect of some trace elements on the lattice parameters of human and synthetic apatites. Calcif. Tissue Res. *22:* 362–367 (1977).

21 Hallsworth, A.S.; Weatherell, J.A.; Robinson, C.: Loss of carbonate during the first stages of enamel caries. Caries Res. *7:* 345–348 (1973).

22 Johansen, E.: Ultrastructural and clinical observations on dental caries; in Sognnaes, Mechanisms of hard tissue destruction. Am. Ass. Advancement of Science, Wash., Publication no. 75, pp. 187–211 (1963).

23   Hallsworth, A.S.; Robinson, C.; Weatherell, J.A.: Mineral and magnesium distribution within the approximal carious lesion of dental enamel. Caries Res. *6:* 156–168 (1972).

24   Ericsson, Y.: The distribution and reactions of F ions in enamel-saliva environment investigated with the radioactive fluorine isotope F-18. Acta odont. scand. *16:* 127–141 (1958).

25   Johansen, E.: The nature of the carious lesion. Dent. Clin. N. Am. *5:* 305–320 (1962).

26   Brudevold, F.; Hein, J.W.; Bonner, J.F.; Nevin, R.B.; Bibby, B.G.; Hodge, H.C.: Reaction of tooth surfaces with 1 ppm of fluoride as sodium fluoride. J. dent. Res. *36:* 661–779 (1957).

27   Nikiforuk, G.: Carbonates and fluorides as chemical determinants of tooth susceptibility and caries; in Mühlemann, König, Caries Symp., Zürich 1961, pp. 62–69 (Huber, Berne 1961).

28   Arends, J.; Jongebloed, W.L.; Schutof, J.: Crystallite diameters of enamel near the anatomical surface. Caries Res. *17:* 97–105 (1983).

29   Cevc, G.; Cevc, P.; Schara, M.; Skaleric, U.: The caries resistance of human teeth is determined by the spatial arrangement of hydroxyapatite microcrystals in enamel. Nature, Lond. *286:* 425–426 (1980).

30   Darling, A.I.: The selective attack of caries on the dental enamel. Ann. R. Coll. Surg. *29:* 354–369 (1961).

31   Helmke, J.G.; Neubauer, G.; Rau, R.: Schmelzstrukturen und Kariesprozess. Dt. zahnärztl. Z. *21:* 1070–1078 (1966).

32   Wachtel, L.W.; Brown, L.R.: In vitro caries: factors influencing the shape of the developing lesion. Archs oral Biol. *8:* 99–107 (1963).

33   Bergman, G.; Linden, L.A.: Effect of an 'internal factor' on enamel decalcification. Archs oral Biol. *11:* 943–945 (1966).

34   Steinman, R.R.; Leonora, J.; Singh, R.J.: The effect of desalivation upon pulpal function and dental caries in rats. J. dent. Res. *59:* 176–185 (1980).

35   Burch, P.R.J.; Jackson, D.: Periodontal disease and dental caries. Some new aetiological considerations. Br. dent. J. *120:* 127–134 (1965).

36   Berndt, A.F.; Stearns, R.I.: Dental fluoride chemistry, Chapter XVI (Thomas, 1978).

37   Bergman, G.: Microscopic demonstration of liquid flow through human dental enamel. Archs oral Biol. *8:* 233–234 (1963).

38   Brabant, H.; Klees, L.: Contribution histologique à l'étude des craquelures de l'émail dentaire humain. Actual. odonto-stomatol. *39:* 359–396 (1957).

39   Robinson, C.; Weatherell, J.A.; Hallsworth, A.S.: Alterations in the composition of permanent human enamel during carious attack; in Leach, Edgar, Council of Europe Workshop 1982. Demineralisation and remineralisation of the teeth, pp. 209–223 (IRL Press, Oxford 1983).

40   Kidd, E.A.M.; Thylstrup, A.; Fejerskov, O.; Bruun, C.: Influence of fluoride in surface enamel and degree of dental fluorosis on caries development in vitro. Caries Res. *14:* 196–202 (1980).

41   Bhussry, B.R.; Hess, W.C.: Aging of enamel and dentin. J. Geront. *18:* 343–344 (1963).

42 Weatherell, J.A.; Robinson, C.; Hallsworth, A.S.: Formation of lesions in enamel using moist acid vapour; in Leach, Edgar, Council of Europe Workshop 1982. Demineralisation and remineralisation of the teeth, pp. 225–241 (IRL Press, Oxford 1983).

43 Backer Dirks, O.; Houwink, B.; Kwant, G.W.: Some special features of the caries-preventive effect of water fluoridation. Archs oral Biol. 4: 187–192 (1961).

44 Goose, D.H.; Roberts, E.E.: Possible influence of fluoridation on tooth crown size. J. dent. Res. 58: 1562–1563 (1979).

45 Lovius, B.B.J.; Goose, D.H.: The effect of fluoridation of water on tooth morphology. Br. dent. J. 127: 322–324 (1969).

46 Mellanby, M.: Diet and the teeth: an experimental study. I. Dental structure in dogs. Med. Res. Counc. Spec. Rep. Ser. 140 (1929).

47 Mellanby, M.: Diet and the teeth: an experimental study. III. The effect of diet and dental structure and disease in man. Med. Res. Counc. Spec. Rep. Ser. 191 (1934).

J.A. Weatherell, MD, Department of Oral Biology, School of Dentistry, University of Leeds, Leeds (UK)

Cariology Today. Int. Congr., Zürich 1983, pp. 231–236 (Karger, Basel 1984)

The Effect of Fluoride on Enamel De- and Remineralization in vitro and in vivo

J.M. ten Cate

Department of Dental Materials Science, University of Amsterdam,
The Netherlands

Introduction

In the oral environment fluoride is present in many forms. Part of it is firmly bound in the apatitic bulk of the mineralized tissues. A second portion is adsorbed onto the mineral phase or present as a non-apatitic precipitate, such as calcium-fluoride (CaF_2). Plaque is known to contain a large amount of fluoride, which in itself can be divided into different categories: free, loosely bound, and firmly bound. Finally small concentrations of fluoride will also be present in the saliva. When considering the working modes of fluoride, it should be realized that fluoride at these various locations and forms will contribute differently. For instance the fluoride bound in apatite is very unlikely to exert an effect on processes in the liquid phase. The well-known caries-preventive effect is the sum of many factors whose relative magnitudes are unknown.

For a long time the primary working mode of fluoride was thought to be its effect on the solubility after incorporation into the tooth enamel. Recently, however, it was argued that this contribution is probably overestimated. As stressed by *Fejerskov* et al. [1981] the percentage of fluoride substituted for OH in the apatite of surface enamel is at most about 10% (for 1 ppm fluoride areas). At such low levels in the enamel the difference in solubility between hydroxyapatite (HAP) and fluoridated hydroxyapatite (F-HAP) is too small to explain the large cariostatic effect. From in vivo data there is no generally accepted relationship between fluoride content in the enamel and caries experience. Teeth from 'high' and from 'low' fluoride areas, although differing in fluoride content seem to behave similarly in artificial caries solutions [*Kidd* et al., 1980; *ten Cate,* unpublished data].

Apart from this one mechanism, fluoride in solution has been shown to influence demineralization, both in rate and appearance, and lesion remineralization, as well as the metabolism of the oral bacteria. In this paper the former two will be discussed to evaluate their importance.

Demineralization

After sugar intake and fermentation to acids in the plaque, enamel is dissolved to such an extent that the acids are neutralized. Reaction with buffering ions diffusing from the saliva is also in part responsible for this process. In between the pH drops the plaque and oral fluid are supersaturated to apatite which means that mineral deposition may occur. This continuous de- and remineralization will gradually transform the outer microns of the enamel. Besides a change in chemical composition, with fluoride being preferentially taken up and carbonate being lost, an increase in crystallinity and crystallite dimensions takes place [*Arends* et al., 1983]. Most likely this is due to the catalytic effect of fluoride on mineral deposition and crystallization. With increased cariogenic challenge there is no balance between mineral loss and uptake during the day and some form of demineralized defect will form, such as a subsurface lesion. From laboratory studies it has become clear that fluoride has a great effect on the rate of demineralization as well as on the histological appearance of the defect formed.

Larsen [1973] showed that enamel is eroded when subjected to demineralizing solutions without fluoride. However, when the solution was supersaturated to fluorapatite (FAP), a surface layer could be seen on the microradiogram. In their model on lesion formation, *Moreno and Zahradnik* [1974] also stress the important role of fluoride for the preservation of the surface layer. In their concept there is a 'quasi equilibrium between 3 minerals (brushite, FAP and the bulk of enamel) and the pore solution'. If FAP or F-HAP were not included in this picture, there is no reason why the surface of the specimen would be dealt with differently by the attacking acids. The effect of fluoride on the rate of demineralization at conditions relevant to the oral situation is given in figure 1 [*ten Cate and Duijsters,* 1983].

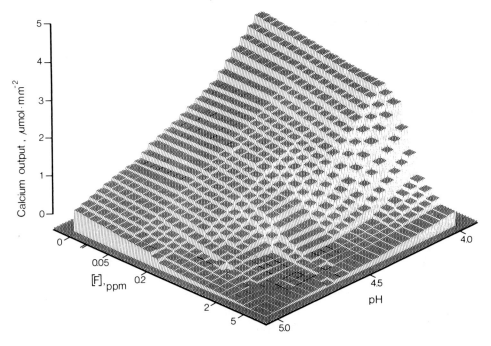

Fig. 1. Calcium output as a function of pH and fluoride concentration in the demineralizing solution initially containing 2.2 mM Ca(NO$_3$)$_2$, 2.2 mM KH$_2$PO$_4$ and 50 mM acetic acid. Reproduced with the permission of the publisher Karger, Basel, from *ten Cate and Duijsters* [1983].

From this it can be concluded that, at any pH likely to be reached during a pH drop, demineralization can be inhibited by fluoride. A second conclusion is that the rate of demineralization seems to be affected to a greater extent when the solution becomes supersaturated to CaF$_2$ (typ. 3 ppm) as opposed to FAP (typ. 0.4 ppm at pH 4.3). An explanation for this could be that the CaF$_2$ deposit, being of different morphology, is a more effective diffusion barrier than FAP, which grows on existing apatitic crystallites and does not affect the surface layer pores. In in vivo experiments it is more difficult to show a similar effect of fluoride on demineralization as described above. In the intra-oral situation a continuous demineralization can never be obtained, since it will always be interrupted by repair periods. From studies with intra-oral devices, however, one can conclude that inhibition of demineralization occurs when fluoride is added during the cariogenic attack.

Ostrom et al. [1977] showed that the enamel was not demineralized when 100 ppm fluoride was included in the 3% sucrose rinse normally used to induce caries. As no effect on microbial content of the plaque was found, it may be concluded that the effect of fluoride is on the processes regarding the solid substrate itself.

Remineralization

A lot of attention has been given to the investigation of the remineralization of defects of the oral calcified tissues, with the majority of the studies dealing with the remineralization of (artificial) white spots. The importance of fluoride in stimulating the deposition mechanism is well documented [*Andresen,* 1921; *Koulourides* et al., 1961; *von der Fehr* et al., 1970]. In recent years it has become clear that although fluoride accelerates apatitic deposition in slurry experiments or in the initial rehardening of porosities, the long-term effects are more complex. This can easily be explained by the working mode of fluoride on apatite precipitation in general. With fluoride present in solution, FAP of F-HAP will precipitate. As a result of their lower solubility product, the driving force for precipitation of these minerals is much greater than for HAP. Consequently precipitation will be less selective, and occur onto the enamel or in the outermost layer as opposed to throughout the porous specimen. This mechanism is in agreement with laboratory experimental findings initially showing an enhancement of the deposition after fluoride treatment. Yet, after 1 day of remineralization the rate of deposition drops even below the control value [*ten Cate and Arends,* 1981; *Boddé,* 1983]. Also from epidemiological data this conclusion can be drawn. In areas with fluoridation of the drinking water one finds a much larger percentage of white spot lesions, compared with non-fluoridated areas. In a longitudinal study only a small percentage of these lesions was found to be converted to either sound surfaces or to cavities [*Pot and Groeneveld,* 1976]. A large percentage of the lesions most likely are of the 'arrested' type, with an inert, fluoride-rich, surface layer covering the lesion body. It should be noted that these data were obtained at a time when fluoride intake from sources other than drinking water was small. In the present day situation fluoride intake is much more frequent and widespread and the speculation seems justified that lesion arrestment now is a major cause for surfaces to remain 'sound', possibly even in areas without fluoridation of the drinking water. If fully substantiated, this conclusion would have great practical implications for the treatment of lesions.

Still, another subject which deserves future investigations regards the possibility to overcome the esthetically unacceptable appearance of white spots. The question is: should this be dealt with either by immersing the lesion with in situ curing resins, which could later on degradate or discolour, or by continuing the survey for rapid remineralizing solutions? Considerable efforts have been given to developing solutions which would give a rapid remineralization in addition to a topical fluoride affect. *Featherstone* et al. [1982] showed that inclusion of mineral constituents into these 'dipping solutions' improved their potential. This area of research seems to be particularly important for patients with impaired salivary function. Whether these rapid remineralizing solutions during their short time of contact will have any effect probably depends on the type of lesion on which they are used. From SEM studies it has become clear that there is a large difference in surface porosities between 'active' and 'arrested' lesions [*Thylstrup and Fredebo,* 1982]. The former type is of particular interest since it would benefit most from remineralization. In vitro as well as in vivo it has been shown that lesions with a 'low' mineral content in the surface layer (softened enamel) can be more easily repaired [*Gelhard,* 1982]. Since diffusion barriers are small in this case, a beneficial effect of remineralizing solutions is also more likely.

References

Andresen, V.: Über Mineralisation und Remineralisation des Zahnschmelzes. Dt. Mschr. Zahnheilk. *39:* 97 (1921).

Arends, J.; Jongebloed, W.L.; Schuthof, J.: Crystallite diameters of enamel near the anatomical surface. Caries Res. *17:* 96–106 (1983).

Boddé, H.E.: The influence of fluoride applications on enamel remineralization; thesis Groningen (1983).

Cate, J.M. ten; Arends, J.: Remineralization of artificial enamel lesions in vitro. IV. Influence of fluorides and diphosphonates on short- and long-term remineralization. Caries Res. *15:* 60–69 (1981).

Cate, J.M. ten; Duijsters, P.P.E.: The influence of fluoride in solution on tooth demineralization. I. Chemical data. Caries Res. *17:* 193–199 (1983).

Featherstone, J.D.B.; Cutress, T.W.; Rodgers, B.E.; Dennison, P.J.: Remineralization of artificial caries-like lesions in vivo by a self-administered mouthrinse or paste. Caries Res. *16:* 235–242 (1982).

Fehr, F.R. von der; Loe, H.; Theilade, E.: Experimental caries in man. Caries Res. *4:* 131–148 (1970).

Fejerskov, O.; Thylstrup, A.; Larsen, M.J.: Rational use of fluorides in caries prevention, a concept based on possible cariostatic mechanisms. Acta odont. scand. *39:* 241–249 (1981).

Gelhard, T.: Remineralization of human enamel in vivo; thesis Groningen (1982).

Kidd, E.A.M.; Thylstrup, A.; Fejerskov, O.; Bruun, C.: The influence of fluoride in surface enamel and degree of dental fluorosis on caries development in vitro. Caries Res. *14:* 196–202 (1980).

Koulourides, T.; Cueto, H.; Pigman, W.: Rehardening of softened enamel surfaces on human teeth by solutions of calcium phosphates. Nature, Lond. *189:* 226–227 (1961).

Larsen, M.J.: Dissolution of enamel. Scand. J. dent. Res. *81:* 518–522 (1973).

Moreno, E.C.; Zahradnik, R.T.: Chemistry of enamel subsurface demineralization in vitro. J. dent. Res. *53:* 226–235 (1974).

Ostrom, C.A.; Koulourides, T.; Hickman, F.; Phantumvanit, P.: Combined effects of sucrose and fluoride on experimental caries and on the associated microbial plaque. J. dent. Res. *56:* 212–221 (1977).

Pot, T.J.; Groeneveld, A.: Het ontstaan en gedrag van de witte vlek; overwegingen aan de hand van klinische waarnemingen. Ned. Tijdschr. T. *83:* 464–471 (1976).

Thylstrup, A.; Fredebo, L.: A method for studying surface coatings and the underlying enamel features in the scanning electron microscope; in Frank, Leach, Surface and colloid phenomena in the oral cavity: methodological aspects, pp. 169–184 (IRL Press, Oxford 1982).

Dr. J.M. ten Cate, Tandheelkundige Materiaalwetenschappen, Universiteit van Amsterdam, Louwesweg 1, NL-1066 EA Amsterdam (The Netherlands)

Cariology Today. Int. Congr., Zürich 1983, pp. 237–244 (Karger, Basel 1984)

Experimental Caries Models and Their Clinical Implications[1]

Leon M. Silverstone

University of Colorado Health Sciences Center, Denver, Colo., USA

Enamel Caries and Its Simulation in vitro

The small lesion of enamel caries is positioned deep to a well-mineralized surface layer and has been shown to consist of four well-recognized histological zones when examined with the polarizing microscope [*Silverstone, 1973*]. *Silverstone* [1977] has presented evidence to show that two of the zones, the surface zone (zone 4) and the dark zone (zone 2), are formed as a result of remineralization phenomena. Thus, the creation of a lesion in human dental enamel is the result of a dynamic series of events and not a process of simple continuing demineralization. The remaining two zones of the carious lesion, the translucent zone (zone 1) and the body of the lesion (zone 3), are produced as a result of demineralization. The two zones created by remineralization phenomena cannot be simulated in vitro when samples of human enamel are exposed to dilute acid solutions. To date, the only technique which is able to create in human enamel lesions which appear histologically indistinguishable from enamel caries is the one employing acidified gels [*Silverstone, 1967, 1968, 1973*). Lesions showing both dark zones and surface zones are created using this technique. In addition, such lesions have irregular advancing fronts comparable to those found in naturally occurring lesions, as opposed to advancing fronts maintaining a direction parallel with the enamel surface as found with acid lesions.

The surface zone of enamel caries has been defined [*Silverstone, 1968*] as the zone at the surface of the lesion which shows a negative birefringence when the ground section is examined in water with the

[1] The support of NIH/NIDR grant DE 04801 is gratefully acknowledged.

polarizing microscope. This definition was arrived at after examining large numbers of lesions of enamel caries and confirming this observation. It is not adequate enough to show a surface layer which appears radiopaque relative to the subsurface region on a microradiograph. The dark zone is defined as the zone at the advancing front of the lesion positioned deep to the body of the lesion and placed superficial to the translucent zone. This zone exhibits positive birefringence when the section is examined in quinoline (n = 1.62) with the polarizing microscope.

There is much evidence to support the contention that acid-softened enamel surfaces can be rehardened and a major contribution has been made in this field by in vitro studies [*Koulourides,* 1968]. Previous experiments on the remineralization of both natural and artificial lesions have shown, in in vitro studies, that both types of lesions can be reduced in size and porosity and, in addition, show higher levels of mineral content and increased microhardness [*Silverstone,* 1973, 1977; *Silverstone* et al., 1981; *Featherstone* et al., 1981; *Arends and Jongebloed,* 1979]. This occurred by the deposition of mineral into the damaged enamel after exposure to a calcifying fluid. Recent in vitro work has concentrated on the remineralizing effect by using different concentrations of various ions in a synthetic calcifying fluid on enamel lesions in vitro. Artificial lesions have been used in preference to natural ones since the lesions can be created having predetermined characteristics. In addition, by creating an artificial lesion over a relatively wide test area, there is sufficient lesion surface to not only have adequate controls, but also to test different remineralization regimens on single lesions. Examination of control sections from a lesion using a range of imbibition media in conjunction with the polarizing microscope makes it possible to study indirectly the ultrastructure of the tissue. Thus, variations in pore volume in test and control regions can be assessed accurately as well as the total amount of oriented mineral in a particular region of a lesion.

*An Artificial Caries Model Simulating in vivo Conditions
More Closely*

The aim of this work was the development of an in vitro model system to simulate more closely the situation in vivo where approximal surfaces are in contact. Then, the production of caries-like lesions and their progression could be studied using 'clinical' techniques in vitro such as a mirror and explorer, and bitewing radiography. These could then be related to histological and microradiographic techniques. Since baselines using sound enamel surfaces were required prior to investigating lesion initiation and progression, an artificial caries technique was employed. This acidified gel technique has been described previously [*Silverstone*, 1968] and is capable of creating lesions in human enamel which appear indistinguishable from natural lesions when examined by histological, microradiographic and ultrastructural techniques [*Silverstone*, 1973, 1977]. Pairs of caries-free human teeth were selected having good interproximal contact. Each pair was then set up in a silicone block such that the tooth crowns were in interproximal contact while the roots were retained within the silicone block. Due to the elastic nature of the silicone, teeth could be removed and then returned so that the identical contact region was reestablished. Teeth were painted with a protective varnish except the area of interproximal contact. These surfaces were photographed at baseline and bitewing radiographs taken with varying kVP, mA and exposure times. Teeth were then exposed to the acidified gel artificial caries medium for lesion formation. After this, tooth surfaces were again photographed and, after replacement into the block, bitewing radiographs retaken. This cycle was repeated so as to follow lesion progression. Single longitudinal sections were obtained through test regions for examination by polarized light and microradiography. After this, tooth segments could still be returned to the silicone block for bitewing radiography. When a lesion was first detected by bitewing radiography, the lesion had penetrated 200 μm into the dentine. This model system appears ideal for studying the effects of various test regimens on both lesion initiation and progression.

Effect of Fluoride on Remineralization

One factor common to many of the results obtained on the remineralization of either enamel caries, artificial caries, or acid-etched enamel is that the presence of fluoride ions enhances greatly the degree of remineralization achieved, and reduces the time period for this mechanism to occur. The aim of this part of the present investigation was to quantitate the effect that fluoride has on the degree of remineralization of enamel lesions in vitro.

Experimental Methods

The synthetic calcifying fluid used in these studies was prepared from synthetic hydroxyapatite having a calcium/phosphate ratio of 1.63. Solutions having two different calcium concentrations were used. These were 1 and 3 mM, the phosphate concentrations remaining at the fixed ratio of 1.62. Sodium chloride at a final concentration of 200 mM was added to the fluids which were adjusted to pH 7.0 using 0.05 mM potassium hydroxide. Fluoride was added to some of the calcifying fluids at concentrations of either 0.05 or 0.50 mM.

Exposure times of specimens to either of the synthetic calcifying fluids were either five or ten consecutive 6-min exposure increments, as well as a single 1-hour exposure. At the completion of a series of exposures, specimens were washed in agitated deionized distilled water for 24 h.

Artificial caries-like lesions were used in the experiments to provide a source of highly reproducible lesions having histological characteristics identical to those of enamel caries. Teeth were then exposed to acidified gelatin gels for the creation of caries-like lesions as described previously. Small naturally occurring lesions of enamel caries were also used in the studies.

After removing teeth from the artificial caries medium, a single central longitudinal section was slit from the tooth to act as a control. Histological features of lesions from control sections were documented both qualitatively and quantitatively using the polarizing microscope. Microradiographs were also taken of the sections using CuKa radiation and employing a step-wedge. The cut faces on the remaining tooth halves were then varnished over so that just the surface above each lesion was exposed for experiment. Tooth halves were then exposed to the synthetic calcifying fluid. One tooth half was exposed to the experimental fluid while the adjacent half of the same tooth was exposed to the identical fluid but containing added fluoride ions. After exposure, tooth halves were washed, the surfaces brushed using water and an automatic toothbrush, and ground sections obtained from each half.

Discussion

When the calcium concentration of the calcifying fluid was adjusted to 3 mM, remineralization was limited to the superficial layers of the lesion. Reducing the calcium level to 1 mM resulted in remineralization occurring throughout the entire depth of the lesion. The addition of fluoride ions to the synthetic calcifying fluid had a marked effect in enhancing remineralization. When the low-calcium fluid was used without the addition of fluoride, a 22% reduction in area of the body of the lesion was obtained. This reduction increased to 72% on the addition of 0.05 mM fluoride (1 ppm). Increasing the fluoride level beyond this concentration had no further effect upon the degree of remineralization achieved.

After exposure to the 3 mM calcium calcifying fluid the surface layer showed clusters of plate-like material growing from the enamel structure. The morphological appearance of this material was similar to dicalcium phosphate dihydrate or octacalcium phosphate crystals. These crystals were never found when the 1 mM calcium calcifying fluid was used. Previous studies on the supersaturation of these calcifying fluids have shown that with the 3 mM fluid several of the more acidic calcium phosphate phases were supersaturated in addition to the apatite phases [*Silverstone and Wefel*, 1981]. The rapid nucleation of these larger acidic calcium phosphates tends to precipitate onto the enamel surface and block the surface pores, thus limiting remineralization to the superficial part of the lesion. With the 1 mM calcium calcifying fluid, only the apatitic phases were supersaturated and remineralization occurred throughout the total depth of the lesion.

Effect of Remineralization on Enamel Crystals

With the introduction of ultrastructural techniques in caries research it was hoped that direct visualization of the diseased tissue would help to resolve some of the problems unresolved by studies at the light microscope level. However, this has not proved to be the case due, in part, to problems associated with preparing ultrathin sections from such a hard tissue, as well as identification of the exact site in the lesion when examining samples at the ultrastructural level. In addition, because of the inevitable oblique transverse cutting of enamel prisms, the crystals too are cut in various oblique transverse planes giving the erroneous appearance that crystals have diameters greater than their true dimensions.

A new microdissection technique has recently produced information on crystal diameters within the various zones of the enamel lesion [*Silverstone*, 1983]. For sound enamel, crystal diameters were found to be in the range 35–40 nm. In the translucent zone of the enamel lesion, crystal diameters were smaller than for sound enamel and varied from 25 to 30 nm. In the dark zone, crystal diameters were significantly greater than sound enamel being 45–100 nm. In the body of the lesion crystal diameters were found to be much smaller, in the range 10–30 nm. In the surface zone, crystal diameters were once again found to be larger than in sound enamel, being in the range 40–75 nm.

This new information with respect to the enamel lesion is of significance because it is the first *direct* evidence of remineralization occurring throughout the prism structure within the enamel lesion. Such crystal growth to produce large single crystals could have resulted from the fusion of remnants of several of the original crystals. Thus, although there is a significant increase in crystal diameter, the total number of crystals within a particular zone is likely to be reduced. Due to the more favorable surface area-to-volume ratio, this effect by itself will result in a reduction in dissolution rate. In addition, crystal growth occurred in the presence of fluoride and so a more stable fluorhydroxyapatite unit is likely to result. These facts help explain previous work where we demonstrated that remineralized lesions were more resistant to lesion progression in vitro relative to control lesions. In addition, the two zones where large crystals have been found, the dark zone and the surface zone, are the two zones of the lesion which are produced as a result of remineralization.

General Discussion

This author believes that one of the main mechanisms whereby fluoride acts in caries prevention (if not the main mechanism) is in promoting remineralization. It has long been known that partially demineralized enamel takes up fluoride preferentially relative to sound enamel. Therefore, small lesions in approximal regions, not diagnosed by conventional techniques of clinical examination and radiography, are able to take up significant amounts of fluoride acting as fluoride ion reservoirs. When conditions favoring demineralization occur, fluoride is released in addition to calcium and phosphate ions. Thus, remineralization occurs and mineral is precipitated back into the lesion. This is the reason why some lesions never progress to the stage where they are diagnosed by conventional techniques.

It is suggested that in order for the submicroscopic crystals in enamel to increase in size relative to those of sound enamel, it is first necessary that the region is partially demineralized. Thus, remineralization can only occur after a bout of demineralization. Therefore, it might be necessary for all proximal surfaces to become carious at the histological level so that they can benefit from remineralization which, in turn, will give the region a degree of resistance towards lesion progression. Since small lesions cannot be diagnosed, their presence remains undisclosed unless they progress to the stage where they are detected by conventional means. The fact that many 'caries-free' proximal surfaces may contain small lesions is highlighted by the fact that this author, in collecting small natural lesions for his research over many years, obtains them by sectioning teeth which appear caries-free proximally even on macroscopic examination.

The phenomenon of remineralization should be emphasized in an effort to prevent the well-meaning clinician from attempting to restore a tooth because there is a small lesion indicated on a bitewing radiograph. A restorative approach is indicated only when there is definite radiographic evidence of lesion progression relative to a previous radiograph. It is essential that the clinician appreciates the true extent of a lesion relative to the size it may appear to be when examined by the relatively insensitive diagnostic techniques available. However, realizing the extent of a lesion, or even the possibility that lesions exist even if they cannot be diagnosed, should in itself encourage the use of a caries-preventive approach. Thus, primary prevention at the clinical level is secondary prevention at the histological level.

The use of fluoride is important in enhancing remineralization, although it does not appear to be necessary to use high concentrations. Recent findings support the frequent supply of low concentrations of fluoride rather than the infrequent application of very high concentrations. The old maxim of 'more is better' does not therefore apply with respect to fluoride levels in enamel and caries susceptibility, in spite of this belief existing for many years. Since it can take 3 or 4 years for a smooth surface lesion to progress to the stage where the dentine is invaded, there is adequate time to intercept the carious process. By employing suitable preventive methods, lesions can be successfully remineralized such that they never progress to the stage where they are diagnosed. Hence, such surfaces will remain 'caries-free' at the clinical and radiographic levels of diagnosis.

Thus, experimental caries models have played a significant role in elucidating mechanisms of breakdown and repair in carious attack upon dental tissues. It should be obvious from this short and rather limited review that much of our knowledge today has been derived from model systems. In addition, because of the sophistication of biomedical research and the expense of clinical trials, model systems will continue to play a significant role in the development of new caries-preventive regimens and their eventual testing at the clinical level.

References

Arends, J.; Jongebloed, W.L.: Crystallite dimensions of enamel. J. Biol. buccale 6: 161–171 (1979).

Featherstone, J.D.B.; Rodgers, B.E.; Smith, M.W.: Physicochemical requirements for rapid remineralization of early carious lesions. Caries Res. 15: 221–235 (1981).

Koulourides, T.: Experimental changes of enamel mineral density; in Harris, Art and science of dental caries research, pp. 355–378 (Academic Press, New York 1968).

Silverstone, L.M.: The histopathology of enamel lesions produced in vitro and their relation with enamel caries; PhD thesis University of Bristol (1967).

Silverstone, L.M.: The surface zone in caries and in caries-like lesions produced in vitro. Br. dent. J. 125: 145–157 (1968).

Silverstone, L.M.: The structure of carious enamel, including the early lesion. Oral Sci. Rev. 3: 100–160 (1973).

Silverstone, L.M.: Remineralization phenomena. Caries Res. 11: suppl. 1, pp. 59–84 (1977).

Silverstone, L.M.: Remineralization and enamel caries: significance of fluoride and effect on crystal diameters; in Leach, Edgar, Demineralization and remineralization of the teeth, pp. 185–205 (IRL Press, Oxford 1983).

Silverstone, L.M.; Wefel, J.S.: The effect of remineralization on artificial caries-like lesions and their crystal content. J. Crystal Growth 53: suppl., pp. 148–159 (1981).

Silverstone, L.M.; Wefel, J.S.; Zimmerman, B.F.; Clarkson, B.H.; Featherstone, M.J.: Remineralization of natural and artificial lesions in human dental enamel in vitro: the effect of calcium concentration of the calcifying fluid. Caries Res. 15: 138–157 (1981).

Leon M. Silverstone, DDSc, PhD, Associate Dean for Research,
University of Colorado Health Sciences Center, Campus Box C-284,
4200 East Ninth Avenue, Denver, CO 80262 (USA)

Cariology Today. Int. Congr., Zürich 1983, pp. 245–258 (Karger, Basel 1984)

Effect of Various Fluorides on Enamel Structure and Chemistry

J. Arends[a], D.G.A. Nelson[a], A.G. Dijkman[a], W.L. Jongebloed[b]

[a] Dental School and [b] Centre for Medical Electron Microscopy,
University of Groningen, The Netherlands

Introduction

Since the introduction of fluorides into dentistry, various methods of fluoride delivery have been employed with the aim of caries prevention. Basically these can be categorized as agents containing either low or high fluoride concentrations. For example, fluoridation of public water supplies is a successful method for delivering low concentrations of fluoride, whereas acidulated phosphate fluoride gels are successful fluoride agents of high concentration.

The chemical diversity of topical fluoride agents is large, and the three main types of fluoride agents used are: (i) inorganic agents: NaF, NH_4F, Na_4SiF_6, SnF_2, TiF_4, etc.; (ii) monofluorophosphate-(MFP-) containing agents: Na_2FPO_3, $(NH_4)_2FPO_3$, etc., and (iii) 'organic fluorides': these contain organic components with ionizable fluoride, e.g. amine fluorides (e.g. Elmex®, Gaba, Basel), silane fluorides (e.g. in Fluor Protector®, Vivadent, Liechtenstein), fluoride-releasing polymers, and many others.

While factors such as agent acidity, the fluoride concentration, the contact period with enamel, its delivery medium (liquid, gel, toothpaste, varnish) are important in determining the enamel-fluoride agent interaction, in nearly all of the above agents the fluoride ion (F^-) is the active ionic species.

Fluoride ions interact with the apatite surfaces of enamel crystallites in four fundamentally different physicochemical ways, depending on the F concentration. They are: (1) non-specific adsorption of fluoride ions, (2) specific adsorption of fluoride ions, (3) dissolution and reprecipitation of fluoridated apatite, and (4) dissolution and reprecipitation of CaF_2. However, dental enamel is a porous material. Therefore diffusion processes are also important in understanding the interaction of fluoride agents and enamel. An important distinction when considering the effect of fluoride is the state of the enamel, which can be either (a) sound or (b) demineralized (i.e. carious, acid-etched or surface-softened enamel). In case b, the enamel structure has been 'opened up' by preferential acid dissolution of interprismatic areas. This increased porosity is considerable in carious enamel, surface-softened enamel [*Arends and ten Cate,* 1981] and less in etched enamel. Crystallite surfaces in acid-treated enamel contain more HPO_4^{2-} groups, which may influence enamel-fluoride interactions.

F^- ions (as well as others) easily penetrate the porous structures of both sound and demineralized enamel and can interact, depending on the local situation (pH and concentrations), with enamel crystallites in the four ways described above. Furthermore, F^- will stimulate remineralization (redepositioning) of mineral at low F levels [*Gelhard,* 1982; *Arends and Gelhard,* 1983a; *Gelhard and Arends,* 1983] and can block or retard remineralization at high fluoride levels [*Boddé,* 1983; *Boddé and Arends,* 1980]. Although acid-treated enamel is of considerable practical interest, our discussion will concentrate mainly on sound enamel. However, most of the concepts mentioned in this work are with some modifications applicable to acid-treated enamel as well. Furthermore, we will limit ourselves to the interactions of fluoride with sound whole enamel and ignore the F effect on dental plaque formation or adhesion. For convenience we shall not specifically take into account the non-stoichiometry of enamel and will consider it as hydroxyapatite as a first approximation.

Fluoride Interactions with Sound Enamel Crystallites
(pH $\approx$ 7, Low F Level < 10 ppm)

1. Diffusion of F in Sound Enamel
Typical enamel structures including prisms, interprismatic regions and the crystallites *in* the prisms are shown in cross-section in figure 1. F^- ions in contact with the outer surface of sound human enamel can diffuse into enamel slowly; the pellicle is not a significant diffusion barrier. At neutral pH, fluoride ions have an apparent diffusion con-

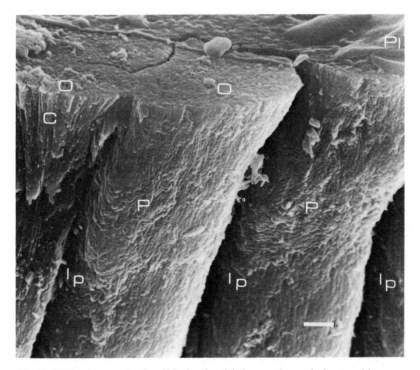

Fig. 1. SEM micrograph of a critical point dried enamel sample fractured in cross-section. O is the outer anatomical enamel surface. P is an enamel prism. C are enamel crystallites. Ip is the interprismatic area. Pl = plaque material. The bar is 1 μm.

stant $D_F \approx 10^{-10}$ cm^{2}s^{-1} in sound enamel [*Flim* et al., 1978]. This corresponds to a F penetration of about 1 μm/min and about 30 μm/day. F$^-$ ions most likely diffuse through interprismatic areas rather quickly with the above D_F value and are then subsequently distributed over and between the enamel crystallites with a much slower process having a D_F value $\approx 10^{-17}$ cm^{2}s^{-1}. Fluoride does not freely diffuse in enamel but interacts strongly with the enamel crystallites lining the interprismatic pores. A schematic picture of F 'diffusion' and adsorption on to the enamel mineral is given in figure 2.

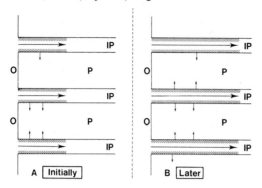

Fig. 2. Schematic representation of F⁻ diffusion in enamel. P is a prism, Ip is an interprismatic area, and F is shown being adsorbed to the crystallites lining the interprismatic areas. O is the outer surface of the enamel. The large arrows indicate diffusion of F through interprismatic areas. The small dashed lines indicate the very slow diffusion of F in intercrystallite regions.

2. F Gradients, Structurally Incorporated F

In sound human enamel, considerable fluoride gradients exist due to local variations in the amount of structurally incorporated F in crystallites. The F content near the outer surface is about 6,000 ppm (0.6%); at a depth of 100 μm it is about 100 ppm or less. The F concentration gradients increase with age after tooth eruption. The origin of high F concentrations near the surface is most likely a combination of the above-mentioned F⁻ diffusion and a superficial de-/remineralization process that incorporates F⁻ into the enamel crystallites. In the oral cavity, enamel is intermittently and locally dissolved by acids produced by microbial fermentation of food, beverages, etc. This occurs rather frequently. The outside of the enamel is in direct equilibrium with the salivary system and mineral dissolved from enamel crystallite surfaces may be redeposited from the saliva. The frequent de-/remineralization cycles are most likely an important source of F in surface enamel (similar to Ostwald ripening of crystals). The effect of F on the enamel structure is probably limited to the outermost few micrometres. Recently *Arends* et al. [1983b] showed that enamel crystallites near the enamel surface are 1.5–2 times larger in diameter than those deep in the enamel. The larger size and consequent lower enamel solubility in acids of crystallites near the surface could be partly related to an enhanced remineralization effect when F⁻ is present.

3. Protective Effect of F⁻, Physicochemical Reasons Why F⁻ Works

F^- influences both the acid solubility of enamel and its dissolution kinetics. They are the thermodynamic and kinetic factors of interest. In the older literature the thermodynamic concept which assumed an equilibrium situation was mainly stressed. Fluorapatite (FAP) is chemically and energetically much more stable than hydroxyapatite (HAP) and the incorporation of fluoride *in* enamel crystallites was considered to make them more stable and thus less soluble. Thus it was assumed that structurally incorporated fluoride was the cause of the protective effect of fluoride. This could occur by two different fluoride interaction mechanisms: (i) Specific exchange of $F^-_{(aq)}$ with $OH^-_{(lattice)}$ could occur, thus causing the interface to behave as FAP. (ii) Dissolution of enamel crystallites followed by reprecipitation of a fluoridated apatite upon reaction with a concentrated fluoride agent would also result in lattice fluoride. It should be kept in mind, however, that chemical stability is not identical to chemical reactivity. At equilibrium we have

$$K_{sp}(FAP) < K_{sp}(HAP) \ll K_{sp}(enamel)$$

(K_{sp} is solubility product).

Kinetically, however, if we have mild buffered sink conditions and k is the dissolution rate,

$$k(FAP) \approx k(\text{fluoridated HAP}) \approx k(HAP) < k(\text{enamel}, CO_3^{2-}\text{-containing}).$$

There are strong recent indications that the amount of fluoride in the lattice is not directly determining the protective effect of F^-. *Nelson* et al. [1983a] showed on pressed hydroxyapatite pellets that the initial dissolution rate is hardly influenced by about 1,000 ppm F^- in the solid, but decreases strongly in the presence of 1 ppm F in the liquid phase.

Arends and Christoffersen [1983] observed that in human and bovine enamel the formation of in vitro lesions can be greatly reduced at pH = 4.5 or 5 if the liquid phase contained a few parts per million F. Structurally incorporated F (in the solid enamel) hardly influenced the dissolution inhibition. Both apatite dissolution inhibition and in vitro caries inhibition in the presence of a few parts per million F^- in solution seem to be associated with the adsorption of fluoride on the outer surface of enamel crystallites. Two different adsorption processes can occur at the interface: non-specific and specific.

(i) Non-specific adsorption describes the fluoride which is preferentially concentrated in the Stern layer compared with the bulk solution, but which has not yet exchanged with a moiety in a surface lattice site. There are good reasons to believe that non-specific adsorption is important for apatite crystallites. The surface of enamel crystallites in aqueous solution is dominated (approximately 80–90% of the available surface) by phosphate ions [*Arends and Jongebloed,* 1977] both in the PO_4^{3-} and HPO_4^{2-} form, although at physiological pH values the protonated form is the most likely. Thus the Stern layer surrounding the crystallite will be calcium-rich. Fluoride ions will be electrostatically attracted into the Stern layer (charge balance being kept by ejection of $HPO_4^{2-}/H_2PO_4^-$ from the Stern layer) where hydrogen bonding of the fluoride with the –OH part of HPO_4^{2-} surface ions takes place (fig. 3a). It is interesting to note that the Stern layer is consequently enriched in Ca^{2+} and F^- ions, suggesting that apatite surfaces can act as a CaF_2 nucleator. Non-specific adsorption must, of course, occur prior to any specific adsorption. An adsorption coefficient $k_{ad}(F^-)$ could be defined for this process:

$$k_{ad}(F^-) = \frac{[F^-_{Stern}]}{[F^-_{bulk}]}$$

where $[F^-_{Stern}]$ is the concentration of fluoride ions in the Stern layer, $[F^-_{bulk}]$ is the concentration of fluoride ions in the bulk solution. We expect $k_{ad} \gg 1$.

(ii) Specific adsorption describes the surface exchange of F^- with OH^- in surface sites. This is known to occur. Specific adsorption can take place at Ca^{2+}, OH^-, HPO_4^{2-} or CO_3^{2-} sites on the crystallite surface. Another example of specific adsorption is the exchange of FPO_3^{2-} ions with surface HPO_4^{2-} ions. Specific adsorption is energetically well defined and results in a larger free energy change than non-specific adsorption. As far as the dissolution kinetics are concerned, the fluoride at the interface (specific and non-specific adsorption), which can be visualized as in figure 4, is the 'chemically active' form of fluoride which results in deceased chemical reactivity.

Primarily the amount of F^- present in the chemisorbed state and in the Stern layer determines dissolution kinetics and acid resistance. This is because fluoride has to be desorbed before proton (acid) attack occurs. Fluoride treatments with agents at low F concentrations (drink-

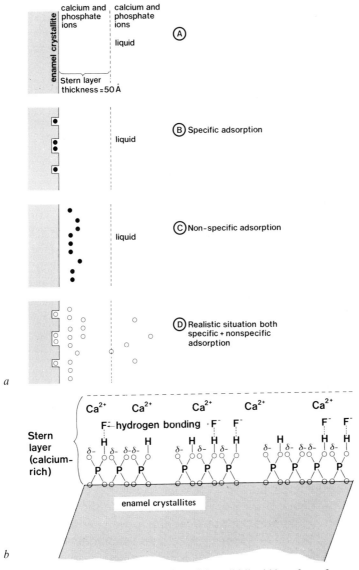

Fig. 3. a Schematic representation of the solid-liquid interface of enamel crystallites. A: The solid enamel (left) is surrounded by the Stern layer, which is inseparable from the solid. B: Specific adsorption of F (●) at special sites near the surface, e.g. one F^- may exchange for an OH site, two for a HPO_4 site. C: Non-specific adsorption in the Stern layer (F = ●). D: Combination of B and C. *b* Schematic representation of the interface of enamel crystallites. The Non-specific F adsorption is shown as hydrogen bonding to phosphate groups covering the surface.

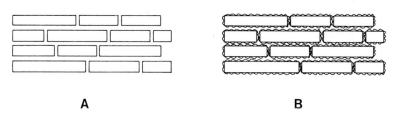

A   B

Fig. 4. Schematic representation of surface enamel treated with a low F agent. This represents *both* specific adsorption (see fig. 3a, B) and non-specific adsorption (fig. 3a, C).

ing water fluoridation, salivary fluoride, F from mouthrinses, fluorides from toothpastes, F leaching away from local application etc.) do not appear to cause new nucleation processes in sound enamel (e.g. complete crystal dissolution and regrowth does not occur) and therefore the effect of low F treatments can be described by these two adsorption processes. The F present at the crystal interface as shown in figure 4 or in the form of a fluoridated apatite can act as a local F reservoir for aqueous F^- ions during de-/remineralization cycles.

MFP and Sound Enamel (pH ≈ 7)

There is convincing evidence that FPO_3^{2-} ions can enter the enamel structure and diffuse as FPO_3^{2-} ions at pH ≈ 7 and 37 °C [*de Rooij,* 1981; *de Rooij and Arends,* 1981]. This is obvious from $^{32}P\text{-}FPO_3^{2-}$ diffusion experiments and also from comparison between $^{32}P\text{-}FPO_3^{2-}$, $^{32}P\text{-}HPO_4^{2-}$ and F^- diffusion profiles. FPO_3^{2-} transport in whole enamel is most likely important for the protective effects of MFP. MFP is hydrolysed by plaque [*Jackson,* 1982] and partly in the saliva, but it is reasonable to assume that in practical applications at least part of the MFP reaches the outer enamel surfaces and subsequently diffuses in. The fastest diffusion coefficient for MFP in whole enamel is about $1.7 \times 10^{-13}\,cm^2s^{-1}$ equivalent to transport distances of several micrometres per day. Experimentally FPO_3^{2-} penetration has been followed up to about 60–70 μm beneath the enamel surface. Diffusion of FPO_3^{2-} (isomorphous with $HO\text{-}PO_3^{2-}$) most likely takes place with $FPO_3^{2-} - HPO_4^{2-}$ exchange as proposed previously by *Ingram* [1972] and *Benton* et al. [1980].

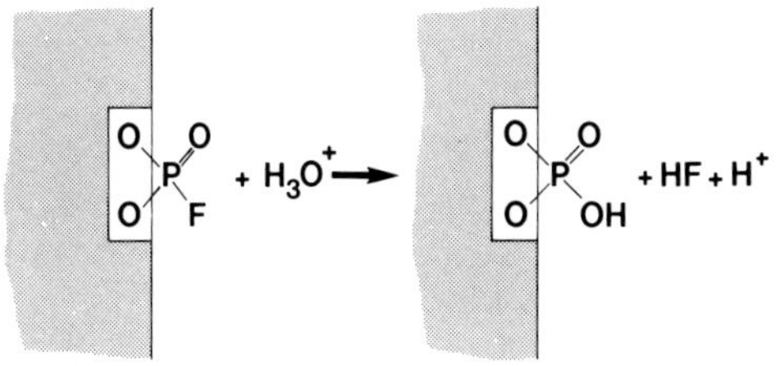

Fig. 5. Schematic representation of the decomposition FPO_3^{2-} to F^- at an enamel crystallite interface.

The MFP could (although transport would take much longer than in the case of pure F^-) also cover crystallite surfaces as depicted in figure 4. Decomposition of FPO_3^{2-} could occur:

(i) If an acid challenge involving H^+ ions took place [*Devonshire and Rowley, 1962; Duff and Stuart, 1982*], hydrolysis would be extremely slow at pH $= 7$, but considerable at acid pH values.

(ii) At the interface of the apatite mineral following chemisorption as shown in figure 5.

The F^- ions released by FPO_3^{2-} decomposition could subsequently be adsorbed at another specific adsorption site or be non-specifically adsorbed. The experimental observation that the heat of adsorption of MFP is about 3–4 times larger than for the adsorption of F^- ions, under identical conditions, is according to the authors, an indication that decomposition at the interface as depicted in figure 5 could indeed take place [*Arends* et al., unpublished]. An important unresolved point is: if MFP ions are adsorbed at the enamel crystallites for long periods, could they act as a *local* F reservoir on the crystallite surfaces and thus generate the protective F^- ion effect locally?

'Organic' Fluorides and Sound Enamel

The name organic fluorides includes several agents with very different chemical formulas and properties, e.g. the amine fluorides [*Mühlemann* et al., 1957], N,N',N'-tris(2 hydroxyethyl)-N-octadecyl-1,3-diamino propanhydrofluoride or fluoridating polyelectrolytes like poly-4 vinyl-N-ethyl-pyridinium fluoride (PEF) [*Bartels* et al., 1982]. These components combine the protective effect of F^- ions with physicochemical protection afforded by long chain aliphatic amines (Elmex) or high molecular polyelectrolytes (PEF). To the authors' knowledge these components have the following general properties:

(i) They form CaF_2 as layers (globules) *on* the surface (F_{on}).

(ii) They fluoridate the underlying enamel by F^- release either directly as described above or through subsequent CaF_2 dissolution.

(iii) The organic components present can influence surface free energies and consequently bacterial adhesion.

Fluoride as a Deposit on the Outer Enamel Surface
(pH Acid or Neutral, High F Levels: > 50 ppm)

When fluoridating agents with an F content of more than 50 ppm (acidic or non-acidic) are in contact for a given period with the outer enamel surface, CaF_2 is mainly formed, often in considerable amounts. The most convenient and commonly employed fluoridating agents are:

(i) 'Non-acidic' type. Neutral F solutions, F tablets, Duraphat®, Elmex, most toothpastes, etc., which have sufficient F content to react with the outer enamel and produce sufficient Ca^{2+} ions by dissolution of the solid so that CaF_2 and some FAP is precipitated.

(ii) 'Acidic' type. These include acidulated phosphate fluoride solutions, Fluor Protector, some toothpastes, and acidic mouthrinses. These produce Ca^{2+} by etching the enamel surface directly because of the low pH and precipitate CaF_2 and FAP on the surface.

The etching properties of the various agents on enamel surfaces are quite different and could be important for the CaF_2 retention and subsequent F^- release.

In all the above situations, CaF_2 is precipitated *on* the enamel. In general, after a single topical F treatment, globular agglomerates of CaF_2 particles (50–150 Å in diameter) are formed [*Nelson* et al., 1983b, c]. In vivo, the globules are soon covered with pellicle through which they slowly dissolve. Recent data of *Dijkman* [1982] and *Dijkman and Arends* [1983] show that F^- ions from CaF_2 deposits are lost with a rate $D_F = 10^{-6}$ cm^{2}s^{-1} in vivo, corresponding to the F^- diffusion constant in water. The data show that the CaF_2 globules slowly dissolve in periods of several weeks. In the experiments mentioned, Fluor Protector, which deposits massive amounts of CaF_2 on the enamel, produced measurable amounts of F *in* the solid enamel during CaF_2 dissolution under in vivo conditions (this has not been found for other agents yet).

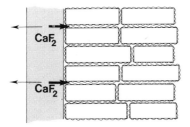

Fig. 6. Schematic representation of CaF_2 on the enamel surface due to the application of a high F agent.

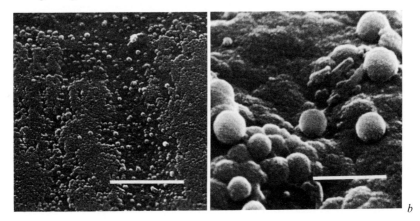

a

b

Fig. 7. SEM micrographs of CaF_2 coatings deposited on intact human enamel surfaces by an acidulated phosphate fluoride gel *(a)* and an acidic silane fluoride polyurethane lacquer *(b)*. Identical magnifications; notice the difference in globule size. The bar is 1 μm.

Fluoride leaches away from CaF_2 precipitated on the surface (fig. 6, 7) and can have the following effects:

(i) It increases the salivary F level.

(ii) It diffuses rapidly through permeable, mineral-deficient, micrometre-size spots into the underlying enamel. These spots which lie parallel to the perikymata have been observed recently [*Haikel* et al., 1983; *Arends* et al., 1983c] and appear to be the initial sites of acid penetration during lesion formation. Thus the layer acts as a source for further inward diffusion of F$^-$ which is subsequently specifically or non-specifically adsorbed on enamel crystallites.

Another effect of CaF_2 deposits recently suggested by *Nelson* et al. [1983b, c] is that CaF_2 can be deposited in natural enamel defects or prism etch pits ($\approx 5 \mu m$ in diameter) produced by topical acidic agents. Both the defects and prism etch pits lie parallel to the perikymata. CaF_2 in these etch pits will not be as easily leached away from the enamel as CaF_2 deposited on smooth surfaces. It is suggested that the surface morphology produced by topical agents is an important factor to consider in clinical fluoridation effectiveness. F^- leaching away from the CaF_2 globules [*Chow*, 1977] on and in the sound enamel surface will of course contribute substantially to the protective effects mentioned in section 3.

Conclusions

Basically there are two types of fluoride interaction with enamel crystallites: adsorption processes when the fluoride concentration is low enough and dissolution/reprecipitation processes when the fluoride concentration is higher. Structurally incorporated fluoride in enamel crystallites is important merely as a reservoir of F^- which can be released into the aqueous environment during a caries challenge. Adsorption processes are the most important type of interaction in reducing enamel crystallite reactivity (dissolution rates). CaF_2 or FAP deposited by topical agents act as temporary fluoride reservoirs which release F^- ions into the aqueous environment where diffusion and adsorption of F on enamel surfaces can subsequently take place. Thus the caries-preventive effects of both low-fluoride and, in part, high-fluoride agents may be due to the same physicochemical process. MFP may be unique in that specific adsorption of FPO_3^{2-} ions occurs, but there is evidence to suggest that decomposition of the FPO_3^{2-} moiety does occur to give F^- ions which can subsequently react with enamel surfaces by adsorption. Because enamel is not a homogeneous reactive material, fluoride action could be especially beneficial at local natural defects which lie parallel to the perikymata. More basic understanding of the processes occurring at the solid/liquid interface is needed because it is at this level that chemical agents appear to be effective in prevention of caries.

Regardless of the modes of action, fluoride must be *retained* in the oral environment to provide lasting benefit, whether this is by topical application (CaF$_2$ formation), or water supply (adsorption of F only) or by long-term structurally incorporated fluoride which can act as a reservoir of F.

References

Arends, J.; Cate, J.M. ten: Tooth enamel remineralization. J. Crystal Growth *53:* 135–147 (1981).

Arends, J.; Christoffersen, J.C.: The influence of fluoride concentration on the progress of demineralization in bovine enamel at pH = 4.5. Caries Res. *17:* 455–457 (1983).

Arends, J.; Gelhard, T.: In vivo remineralization of human enamel; in Leach, Edgar, Demineralization and remineralization of teeth, pp. 1–16 (IRL Press, Oxford 1983a).

Arends, J.; Jongebloed, W.L.: The enamel substrate-characteristics of the enamel surface. Swed. dent. J. *1:* 215–244 (1977).

Arends, J.; Jongebloed, W.L.; Schuthof, J.: Crystallite diameters of enamel near the anatomical surface. Caries Res. *17:* 97–106 (1983b).

Arends, J.; Jongebloed, W.L.; Schuthof, J.: Ultrastructure of de- and remineralization; in Leach, Edgar, Demineralization and remineralization of teeth, pp. 155–163 (IRL Press, Oxford 1983c).

Bartels, T.; Kelders, H.; Arends, J.: Fluoridation of human enamel by fluoride-containing polyelectrolytes. Caries Res. *16:* 57–63 (1982).

Benton, D.P.; Bullock, J.I.; Danil de Namur, A.F.; Ingram, G.S.: Calorimetric studies of the interaction between hydroxyapatite and certain ions in aqueous solutions. Caries Res. *14:* 110–114 (1980).

Boddé, H.E.: The influence of fluoride applications on enamel remineralization; thesis University Groningen (1983).

Boddé, H.E.; Arends, J.: Remineralization of artificial carious lesions (Abstract). Caries Res. *15:* 198 (1980).

Chow, L.C.: Chemistry of topical fluorides. Caries Res. *11:* suppl. 1, pp. 191–197 (1977).

Devonshire, L.N.; Rowley, H.H.: Kinetics of hydrolysis of fluorophosphates. I. Mono-fluorophosphoric acid. Inorg. Chem. *1:* 680–683 (1962).

Dijkman, T.: Topical fluoride applications on human enamel; thesis University Groningen (1982).

Dijkman, A.G.; Arends, J.: Topical fluoridation of sound enamel in vivo. Kariesprophylaxe (in press, 1983).

Duff, E.J.; Stuart, J.L.: Acid hydrolysis of aqueous sodium monofluorophosphate solutions. Caries Res. *16:* 361–366 (1982).

Flim, G.J.; Kolar, Z.; Arends, J.: Diffusion of fluoride ions in dental enamel at pH = 7. J. Bioeng. *2:* 93–102 (1978).

Gelhard, T.: Remineralization of human enamel in vivo; thesis University Groningen (1982).

Gelhard, T.; Arends, J.: In vivo enamel remineralization. Caries Res. (in press, 1983).

Haikel, Y.; Frank, R.M.; Voegel, J.C.: SEM of the human enamel surface layer of incipient carious lesions. Caries Res. *17:* 1–14 (1983).

Ingram, G.S.: The reaction of MFP and apatite. Caries Res. *6:* 1–15 (1972).

Jackson, L.R.: In vitro hydrolysis of MFP by dental plaque microorganisms. J. dent. Res. *61:* 953–956 (1982).

Mühlemann, H.R.; Schmid, H.; König, K.G.: Enamel solubility reduction with inorganic and organic fluorides. Helv. odont. Acta *1:* 23–33 (1957).

Nelson, D.G.A.; Featherstone, J.D.B.; Duncan, J.F.; Cutress, T.W.: Effect of carbonate and fluoride on the dissolution behaviour of synthetic apatites. Caries Res. *17:* 200–211 (1983a).

Nelson, D.G.A.; Jongebloed, W.L.; Arends, J.: Morphology of enamel surfaces treated with topical fluoride agents: SEM considerations. J. dent. Res. (in press, 1983b).

Nelson, D.G.A.; Jongebloed, W.L.; Arends, J.: Crystallographic structure of enamel surfaces treated with topical fluoride agents: TEM and XRD considerations. J. dent. Res. (in press, 1983c).

Rooij, H. de: Diffusion of phosphate and monofluorophosphate ions in bovine enamel; thesis University Groningen (1981).

Rooij, H. de; Arends, J.: Diffusion of MFP in whole bovine enamel at pH = 7. Caries Res. *15:* 363–368 (1981).

Prof. Dr. J. Arends, Materia Technica, Dental School, Ant. Deusinglaan 1,
NL-9713 AV Groningen (The Netherlands)

Cariology Today. Int. Congr., Zürich 1983, pp. 259–268 (Karger, Basel 1984)

Diffusion Phenomena and Enamel Caries Development[1]

J.D.B. Featherstone

Eastman Dental Center, Rochester, N.Y., USA

Introduction

The transport, or diffusion, of acid into enamel and the diffusion of mineral out of enamel are necessary prerequisites for the progress of enamel caries. The relative importance of these diffusion processes and other related chemical events still remains in question. Several workers have made important contributions in recent years to our understanding of the chemical mechanisms of enamel dissolution and the caries process by proposing models based on their in vitro studies with dental enamel [*Gray*, 1966, 1977; *Moreno and Zahradnik*, 1974; *Larsen*, 1973; *Brown*, 1974; *Van Dijk* et al., 1979; *Featherstone* et al., 1979; *Cussler and Featherstone*, 1981; *Arends*, 1982; *Moreno and Margolis*, 1983; *Featherstone and Cussler*, 1983]. There is a voluminous literature on calcium phosphate chemistry, and specifically apatite reactions. Phosphate chemistry is highly relevant to the caries process [*Nancollas*, 1982]. However, the present paper will be limited to diffusion aspects of enamel caries.

The physical and chemical composition of enamel determines the diffusion steps which can occur. Enamel is definitely not a solid impermeable mass of hydroxyapatite. It is a complex porous solid, composed of long thin crystals of hydroxyapatite-like mineral surrounded

[1] The support of NIH/NIDR Grant DE 05510 is gratefully acknowledged. Partial support was provided by New York State Health Research Council Grant 13-032. The expert assistance of *M. Shariati, R. Glena, S. Pearson* and *C. Shields* is acknowledged in these studies.

by a matrix of water and organic material. The crystals are not pure
hydroxyapatite and are best considered as a much more reactive
carbonated-apatite with numerous cation impurities replacing some of
the calcium ions in the structure. These crystals are about 40 nm in
diameter running from the outer enamel surface to the dentine, rather
than short discrete crystals, and these run nearly perpendicular to the
surface [*Orams* et al., 1976]. The so-called enamel prisms, or rods, are
comprised of crystals clustered together, about 100 across, to give a rod
diameter of about 4 μm. This inorganic phase makes up about 95% by
weight but only about 85% by volume of enamel.

Among all crystals and rods is a water/organic phase which occupies a few percent by weight but up to 15% by volume. Ions or
molecules can diffuse through this matrix in their aqueous state. The
organic content of mature dental enamel is approximately 1% by
weight [*Jenkins,* 1978] but this translates to about 3% by volume.
Approximately equal amounts of protein [*Robinson* et al., 1977] and
lipid [*Odutuga and Prout,* 1974] are present.

In the caries process acid is produced by bacteria in the plaque on
the tooth surface. Before this acid can react and dissolve the
carbonated-apatite crystals within the enamel the acid has to diffuse to
the crystal surfaces through the porous water/organic matrix and compete with the protein and lipid for active sites at the crystal surfaces.
Similarly, calcium and phosphate have to diffuse out through this
matrix before demineralization is complete.

Several investigators have measured the diffusion of ions and molecules into or through enamel and a selection of these studies are
relevant to the present discussion. *Braden* et al. [1971] used radioactive
sodium and fluoride to show that the uptake of these ions into enamel
was diffusion controlled. *Van Dijk* et al. [1983] have recently compared
some of the diffusion literature relating to the caries process in an
attempt to explain various differences. Table I compares selected diffusion coefficients to illustrate our present state of knowledge. It is
obvious that a diffusion coefficient in the order of 10^{-8} cm^2/s is
appropriate for the diffusion of nonreacting species through enamel.
The net apparent diffusion coefficient for the overall caries process was
estimated at about 10^{-9} cm^2/s or less. These values are 100- to 10,000-
fold smaller than those for simple diffusion in water where there are no
pores or organic material to restrict movement. Similarly these values
are about 100- to 1,000-fold smaller than values for diffusion through

Table I. Selected diffusion coefficients (D) for the diffusion of ions and molecules through enamel and related media: in some cases values have been estimated from data in the publications referred to

Species	Diffusion matrix	D, cm^2/s	Reference
Ca^{2+}	bovine enamel, pH 7	3×10^{-12}	*Flim and Arends*, 1977a
Rb$^+$	bovine enamel	4×10^{-8}	*Borggreven* et al., 1977
Sorbitol	bovine enamel	1×10^{-8}	*Borggreven* et al., 1977
H$_2$O	human enamel	1×10^{-8}	*Moreno and Burke*, 1974
HPO$_4^{2-}$	bovine enamel, pH 7	2×10^{-12}	*de Rooij* et al., 1980
F$^-$	bovine enamel, pH 7	3×10^{-10}	*Flim* et al., 1978
Cl$^-$	bovine enamel	2×10^{-8}	*Borggreven* et al., 1977
Ca^{2+}	gelatin/water	1×10^{-7}	*Oldershaw* et al., 1981
Ca^{2+}	lipid membrane	3×10^{-9}	*Oldershaw* et al., 1981
Acetate lactate	dental plaque	5×10^{-6}	*McNee* et al., 1981
Ions, small molecules	water	10^{-6}–10^{-5}	*Crank and Park*, 1968
Combined net demineraliza-tion during artificial caries	human enamel	$\sim 10^{-9}$	*Featherstone* et al., 1979

plaque. Thus the diffusion processes in plaque are many times faster than those in enamel. It is also obvious that calcium, phosphate and fluoride which are part of, and also react with, enamel mineral, have much smaller measured diffusion coefficients. This very strongly reflects their interaction with enamel crystals. It is also of note that protein and lipid markedly restrict calcium movement by several orders of magnitude. One of the questions, therefore, which remains is just what the role of the organic matrix is and how important it is.

Another very fundamental question is whether the rate of the subsurface demineralization process is determined by diffusion, by surface-controlled reactions, or both. We have speculated that the diffusion processes are slow relative to the crystal dissolution reaction, and that this holds for a wide variety of porous solids [*Cussler and Featherstone*, 1981]. The composition of the solid crystals and the concentrations of the ions in solution markedly affect the type of dissolution and whether subsurface dissolution occurs as well as precipitation in the 'surface layer'.

Chemical reaction rates and diffusion rates are governed by activation energies, and measurement of these will give information as to

which process is rate determining. No previous reports of the measurement of apparent activation energy for artificial carious lesion formation were available. The aim of the experimental work reported in the
present review was to estimate the overall activation energy for lesion
formation. This information, together with recently reported studies
and the earlier literature, gives a better understanding of the role of
diffusion in the caries process.

Materials and Methods

Temperature Effect on Lesion Formation
The crowns of 32 molars and premolars with caries-free surfaces were removed from
the roots, brushed with warm detergent solution, rinsed in deionized water, and air dried.
Each crown was varnished leaving two narrow windows and immersed individually in
40 ml of 0.1 mol/l lactate buffer, pH 4.5, containing 0.1 mmol/l diphosphonate (MHDP),
for one period of 2, 7, 14 or 21 days at one of 25, 37, 45 or 56 °C. These conditions
produced subsurface caries-like lesions [*Featherstone* et al., 1979]. At the end of each test
the teeth were sectioned through the lesion centers, embedded, and depths measured as
described previously [*Featherstone and Rodgers*, 1981]. The progression of depth versus
square root of time was linear. Lesion rates were calculated by linear regression from this
data and an Arrhenius plot of ln (slope)^2 vs. 1/T (where T = absolute temperature) was
used to calculate the apparent activation energy, E_a.

Acetic, Propionic and Lactic Acid Effect on Lesion Rate
Subsurface caries-like lesions were produced in human tooth crowns as described
previously and above [*Featherstone and Rodgers*, 1981] using buffers all at pH 5.0 of
acetate (0.02, 0.04 mol/l), propionate (0.01, 0.02 mol/l), lactate (0.02, 0.04 mol/l) together
with MHDP at 0.1 mmol/l, each singly, and in double and triple combinations over
immersion periods of 2, 7, 14, 21, 30 days at 37 °C. Details are reported elsewhere
[*Shariati and Featherstone*, 1983]. The data is briefly summarized here since it is of central
importance to diffusion and dental caries.

Results

Activation Energy – Temperature Dependence of Lesion Rates
The rate of artificial lesion formation increased with temperature
(fig. 1) but not markedly. A plot of ln (slope)^2 vs. 1/T was linear and
yielded an apparent activation energy of 13 kJ/mol for artificial carious
lesion formation. The (slope)^2 was used as this is directly proportional
to the diffusion coefficient and gives a direct rate parameter.

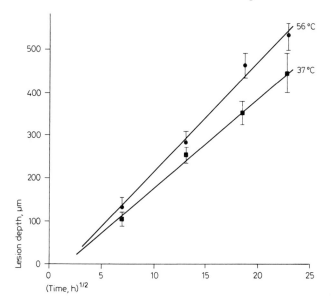

Fig. 1. Lesion depth versus square root of time for 0.1 mol/l lactate, 0.1 mmol/l MHDP, pH 4.5 at 37 and 56 °C. Error bars are standard deviations.

Effect of Acetic, Propionic and Lactic Acids on Lesion Rates

Figure 2 illustrates typical lesion rate profiles for the acid mixtures shown, all at pH 5.0. Full details have been reported elsewhere [*Shariati and Featherstone,* 1983]. Total acid concentration, not pH alone, affected lesion formation rate. The rate of formation was a function of a combination of calculated unionized acid concentration and acid dissociation constant, as reported previously for single acids and simple mixtures [*Featherstone and Rodgers,* 1981]. Significantly, the linear regression lines fitted to the data all cut the time axis at 2–4 h (fig. 1, 2) indicating a lag time before a true diffusion process, linear with (time)$^{1/2}$, takes over. This is discussed further below.

Discussion

Table II compares activation energies for various processes involv-ing diffusion and/or surface control. It is obvious that subsurface

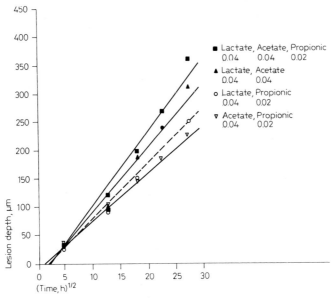

Fig. 2. Lesion depth versus square root of time for acid buffer mixtures at the concentrations shown (mol/l), pH 5.0, with 0.1 mmol/l MHDP, 37 °C. Each point is the mean depth for four lesions. Solid lines are calculated linear regression lines.

demineralization of human enamel as assessed in the present study has an activation energy, E_a, which places it clearly in the diffusion-controlled category. Remineralization of etched enamel is apparently largely surface controlled, whereas subsurface remineralization is apparently intermediate between surface reaction controlled and diffusion controlled.

The obvious corollary of this is that in the demineralization process the diffusion of acid into the enamel and the diffusion of mineral out through the interprismatic and intercrystalline water/organic phase is extremely important. We have now produced considerable evidence that rate of lesion formation is a function of calculated unionized concentration of each organic acid and also its ability to dissociate inside the enamel to produce H^+ ions to attack the carbonated-apatite crystals. One interpretation of this is that higher concentrations of unionized acid (HA, HL, etc.) provide greater capacity for the external environment to continually remain as a source of H^+ ions. Alternative-

Table II. Activation energies, E_a, for various processes illustrating the values attribuable to diffusion or surface-controlled processes

System	E_a, kJ/mol	Reference
Ca^{2+}/water diffusion	19	*Hollingshead and Gordon,* 1941
Ca^{2+}/bovine enamel	68, first process	
	125, second process	*Flim and Arends,* 1977b
Water/human enamel	19–58	*Burke and Moreno,* 1975
Remineralization/enamel	67, etched enamel	
	30, lesion enamel	*ten Cate,* 1978
Surface-controlled reactions	45–80	*Marshall and Nancollas,* 1969
Diffusion-controlled reactions	8–25	*Bircumshaw and Riddirord,* 1952
Artificial carious lesions/lactate	13	*Featherstone,* present study

ly it is possible that the protein/lipid content of enamel provides a porous structure among the charged apatite crystals through which the unionized form of each acid can preferentially diffuse, as it does through other body membranes. The acid molecules will always dissociate as they diffuse, providing a continual source of H^+ ions at every point which the acid molecules reach. We have shown that lactic acid potentiates the action of acetic and propionic acids, which in themselves are effective demineralizers.

The lipid component of enamel may be very important as an inhibitor of demineralization. In a recent study we extracted lipid from human enamel and found that lesion progress more than doubled compared with normal enamel [*Featherstone and Rosenberg,* 1983]. This fits extremely well with greatly reduced diffusion coefficients for the diffusion of species through lipid-like membranes (table I). In experiments using powdered apatite suspensions in gelatin gels we have produced subsurface demineralization [*Featherstone and Cussler,* 1983] with a reprecipitated surface layer using hydrochloric acid or acetic acid. In this case, with no lipid present, the unionized acid form appeared to play no part. The pattern of dissolution and precipitation follows an overall theory developed for porous solids [*Cussler and Featherstone,* 1981]. In these experiments the first stages observed were dissolution of the surface apatite in contact with the acid. This soon gave way to partial dissolution of the apatite and was subsequently followed by precipitation at the gel surface and partial dissolution below the surface.

In the weak acid/enamel lesion experiments briefly reported above a lag phase was observed prior to subsurface dissolution, diffusion control, and surface layer formation occurring. This initial stage appears to be caused by partial dissolution of crystals at the enamel surface. Recently, *Haikel* et al. [1983] suggested that existing pores and holes in the enamel surface are the points of initiation of the caries process. However, *Thylstrup and Featherstone* [1983a, b] have demonstrated by SEM that the surface enamel of artificial carious lesions is opened up in the first minutes or hours and is subsequently partially closed up by remineralization giving an appearance similar to normal unattacked enamel. The appearance of the very early stages of lesion formation is very similar to the surface enamel in active natural carious lesions. This period of initial attack at the surface coincides with the lag phase reported above. Hence it appears that there is an initial opening up of the enamel, even with pellicle or an inhibitor like MHDP present, followed by subsurface diffusion, acid attack, remineralization near the surface, and subsequent lesion progression.

As demineralization proceeds more crystals dissolve leaving larger open pores in the water/organic matrix and giving the calcium and phosphate a relatively easy path out of the lesion, hampered by the desire to precipitate along the way depending on concentrations of calcium, phosphate, fluoride, and pH at any point. Mineral loss from the lesion can continue as long as sufficient acid is available and/or conditions of undersaturation exist.

Reversal of these diffusion and dissolution processes lead to remineralization and arrestment or reversal of the overall demineralization phenomenon. If fluoride is present at the time of acid challenge it will diffuse with the acid and may markedly inhibit the dissolution step at the crystal surface [*Featherstone,* unpubl. data]. If present during a possible remineralization phase it enhances crystal growth and hence makes the overall remineralization process more rapid and more effective. These two aspects of fluoride action are extremely important in its ability to reduce or prevent caries. As our understanding of the diffusion and reaction processes continues to improve it may be possible to employ fluoride and other agents even more effectively in caries prevention.

References

Arends, J.: Mechanism of dental caries; in Nancollas, Biological mineralization and demineralization, pp. 303–325; Dahlem Konferenzen, 1982 (Springer, Berlin 1982).

Bircumshaw, L.L.; Riddiford, A.C.: Transport control in heterogenous reactions. Q. Rev. 6: 157–185 (1952).

Borggreven, J.M.P.; Van Dijk, J.W.; Driessens, F.C.M.: A quantitative radiochemical study of ionic and molecular transport in bovine dental enamel. Archs oral Biol. 22: 467–472 (1977).

Braden, M.; Duckworth, R.; Joyston-Bechal, S.: The uptake of ^{24}Na by human dental enamel. Archs oral Biol. 16: 367–374 (1971).

Brown, W.E.: Physicochemical mechanisms of dental caries. J. dent. Res. 53: 204–216 (1974).

Burke, E.J.; Moreno, E.C.: Diffusion fluxes of tritiated water across human enamel membranes. Archs oral Biol. 20: 327–332 (1975).

Crank, J.; Park, G.S.: Diffusion in polymers (Academic Press, London 1968).

Cussler, E.L.; Featherstone, J.D.B.: Demineralization of porous solids. Science 213: 1018–1019 (1981).

de Rooij, J.F.; Kolar, A.; Arends, J.: Phosphate diffusion in whole bovine enamel at pH 7. Caries Res. 14: 393–402 (1980).

Featherstone, J.D.B.: Diffusion phenomena during artificial carious lesion formation. J. dent. Res. 50: 48–51 (1977).

Featherstone, J.D.B.; Cussler, E.L.: Subsurface demineralization in porous apatite-gel suspensions. Abstr. ORCA, Dublin 1983.

Featherstone, J.D.B.; Duncan, J.F.; Cutress, T.W.: A mechanism for dental caries based on chemical processes and diffusion phenomena during in vitro caries simulation in human tooth enamel. Archs oral Biol. 24: 101–112 (1979).

Featherstone, J.D.B.; Rodgers, B.E.: Effect of acetic, lactic, and other organic acids in the formation of artificial carious lesions. Caries Res. 15: 337–385 (1981).

Featherstone, J.D.B.; Rosenberg, H.: Lipid effect on the progress of artificial carious lesions in dental enamel Caries Res. (in press, 1983).

Flim, G.J.; Arends, J.: Diffusion of ^{45}Ca in bovine enamel. Calcif. Tissue Res. 24: 59–64 (1977a).

Flim, G.J.; Arends, J.: The temperature dependence of ^{45}Ca diffusion in bovine enamel. Calcif. Tissue Res. 24: 173–177 (1977b).

Flim, G.J.; Kolar, Z.; Arends, J.: Diffusion of fluoride ions in dental enamel at pH 7. J. Bioeng. 2: 93–102 (1978).

Gray, J.A.: Kinetics of enamel dissolution during formation of incipient caries-like lesions. Archs oral Biol. 11: 397–421 (1966).

Gray, J.A.: Chemical events during carcinogenesis; in Proc. Symp. on Incipient Caries of Enamel, University of Michigan 1977.

Haikel, Y.; Frank, R.M.; Voegel, J.C.: Scanning electron microscopy of the human enamel surface layer of incipient carious lesions. Caries Res. 17: 1–13 (1983).

Hollingshead, E.A.; Gordon, A.R.: The differential diffusion constant of calcium chloride in aqueous solution. J. chem. Phys. 9: 152–153 (1941).

Jenkins, G.N.: The physiology and biochemistry of the mouth (Blackwell Scientific Publications, Oxford 1978).

Larsen, M.J.: Dissolution of enamel. Scand. J. dent. Res. *81:* 518–522 (1973).

Marshall, R.W.; Nancollas, G.H.: The kinetics of crystal growth of dicalcium phosphate dihydrate. J. phys. Chem. *73:* 3838–3844 (1969).

McNee, S.G.; Geddes, D.A.M.; Sweeney, D.; Weetman, D.A.; Beeley, J.A.: Permeability of dental plaque. Caries Res. *15:* 203 (1981).

Moreno, E.C.; Burke, E.J.: A diaphragm cell and the procedure for studying isothermal diffusion in dental enamel. Archs oral Biol. *19:* 417–420 (1974).

Moreno, E.C.; Margolis, H.C.: Physical chemical aspects of enamel demineralization. J. dent. Res. *62:* 163 (1983).

Moreno, E.C.; Zahradnik, R.T.: Chemistry of enamel subsurface demineralization in vitro. J. dent. Res. *53:* 226–235 (1974).

Nancollas, G.H.: Biological mineralization and demineralization. Dahlem Konferenzen (Springer, Berlin 1982).

Odutuga, A.A.; Prout, R.E.S.: Lipid analysis of human enamel and dentine. Archs oral Biol. *19:* 729–731 (1974).

Oldershaw, M.D.; Featherstone, J.D.B.; Rosenberg, H.: Lipid effect on ionic transport in relation to enamel demineralization and remineralization. J. dent. Res. *60A:* abstr. 819 (1981).

Orams, H.J.; Zybert, J.J.; Phakey, P.P.; Rachinger, W.A.: Ultrastructural study of human dental enamel using selected area argon ion-beaming thinning. Archs oral Biol. *21:* 659–661 (1976).

Robinson, C.; Fuchs, P.; Weatherell, J.A.: The fate of matrix proteins during the development of dental enamel. Calcif. Tissue Res. *22:* suppl., pp. 185–190 (1977).

Shariati, M.; Featherstone, J.D.B.: Importance of acid type in dental caries. J. dent. Res. *62:* 187 (1983).

ten Cate, J.M.; Arends, J.: Remineralization of artificial enamel lesions in vitro. II. Determination of activation energy and reaction order. Caries Res. *12:* 213–222 (1978).

Thylstrup, A.; Featherstone, J.D.B.; Fredebo, L.: Surface morphology and dynamics of early enamel caries development; in Leach, Demineralization and remineralization of teeth (IRL Press, London 1983a).

Thylstrup, A.; Featherstone, J.D.B.; Holmen, L.; Fredebo, L.: Structural and chemical changes during development of artificial caries. Abstr. ORCA, Dublin 1983b.

Van Dijk, J.W.E.; Borggreven, J.M.P.M.; Driessens, F.C.M.: Chemical and mathematical simulation of caries. Caries Res. *13:* 169–180 (1979).

Van Dijk, J.W.E.; Borggreven, J.M.P.M.; Driessens, F.C.M.: The diffusion in tooth enamel in relation to the caries process (in press, 1983).

J.D.B. Featherstone, PhD, Eastman Dental Center,
625 Elmwood Avenue, Rochester, N.Y. (USA)

Cariology Today. Int. Congr., Zürich 1983, pp. 269–278 (Karger, Basel 1984)

Fluoride in Body Fluids –
Cariostatic and Toxicologic Aspects[1]

Jan Ekstrand[a], Gary M. Whitford[b]

[a] Department of Cariology, School of Dentistry, Karolinska Institutet, Huddinge, Sweden; [b] Department of Oral Biology-Physiology, School of Dentistry, Medical College of Georgia, Augusta, Ga., USA

Introduction

One of the first hypotheses to account for the cariostatic effect of fluoride was that fluoride incorporated into the enamel mineral during its formation rendered the tissue more resistant to acid attack. While this explanation may account for a portion of the protection, more recent research findings have raised doubt about its preeminence. For example, most studies on the relationship between surface enamel fluoride concentrations and susceptibility to dental caries have not yielded statistically significant associations [*Poulsen and Larsen*, 1975; *Richards* et al., 1977; *Mellberg and Singer*, 1977]. It is also known that, among persons born and raised in an area with fluoridated water, a decrease in fluoride intake due to defluoridation or to moving into an area without water fluoridation results in an increase in the caries rate [*Klein*, 1948; *Russel*, 1949; *Lemke* et al., 1970; *Kunzel*, 1980].

There is evidence that the dynamically important fluoride in the oral environment is that of the oral fluids. These include the saliva, gingival crevicular fluid and the fluid of dental plaque. The fluoride levels of the former two fluids are directly related to those of plasma [*Ekstrand* et al., 1977; *Whitford* et al., 1981]. They are probably an important source of fluoride for plaque fluid. Thus, knowledge of the systemic metabolism and pharmacokinetics of fluoride appears to be

[1] Supported by Grants DE-04332 and DE-06113 from NIDR, NIH. Swedish Medical Research Council project No. 6002, and the Swedish Patent Revenue Research Fund.

relevant to understanding the cariostatic action of the ion. There is no question that such knowledge is essential to the complete understanding of dental fluorosis and fluoride toxicity in general.

It is the purpose of this paper to discuss the current status of what is known of fluoride in the body fluids and the factors that can influence these concentrations. Where possible, the relationships of these concentrations to fluoride cariostasis and dental fluorosis will be identified.

Fluoride in Plasma

Using his HMDS-facilitated diffusion method, *Taves* [1968] established that the plasma concentration of ionic fluoride is approximately 1 μM (0.019 ppm) among persons consuming drinking water containing 1.0 ppm fluoride. Prior to this, the generally accepted value was about ten times higher [*Singer and Armstrong,* 1960]. The higher values were due to analytical problems that were later resolved.

In spite of the fact that adequate analytical methods are now available, the literature cites a wide range of values for average or 'normal' plasma fluoride concentrations [*Guy,* 1979]. It is apparent that some of the disagreement can be explained by analytical problems. There may, in some cases, be substantial and long-term differences in fluoride intake among different groups of subjects. In addition, there are several physiologic variables that can influence plasma fluoride levels. *Ekstrand and Ehrnebo* [1979] have identified interaction phenomena that can result in decreased fluoride bioavailability. Recent data from animal studies have shown that the rate of fluoride absorption from the stomach is a function of gastric acid secretion and the acidity of the ingested solution as well [*Whitford,* 1983]. When gastric acid secretion or the acidity of the gastric contents is high, the absorption rate is increased. This results in very early and high peak plasma levels (e.g., at 5 min) and relatively lower levels a few hours later compared to the levels found when the acidity of the stomach is low. The rate of fluoride clearance from plasma by the kidneys is dependent on the pH of the urine [*Whitford* et al., 1976; *Whitford and Pashley,* 1979; *Ekstrand* et al., 1980]. Thus, for several hours following the ingestion of fixed amounts of fluoride, persons with a relatively acidic urine show higher plasma fluoride levels than do persons with more alkaline urine. Indeed, low urinary pH values may double the plasma half-life [*Ekstrand* et al., 1980]. The volume of distribution of fluoride in the soft tissues of body is a function of the magnitude of the pH gradient across cell membranes. When the gradient is reduced, as in respiratory or metabolic acidosis, relatively less fluoride will be found in the plasma and vice versa. These redistributions appear to be due to the diffusion equilibrium of hydrogen fluoride [*Whitford*, 1983].

Other studies have identified additional factors that should be considered when comparing plasma fluoride levels as reported by different investigators. Examples of such factors are: the time of blood sampling after fluoride ingestion [*Ekstrand*, 1983]; fasting or nonfasting conditions [*Ekstrand*, 1983]; blood sampling frequency [*Ekstrand*, 1978]; the age of the subject [*Whitford*, 1983]; previous fluoride exposure [*Ericsson* et al., 1973]; the site chosen for taking the blood sample [*Whitford*, 1983].

Each of the above factors can influence the observed concentrations of fluoride in plasma. Several of them will also affect the fluoride concentrations of the oral fluids.

Fluoride in Oral Fluids and the Possible Relation to Dental Caries

The impact of elevated fluoride levels in saliva and gingival crevicular fluid on dental caries has not received detailed research attention. Several animal studies, however, have suggested the potential importance of these concentrations (table I).

Larson et al. [1977] showed that gastric intubation of fluoride for 8 weeks to rats on a caries diet had a cariostatic effect on erupted molars although the effect was not as good as when the same amount of fluoride was given via drinking water. *Whitford and Schuster* [1982] conducted a similar study for the same period of time but administered fluoride constantly via miniature infusion pumps. They noted the same degree of caries reduction and also reported a slight elevation in the saliva fluoride levels compared to controls. These results confirm the results of *Bowen* [1973] who demonstrated that gastric intubation of fluoride resulted in an increase in saliva and plaque fluoride contents of monkeys.

Mirth et al. [1982], who scored caries in rats after both waterborne fluoride and administration of 0.2 mg/day via constant infusion for 32 days, did not note any effect of the systemically administered fluoride.

Table I. Caries in relation to systemic and waterborne fluoride in rats

Larson et al., 1977 8-week study	F in drinking water		F via gastric intubation
	control	5 ppm	5 ppm
Caries score[1]	11.6	0.3	4.2

Whitford and Schuster, 1982 8-week study	F in drinking water			F via infusion pump
	control	10 ppm (0.4 mg/day)	25 ppm (1.1 mg/day)	0.14 mg/day
Caries score	18.1	8.8	5.3	13.9
Terminal plasma F, μM	0.1	3.0	6.7	1.5
Whole saliva F, μM	0.03	1.0	2.2	0.5

Mirth et al., 1982 32-day study	F in drinking water		F via infusion pump		F via slow release device	
	control	10 ppm	control	0.2 mg/day	control	0.15 mg/day
Caries score	12.8	3.6	11.3	12.6	9.7	3.6

Caries score according to Keyes.

[1] Mean of first and second molar smooth surface.

In their study they also included one group of rats who received fluoride in the oral environment by intraoral slow-releasing devices. The caries reduction was the same as for the group who only received fluoride (10 ppm) via the drinking water (table I).

These studies suggest that the fluoride of the oral fluids can have an important role in the cariostatic action of the ion. It is likely that there are multiple mechanisms involved in the effect including the promotion of enamel remineralization, alterations in the rate and nature of pellicle formation on surface enamel, and inhibition of plaque bacterial metabolism and acid production.

One hypothesis regarding the latter effect is that during periods of plaque metabolism when the pH of plaque fluid is falling, local fluoride concentrations in the extracellular fluid increase to levels that can inhibit further acid production. The additional fluoride apparently derives mainly from extracellular mineral precipitates within the plaque although the surface enamel itself may be a source as well. At the same time, the pH gradient between plaque fluid and the intracellular fluids of plaque microorganisms increases thus establishing a steep diffusion gradient for hydrogen fluoride. Having entered the intracellular spaces where the pH is relatively high, the molecule would dissociate to release ionic fluoride and a proton. Ionic fluoride, because of its limited ability to permeate the cell membrane and wall, becomes trapped and accumulates to inhibitory concentrations [*Whitford* et al., 1977]. As acid production subsides, the pH gradient collapses owing to oral fluid buffers. Thus, fluoride would diffuse again as hydrogen fluoride, from the cells back into the extracellular fluid of plaque where it would be available for remobilization during the next exposure to metabolizable substrate.

Plasma Fluoride Levels and Enamel Fluorosis

The only established adverse effect of the long-term ingestion of water containing fluoride at 1 ppm is a low incidence of mild to very mild enamel fluorosis. This condition can develop only if fluoride is ingested during enamel formation and, at this level of involvement, it does not present a public health problem. According to Dean's findings with US subjects [*Dean, 1938*], the degree and prevalence of enamel fluorosis begins to become a public health problem when the main source of fluoride is water containing 1.6–1.8 ppm. The margin of safety for this disturbance in enamel mineralization is, therefore, low. It indicates the need to monitor fluoride intake from all sources, to carefully control the fluoride levels of fluoridated communal water supplies, and to identify the major factors that influence fluoride retention by individuals. It is noteworthy that, unlike Dean's subjects, children now have access to a variety of fluoride-containing products in both fluoridated and nonfluoridated communities. In some other countries, where nutritional or other factors may have affected susceptibility or fluoride balance, regions of endemic fluorosis exist in spite of the apparent absence of excessive fluoride intake [*Leatherwood* et al., 1965; *Nanda* et al., 1974]. The findings of *Whitford and Reynolds* [1979], who reported that a mild but chronic dietary-induced acidosis approximately doubled fluoride retention in rats, may be relevant to understanding the occurrence of fluorosis in the absence of excessive fluoride intake.

In their review of dental fluorosis, *Fejerskov* et al. [1977] discussed several possible mechanisms including direct effects of fluoride on ameloblasts, disturbances in nucleation and crystal growth, and alterations in calcium homeostasis. The authors correctly pointed out that most of the research on enamel fluorosis has been done with unusually high doses of fluoride. It is important to bear this in mind when evaluating the literature because there is little doubt that many of the reported effects of high fluoride doses on ameloblasts or developing enamel do not occur in humans consuming water containing fluoride at levels found in areas of endemic fluorosis.

It seems likely that the development of enamel fluorosis among groups of humans with different fluoride intake levels is a sigmoidal function of the average plasma fluoride level. This relationship has received insufficient research attention perhaps because of former difficulties in accurately determining plasma fluoride concentration. This is no longer a serious obstacle and work is needed to build on the findings of *Angmar-Månsson* et al. [1976]. They found that once-daily peak plasma fluoride levels of 10 μM (0.19 ppm) for 1 week, produced by single daily injections, caused disturbed mineralization patterns in the developing enamel of rat incisors. This was confirmed by *Angmar-Månsson and Whitford* [1982] and, further, it was found that during a week of twice-daily injections that produced peak plasma levels of about 5 μM (so that the total daily dose was the same as in the single daily injection group), there was no evidence of fluorosis. These find-ings indicated that, when the exposure period is brief and involving intermittent doses, there is a critical plasma fluoride threshold that must be exceeded if dental fluorosis is to develop. The threshold level may be a function of the duration of the exposure period, however. Thus, 5-μM peaks may have produced fluorosis if the doses had been given for 2 weeks, for example. By extension, it was predicted that a single dose of sufficient magnitude would produce rat incisor enamel fluo-rosis. This was confirmed with single doses of 0.75 mg/kg body weight and higher [Angmar-Månsson and Whitford, 1983]. Such doses of fluo-ride are associated with the clinical use of topical fluoride gels in children [Ekstrand et al., 1981; LeCompte and Whitford, 1982]. Further-more, it has recently been shown that the plasma fluoride concentration in small children (4–5 years) after swallowing 0.5 mg fluoride as NaF tablets or toothpaste are close to 5 µM within 30 min after intake. The fluoride levels were back to normal within a few hours [Ekstrand et al., 1983]. In the single-dose rat studies, the incisors were removed for examination by microradiography after the incisor enamel had com-pletely renewed itself. That is, the enamel was formed while circulating plasma fluoride levels were within the normal range of 0.5–1.5 µM. One explanation for this paradoxical finding is that the fluoride initially taken up by the bone supporting the developing enamel was slowly released during the following weeks resulting in prolonged and locally high fluoride levels.

In animals whose plasma fluoride levels were continuously elevated at 3–5 µM for 1 week (by subcutaneously implanted miniature infusion pumps), fluorosis was found in most of the incisors [Angmar-Månsson and Whitford, 1982]. These latter conditions would be more akin to the plasma fluoride levels of humans in areas of endemic enamel fluorosis. That is, they would be slightly elevated but relatively constant for long periods of time [Guy et al., 1976; Ekstrand, 1978].

The intriguing hypothesis of Weatherell et al. [1977] may be re-levant to the developing of enamel fluorosis in endemic regions where plasma fluoride levels of children at risk would rarely, if ever, exceed 2 or 3 µM. In experiments with rats, they showed that enamel fluoride levels decline as the tissue matures. They suggested that, due to a local redistribution, the ion accumulated in the younger, maturing enamel. This hypothesis has been supported by studies in other species [Speirs, 1975; Weatherell et al., 1977].

These findings indicate that enamel fluorosis can be produced by single high fluoride doses, multiple but lower doses, and by low-level but continuous exposure. Intermittent high plasma fluoride peaks can, but do not necessarily, cause enamel fluorosis. It may be that there are several sites of action and mechanisms involved in the development of dental fluorosis. However, the simplest explanation is that the production of the defective mineral is associated with elevated fluoride concentrations at some as yet unidentified critical site and that there are several dosage schedules that can achieve these levels.

References

Angmar-Månsson, B.; Ericsson, Y.; Ekberg, O.: Plasma fluoride and enamel fluorosis. Calcif. Tissue Res. *22:* 77–84 (1976).

Angmar-Månsson, B.; Whitford, G.M.: Plasma fluoride levels and enamel fluorosis in the rat. Caries Res. *16:* 334–339 (1982).

Angmar-Månsson, B.; Whitford, G.M.: Single fluoride doses and enamel fluorosis in the rat. Caries Res. *17:* 172, abstr. 45 (1983).

Bowen, W.H.: The effect of single daily doses of fluoride on saliva, plaque and urine in monkeys *(Macaca fasicularis)*. J. Int. Ass. Dent. Child. *4:* 11–14 (1973).

Dean, H.T.: Endemic dental fluorosis and its relation to dental caries. Publ. Hlth Rep. *53:* 1443–1452 (1938).

Ekstrand, J.: Relationship between fluoride in the drinking water and the plasma fluoride concentrations in man. Caries Res. *12:* 123–127 (1978).

Ekstrand, J.: The use of pharmacokinetics models and techniques in fluoride research. Proc. Int. Fluoride Symposium, Logan 1982 (Pergamon Press, Salt Lake City, in press, 1983).

Ekstrand, J.; Alvan, G.; Boreus, L.; Norlin, A.: Pharmacokinetics of fluoride in man after single and multiple oral doses. Eur. J. clin. Pharmacol. *12:* 311–317 (1977)

Ekstrand, J.; Ehrnebo, M.: Influence of milk products on fluoride bioavailability in man. Eur. J. clin. Pharmacol. *16:* 211–215 (1979).

Ekstrand, J.; Ehrnebo, M.; Whitford, G.M.; Järnberg, P.O.: Fluoride pharmacokinetics during acid-base balance changes in man. Eur. J. clin. Pharmacol. *18:* 189–194 (1980).

Ekstrand, J.; Koch, O.; Lindgren, L.E.; Petersson, L.G.: Pharmacokinetics of fluoride gels in children and adults. Caries Res. *15:* 213–220 (1981).

Ekstrand, J.; Koch, G.; Petersson, L.G.: Plasma fluoride concentrations in pre-school children after ingestion of fluoride tablets and toothpaste. Caries Res. *17:* 379–384 (1983).

Ericsson, Y.; Gydell, K.; Hammarskiöld, T.: Blood plasma fluoride: an indicator of skeletal fluoride content. Int. Res. Commun. Syst. *33* (1973).

Fejerskov, O.; Thylstrup, A.; Larsen, M.J.: Clinical and structure features and possible pathologic mechanisms of dental fluorosis. Scand. J. dent. Res. *85:* 510–534 (1977)

Guy, W.S.: Inorganic fluoride in human blood; in Johansen, Taves, Olsen, Continuing evaluation of the use of fluorides. Am. Ass. Adv. Sci., Wash. Select. Symp. 11, pp. 125–148 (Westview Press, Boulder 1979).

Guy, W.S.; Taves, D.R.; Brey, W.S., Jr.: Organic fluorocompounds in human plasma: prevalence and characterization; in Biochemistry involving carbon-fluorine bond. Am. Chem. Soc. Symp. Ser. No. 28, pp. 134–177 (1976).

Klein, H.: Dental effects of accidentally fluorinated water. I. Dental caries experience in deciduous and permanent teeth of school age children. J. Am. dent. Ass. *36:* 443–453 (1948).

Kunzel, W.: Effect of an interruption in water fluoridation on the caries prevalence of the primary and secondary dentition. Caries Res. *14:* 304–310 (1980).

Larson, R.H.; Mellberg, J.R.; Senning, R.: Experiments on local and systemic action of fluoride in caries inhibition in the rat. Archs oral Biol. *22:* 437–439 (1977).

Leatherwood, E.C.; Burnett, G.W.; Chandravejjsmarn, R.; Sirikaya, P.: Dental caries and dental fluorosis in Thailand. Am. J. Publ. Hlth *55:* 1792–1799 (1965).

LeCompte, E.J.; Whitford, G.M.: Pharmacokinetics of fluoride from APF gel and fluoride tablets in children. J. dent. Res. *61:* 469–472 (1982).

Lemke, C.W.; Dohertz, J.M.; Aria, M.C.: Controlled fluoridation: the dental effects of discontinuation in Antigo, Washington. J. Am. dent. Ass. *80:* 782–786 (1970).

Mellberg, J.R.; Singer, L.; Assimilation of fluoride by enamel throughout the life of the tooth; discussion. Caries Res. *11:* suppl. 1, pp. 101–105 (1977).

Mirth, D.B.; Adderly, D.D.; Amsbaugh, S.M.; Monell-Torrens, E.; Bowen, W.H.: Evaluation of oral and systemic controlled release fluoride in rats. J. dent. Res. *61:* 324, abstr. 1332 (1982).

Nanda, R.S.; Zipkin, L.; Doyle, J.; Horowitz, H.S.: Factors affecting the prevalence of dental fluorosis in Lucknow, India. Archs oral Biol. *19:* 781–792 (1974).

Poulsen, S.; Larsen, M.J.: Dental caries in relation to fluoride content of enamel in the primary dentition. Caries Res. *9:* 59–65 (1975).

Richards, A.; Larsen, M.J.; Fejerskov, O.; Thylstrup, A.: Fluoride content of buccal surface enamel and its relation to dental caries in children. Archs oral Biol. *22:* 425–428 (1977).

Russel, A.L.: Dental effects of exposure to fluoride-bearing Dakota sandstone waters at various ages and for various lengths of time. J. dent. Res. *28:* 600–612 (1949).

Singer, L.; Armstrong, W.D.: Regulation of human plasma fluoride concentration. J. appl. Physiol. *15:* 508–510 (1960).

Speirs, R.: Fluoride incorporation into developing enamel of permanent teeth in the domestic pig. Archs oral Biol. *20:* 877–883 (1975).

Taves, D.R.: Determination of submicromolar concentrations of fluoride in biological samples. Talanta *15:* 1015–1023 (1968).

Weatherell, J.; Deutsch, D.; Robinson, C.; Hallsworth, A.S.: Assimilation of fluoride by enamel throughout life of the tooth. Caries Res. *11:* suppl. 1, pp. 88–115 (1977).

Whitford, G.M.: Physiologic determinants of plasma fluoride concentrations. Proc. Int. Fluoride Symp., Logan 1982 (Pergamon Press, Salt Lake City, in press, 1983).

Whitford, G.M.; Pashley, D.H.: The effect of body fluid pH on fluoride distribution, toxicity and renal clearance; in Johansen, Taves, Olsen, Continuing evaluation of the use of fluorides. Am. Ass. Adv. Sci., Wash. Select. Symp. 11, pp. 187–221 (Westview Press, Boulder 1979).

Whitford, G.M.; Pashley, D.H.; Pearson, D.E.: Fluoride in gingival crevicular fluid and a new method for evaporative water loss corrections. Caries Res. *15:* 399–405 (1981).

Whitford, G.M.; Pashley, D.H.; Stringer, G.I.: Fluoride renal clearance. A pH-dependent event. Am. J. Physiol. *230:* 527–532 (1976).

Whitford, G.M.; Reynolds, K.E.: Plasma and developing enamel fluoride concentrations during chronic acid-base disturbances. J. dent. Res. *58:* 2058–2065 (1979).

Whitford, G.M.; Schuster, G.S.: Systemic versus waterborne fluoride and dental caries. J. dent. Res. *61:* 324, abstr. 1331 (1982).

Whitford, G.M.; Schuster, G.S.; Pashley, D.H.; Venkateswarlu, P.: Fluoride uptake by *Streptococcus mutans* 6715. Infect Immunity *18:* 680–687 (1977).

Dr. J. Ekstrand, Department of Cariology, School of Dentistry, Karolinska Institutet, Box 4064, S-141 04 Huddinge (Sweden)

Prevention and Therapy – Where from Here?

Moderator: H. Löe, Bethesda, Md., USA

Cariology Today. Int. Congr., Zürich 1983, pp. 279–284 (Karger, Basel 1984)

How Should Prevention Be Achieved?

K.G. König

Institute of Preventive and Community Dentistry, University of Nijmegen, The Netherlands

A large arsenal of effective dental preventive methods is available, but only a fraction of the tools and measures is widely used. During the last decades efforts to implement prevention were directed mainly to the community and group level, as exemplified by water fluoridation and school programs. At these levels a certain saturation seems to have been reached. Those communities where, e.g., water fluoridation made a chance have already got it; on the other hand communities in which fluoridation was not accepted, or where it was not feasible for technical reasons, most likely will not get it in the near future. 'Saturation' with public preventive methods, therefore, does not mean that there is no need for further action; it only means that all political and technical possibilities have been exhausted without success. In spite of considerable progress made by preventive dentistry on the community level and a remarkable decrease of caries rates among children of developed countries – even in non-fluoride areas [*Glass,* 1982] –, there are many groups and individuals at risk for which the right approach still has to be found and elaborated.

One possibility is individual prevention initiated and monitored by professionals in the private office. In contrast to implementation on the community and group level initiated by Public Health Authorities (backed up by WHO resolutions and documentations), no standard strategies have been generally accepted for implementation of individual preventive schemes. Individual prevention depends largely on the incidental personal 'philosophy' and motivational capacities available in a dental office.

Obviously, there is no lack of *standard technical procedures* for adequately applying fluoride preparations, teaching oral hygiene, giving dietary advice, and providing other special measures. However, technicalities is only one aspect of individual prevention; the other, still widely disregarded aspect is the bulk of *psychological problems* jeopardizing patient cooperation, and the present paper is dealing with a detail of this aspect.

The reasons for attention to patient behaviour, information, acceptance, and motivation are obvious. The time an average dental-minded patient spends in his dentist's chair per year will scarcely exceed a total of 2 h, and the total time he spends for preventive activities can be assumed to be no more than 1 h. During this hour (or fractions of it repeatedly) the dentist can actively intervene. However, since plaque bacteria do not sleep, during 8,759 of the 8,760 h of a year attacking forces threatening periodontal and dental health can only be kept under control by the patient himself. Therefore, the patient certainly must know what to do to keep his oral structures healthy, he must be motivated to do it continuously and to accept certain inconveniences inherent in a behaviour preserving oral health.

Without knowledge of self-applied preventive measures, acceptance and motivation by the patient, he or she cannot and will not put into effect his necessary own contribution to his individual prevention scheme.

Mühlemann [1977] is one of the few European dental experts who paid full attention not only to the technical, but also to the psychological side of individual prevention. The elements of *Mühlemann's* approach to the problem cover factual information on disease symptoms, aims and techniques of (daily) home care, and importance of recall visits. *Mühlemann* suggested a formal contract on duties and rights to be signed by the patient (not the dentist) which was even to include – for countries which have a social security or health insurance system – the party involved in financing treatment costs as the third partner.

Some doubts whether such a contract alone will work satisfactorily seem to have been present from the beginning, because *Mühlemann* [1977] himself states clearly: 'Patients (often unconsciously) do not appreciate scientific demonstrations of the lack of cleanliness in their mouths. Intimidation and/or punishment for oral neglect is not an appropriate tool to enhance cooperation with the dentist. The never-ending challenge of the patient to comply with professional recommendations is too much of a unidirectional, onesided act.' To exclude these adverse mechanisms it seems necessary to look into possibilities to eliminate anything intimidating, threatening, and unidirectional from any such contract.

Modern textbooks describe the 'psychological contract' as a relationship between members of a task-oriented group formed for the purpose of jointly accomplishing certain specific tasks [*Dworkin* et al., 1978]. In our case the task is to transfer knowledge about prevention from the dentist and his team to the patient, help him to acquire a positive attitude, and guide him in developing a behaviour instrumental in effectively performing preventive measures in everyday life. Psychologists advise not to put this contract in the form of a written, legally binding agreement specifying criteria and procedures for all aspects of the relationship, because this would interfere with the vitality of the relationship. On the contrary, the psychological contract should be dynamic, adaptive, and constantly open for renegotiation. *Visser* [1981] has developed a contract as a framework covering the main aspects of the dentist-patient relationship. *Visser* described the basic idea of the contract as follows: 'The well-informed patient himself determines, by the care he invests in his oral health, and in keeping with his individual oral and general condition, the level of dental treatment and thereby the prognosis.'

Implications of the contract for the dentist and his team are (1) relations between preventive and curative/restorative activities are made explicit by repetitive feedback; (2) the patient is learning to assume an active role in the relationship and recognizes his responsibilities; (3) the dentist accepts and respects the expectations and decisions of the patient and agrees to render his service at the level agreed upon; (4) the dentist accepts his role as guide and teacher, developing a message taking into account the given individual dental and oral situation, kind of therapy, preventive measures, and prognosis; (5) a favourable starting position for changes of behaviour is created for the patient; (6) the negotiations aim at openness and mutual confidence, and (7) repeated talks adapt the contract to assume a definite form – in this process the wall of misunderstandings between professionals and layman is removed.

One aspect regarding 'openness' in the dentist-patient relationship has received little attention so far in the dental literature, although every psychologist and many lay people are fully aware of the problem. We are not dealing here with the dentist-patient relationship per se, but with a sideline: the discrepancies between the conscious and the subconscious within the personality of the patient which interfere with the dentist-patient relationship. *Mühlemann* [1977] shortly touches the point by stating that 'patients (often unconsciously) do not appreciate scientific demonstration . . .' – they handle, with virtuosity, all Freudian defense mechanisms which can protect them against discovering their real situation and behaviour: repression, rationalization, and denial of reality.

Obviously, the dentist is not and should not assume the role of a psychiatrist. However, his strategy of motivating patients and making them adopt a better health-promoting behaviour may and in my opinion in the case of adult patients should always take into account the existence and the mechanisms of the subconscious.

An article in this context cannot be exhaustive. As an example let us assume the situation which usually prevails before the dentist starts his attempts to change a patient's habitual eating pattern. In this situation dentists usually try to retrieve anamnestically or by asking the patient to run a diary, how the patient's eating pattern looks like. As a result the dentist will be confronted with two possibilities: (1) a naive patient will tell or write the truth, and the dentist can 'demonstrate scientifically' that the patient takes in-between sweets much too often and is misbehaving grossly; (2) the sophisticated patients (that is the majority) will be reigned by defense mechanisms, and their true behaviour will not be revealed.

In the first case (a minority of adults) the patient will be offended, perhaps even deeply hurt; nevertheless, there is a good chance that in an ideal dentist-patient relationship dominated by mutual understanding and confidence the damage can be restored, but the question is: Was this necessary, if the patient could very easily and subtly have discovered this himself, without being forced to blush and feeling ashamed? The risk of getting demotivated certainly is not negligible.

In the second case of sophisticated patients, the majority will never confess their sins, and their 'lies' will presumably never be discovered by themselves, because their defense mechanisms most likely will be reinforced rather than diminished or abolished.

With an adequate strategy it is possible to minimize these hazards endangering a good, open patient-dentist relationship. The underlying idea is that eating habits as well as hygiene patterns belong to the strictly private life of an individual. Therefore, the dentist fully respecting the privacy of his patient will act wisely by building for him a golden bridge for retreat which will not damage his self-respect. The dentist can mention how many deviations from normality may occur in the busy social life of modern man: parties, birthdays, stress situations, travel, and so forth. The advice, therefore, is to practice for a few days on scribbling-paper before 'official records' are entered into the dietary history diary. Discovering the high frequency of abnormal situations, the unobserved patient is not forced to practice repression or denial of reality, but will 'choose' the innocent defense mechanism of rationalization: the sweets orgy at Aunt Clementine's birthday last Sunday, the trip to New York on Monday – these were exceptional days not representative for his normal pattern of food intake. Before the patient has to admit that his whole life is a series of such exceptions, he may make up his mind to live a more 'normal life' from then on, and – before he actually starts to write down his food intake for the records – he has made a good start in the direction of a more healthy eating pattern. There is nothing dishonest about this, because that is the way the subconscious functions, and the mechanism is absolutely normal. Still, the patient may evade the truth, but the approach described may increase the chances that a patient, not intimidated by the presence of the dentist/health professional, choses to let a lot of his discoveries from the subconscious emerge into the realm of his consciousness – without having to be ashamed of anybody. Let us keep in mind that the preponderance of powerful defense mechanisms made *S. Freud* choose for a non-directive approach in his psychoanalytical method.

This strategy of a non-directive approach in trying to implement dental mindedness also implies that it may be better to leave much of the refresher counseling to members of the dental team who usually are approached by the patient without shyness. This means that enquiries, explications, and corrections should be dealt with by the hygienist or other auxiliaries in charge rather than the academically trained dentist. The feasibility of this procedure has been demonstrated [*Hetland* et al., 1982].

In conclusion, it may be stated that there is no lack of technically mature preventive tools, for mass and group application, but also for individual measures. What is needed in the future is broader individual acceptance (by mediators as well as individuals of the target group) for patient-applied methods and an improved psychological approach to get them implemented in everyday practice. Large-scale multidisciplinary research into these problems is necessary.

References

Dworkin, S.F.; Ference, T.P.; Giddon, D.B.: Behavioral science and dental practice (Mosby, St. Louis 1978).

Glass, R.L.: The First International Conference on the Declining Prevalence of Dental Caries. J. dent. Res. *61:* 1301–1383 (1982).

Hetland, L.; Midtun, N.; Kristoffersen, T.: Effect of oral hygiene instructions given by paraprofessional personnel. Community Dent. oral Epidemiol. *10:* 8–14 (1982).

Mühlemann, H.R.: Psychological and chemical mediators of gingival health. J. prev. Dent. *4:* 6–17 (1977).

Visser, R.S.H.: Relatie tandarts-patiënt; in Handboek voor de tandheelkundige praktijk, chapter A1–2 (Bohn, Scheltema en Holkema, Utrecht 1981).

Prof. K.G. König, University of Nijmegen, Department of Preventive and Community Dentistry, PO Box 9101, NL–Nijmegen (The Netherlands)

Cariology Today. Int. Congr., Zürich 1983, pp. 285–292 (Karger, Basel 1984)

Vaccination, a Dead Issue?

Bo Krasse, Barry C. McBride

Department of Oral Biology, University of British Columbia, Vancouver, B. C., Canada

Introduction

Caries vaccines and mucosal defence mechanisms have been thoroughly reviewed in recent publications [13, 14]. These reviews illustrate the tremendous effort devoted to research in the area. However, the title chosen by the editor of this symposium 'A Dead Issue' appears to reflect a growing pessimism concerning the possibility of producing an effective caries vaccine. What has happened to dull the enthusiasm for developing an immunological approach for the control of dental caries? The basic need has not changed. It would be beneficial to develop a safe reliable economical means to control the disease. By analogy to other microbial diseases it would appear reasonable to assume that periodic immunization would provide protection against colonization by cariogenic microorganisms and, therefore, offer a high level of protection against dental caries. Analysis of the unique characteristics of the disease may explain why a successful vaccine has not been developed.

Unlike smallpox or measles the etiologic agent is part of the indigenous flora. Only a certain percentage of dental caries is due to *Streptococcus mutans* and consequently an *S. mutans* vaccine would only provide partial protection. The organism is acquired during infancy and generally remains with us for life. The implication is that the immune system must respond to the bacteria on a daily, not a periodic basis. It is possible that constant exposure to an antigen leads to the development of tolerance or to immune exclusion.

Dental caries is a disease process which develops on a nonliving body surface. The formation of a lesion involves destruction of tissue, but does not bring the organism into contact with the immune system, and consequently there is no stimulation of immunoglobulin synthesis.

In other words the immune system cannot differentiate between a healthy and a diseased state.

Cariogenic organisms primarily reside on body surfaces which are isolated from the activity of phagocytic cells and complement. Antibodies will work by preventing colonization, e.g., by interfering with adherence to pellicle or plaque.

The hard tissue does not shed, and consequently the tooth is colonized by a population which is relatively stable and does not have to continually recolonize as is the case of organisms growing on an epithelial surface.

The microbial heterogeneity of the oral system poses problems not normally encountered in diseases which have been effectively controlled by vaccination. The latter are usually an interaction of the host with a single organism, whereas in the former the tooth is populated by a large mixed population of organisms. Some of these organisms may combine by nonimmunogenic mechanisms with antibody, and others will share cross-reacting antigens. The net effect will be a reduction of the antibody available for reaction with S. mutans. Antibody may even promote adherence by binding to the tooth [10]. This mechanism might explain why immunization also can cause an increased caries incidence [3].

Mechanism of Action

Despite the limitations discussed above, a number of animal experiments have indicated that immunization against S. mutans is feasible. An important question is how is this protection conferred. Theoretically it could be achieved by immune components from serum and by sIgA antibodies in salivary secretions.

When the teeth erupt, local inflammation is common [19], and during this process serum antibodies directed against S. mutans could stimulate opsonization and phagocytosis. Such antibodies could also inhibit the initial adherence of S. mutans to the teeth. In vitro, an inhibitory effect of serum antibodies both on adherence and on glycosyl transferase has been demonstrated. In animal experiments a lower number of S. mutans has been found in plaque material from immunized animals than from control animals. Thus, parenteral immunization directed against S. mutans could favor the establishment of a noncariogenic microflora on teeth. Such indigenous flora could prevent or delay the colonization of pathogenic *S. mutans*. As the teeth are highly susceptible to dental caries immediately after eruption, a delay in colonization of *S. mutans* might be the explanation for the caries reduction observed in experiments on primates.

The immune components from serum enter the oral cavity via the gingival crevicular fluid. Consequently, specific serum antibodies could influence the colonization of *S. mutans* in the gingival domain.

The other possible mechanism by which immunization could work is via salivary IgA antibodies. Such antibodies have been found to protect experimental animals against both *S. mutans* infection and dental caries.

Salivary IgA antibodies in human saliva have been found to inhibit the attachment of *Streptococcus sanguis* to epithelial cells, but a corresponding inhibitory effect was not found in recent adherence experiments with *S. mutans* and hydroxyapatite [7]. In the latter study it is possible that the sIgA preparation did not contain antibodies directed towards relevant cell wall adhesins.

Some findings in humans support the concept that salivary IgA antibodies could interfere with the establishment of *S. mutans* and protect against dental caries. For example, after challenge with streptomycin-resistant *S. mutans* these microorganisms were more rapidly eliminated from the oral cavity of persons with a higher antibody activity than from persons with lower antibody activity [4, 8]. The observation that IgA-deficient subjects show higher levels of caries than normal controls supports the view that salivary IgA antibodies could have a caries-protective effect [9].

In animals active immunization with whole cells, cell wall proteins, and glucosyltransferase has resulted in the production of serum and salivary antibodies as well as protection against *S. mutans* infection and dental caries. There is, however, a definite difference in response between rodents and primates (table I). Both parenteral and peroral immunization is effective in the rodent models, but in primates a salivary IgA response has not yet been obtained after peroral immunization [11, 20]. In humans this route of immunization has resulted in a salivary IgA response in some studies [4, 13] but not in others [2, 8]. Thus, despite a great deal of effort and a number of positive animal experiments, a series of critical questions remain unanswered.

Before we can decide whether the issue is 'dead' or 'alive', we must have answered the following questions:

Table I. Effect of vaccination against *S. mutans* in rodents, primates, and humans

Immunization route	Antibody		Reduction	
	serum	saliva	*S. mutans*	caries
Rodents				
Parenteral	+	+	+	+
Peroral	+	+	+	+
Primates				
Parenteral		+	+	+
Peroral	–	–		
Intraductal	+	+	+	
Humans				
Peroral		±	±	

± = Positive effect in some studies, but not in others.

(1) Which antigen will provide the most effective protection? Possibly the answer is a combination of purified antigens representing the different adhesins and enzymes responsible for colonization. It is essential that the antigens will not cross-react with human tissue.

(2) Will sIgA or IgG, or a combination of antibodies, be required for protection? IgG may be effective during tooth eruption, but a combination of IgG and sIgA may be necessary for protection of erupted teeth.

(3) How do we stimulate man to secrete specific IgA, and will immunity last for long enough periods to be practical? A combination of parenteral and peroral immunization may be necessary [17]. It is possible that adjuvants will promote the adsorption of antigen either in the gut [6] or through retrograde transfer into the minor salivary glands [15, 18].

(4) Do strains of *S. mutans* differ markedly in their cariogenicity? If there is a wide spectrum of pathogenecity, it will be necessary to define what creates virulence and identify those antigens unique to this state. For example, recent studies have indicated that freshly isolated strains of *S. mutans* possess antigens which are lost upon subculture. Loss of these antigens correlates with a decreased ability to adhere to saliva-coated hydroxyapatite [12, 16, 21].

Discussion

Given that *S. mutans* is not the only cariogenic microorganism and that a series of other factors influence the development of the disease, the question arises as to what extent successful vaccination against *S. mutans* could reduce the incidence of dental caries.

In a recent study it was found that children who had become infected with *S. mutans* before the age of 2 years had 10.6 dmfs at 4 years of age. For children in whom *S. mutans* had not been detected the corresponding dmfs figure was 0.3 [1]. In a study on 13- to 14-year-old children who were followed for 3 years, the children who had $> 10^6$ *S. mutans* per milliliter saliva developed 4–5 times as many new carious lesions as those who were not infected [21].

These studies were made in Scandinavia where most children are exposed to various caries-preventive programs from an early age. The figures thus indicate that a considerable caries reduction could be obtained, if colonization of *S. mutans* were prevented or reduced at the time of eruption of both deciduous and permanent teeth. This means that successful vaccination directed against *S. mutans* could be a valuable adjunct to other caries-preventive measures.

Antimicrobial treatment of highly infected individuals drastically reduces the number of *S. mutans* in plaque and saliva, and this effectively reduces the caries risk. After antimicrobial treatment, however, the number of *S. mutans* often rises again and sometimes to values which are higher than those before the treatment. One explanation for this reoccurrence could be that antibodies directed against *S. mutans* disappear over time in the oral fluids due to lack of local stimulation and the short memory of the IgA antibody system. This means that vaccination could be supplemental to antimicrobial treatment in persons highly infected with *S. mutans*.

Vaccination could also be a valuable adjunct for handicapped persons and persons with a reduced salivary secretion rate. As with influenza and pneumococcal vaccines, a caries vaccine in the Western world might be of greatest value to persons at a high risk. In addition, vaccination would probably be more acceptable than trying to alter either human behavior or the social environment. The difficulties in changing sucrose consumption and in introducing water fluoridation illustrate this problem with regard to dental caries.

In Third World countries on the other hand, the situation is quite

different. There a rapid increase in caries has been observed in children
and adolescents. The low dentist to population ratio and the lack of
organized dental health care limit the possibilities of utilizing conventional caries-preventive methods. The existence of basic medical health
care systems might, however, form a basis for the use of a caries
vaccine. Thus, it is obvious that vaccination against dental caries could
be of great value for selected groups at a high caries risk in some
societies and as a general public health measure in others.

The benefit of a caries vaccine must, of course, be weighed against
the risks. A primary requirement for a vaccine as for drugs in general
is that it be safe. Streptococcal vaccines seem to present special problems, as vaccines against beta-hemolytic streptococci are not yet available. The diseases caused by these microorganisms are considerably
more severe than dental caries, and, consequently, a vaccine against
hemolytic streptococci ought to be more desirable than a vaccine
against *S. mutans*. Dental caries is, however, still a serious sociomedical
problem, and the inclusion of a caries vaccine into the armamentarium
of caries-preventive measures might be attractive for the public health
authorities in many countries.

Thus, research towards development of a caries vaccine seems to
be justified from the public health point of view. There are, however,
other reasons which make the research in this area active and vigorous.
The search for answers to the questions posed above has led to an
increased understanding of how the secretory IgA antibody system
works. We have also made a number of observations which support the
concept that research of a more basic character often leads to information which is essential for solving other important health problems [5].

Our conclusion must, therefore, be that vaccination against dental
caries is not a dead issue. It is a difficult problem, and vaccination may
turn out to be impractical in humans, but the issue as such is relevant
and highly vital.

References

1   Alaluusua, S.; Olli-Veikko, R.: Longitudinal study of *Streptococcus mutans* estab-
     lishment and dental caries experience in children from 2 to 4 years old. Scand. J.
     dent. Res. (submitted 1983).
2   Bonta, C.Y.; Linzer, R.; Emmings, F.; Evans, R.T.; Genco, R.J.: Human oral

infectivity and immunization studies with *Streptococcus mutans* strain B13. J. dent. Res. *51:* suppl. 17, p. 143 (1979).

3 Burckhardt, J.J.; Guggenheim, B.: Increased smooth surface caries incidence in gnotobiotic rats immunized with *Actinomyces viscosus*. Caries Res. *14:* 56–59 (1980).

4 Cole, M.F.; Emilson, C.G.; Ciardi, J.E.; Bowen, W.H.: Induction of secretory immunity against *Streptococcus mutans* in human subjects (Abstract). J. dent. Res. *60:* 509 (1981).

5 Comroe, J.H.; Dripps, R.D.: Scientific basis for the support of biomedical sciences. Science *192:* 105–108 (1976).

6 Evans, R.T.; Riepenhoff-Talty, M.; Suzuki, H.; Linzer, R.; Ogra, P.L.; Genco, R.J.: Characterization of liposome-antigen mixtures used to induce secretory immune responses. J. dent. Res. *62:* 193 (1983).

7 Gahnberg, L.; Olsson, J.; Krasse, B.; Carlen, A.: Interference of salivary immuno-globulin A antibodies and other salivary fractions with adherence of *Streptococcus mutans* to hydroxyapatite. Infect. Immunity *37:* 401–406 (1982).

8 Gahnberg, L.; Krasse, B.: Salivary immunoglobulin A antibodies and recovery from challenge of *Streptococcus mutans* after oral administration of *Streptococcus mutans* vaccine in humans. Infect. Immunity *39:* 514–519 (1983).

9 Legler, D.W.; McGhee, J.K.; Lynch, D.P.; Mestecky, J.F.; Schaefer, M.E.; Carson, J.; Bradley, E.L., Jr.: Immunodeficiency disease and dental caries in man. Archs oral Biol. *26:* 905–910 (1981).

10 Liljemark, W.F.; Blomquist, C.G.; Ofstehage, J.C.: Aggregation and adherence of *Streptococcus sanguis:* role of human salivary immunoglobulin A. Infect. Immunity *26:* 1104–1110 (1979).

11 Linzer, R.; Evans, R.T.; Emmings, F.G.; Genco, R.J.: Use of combined immuniza-tion routes in induction of a salivary immunoglobulin A response to *Streptococcus mutans* in *Macaca fascicularis*. Infect. Immunity *31:* 345–351 (1981).

12 McBride, B.C.; Shim, M.; Olsson, J.; Krasse, B.: Chemical and immunological differences between cell surfaces of hydrophilic and hydrophobic strains of *Strepto-coccus mutans* (submitted).

13 McGhee, J.R.; Michalek, S.M.: Immunobiology of dental caries: microbial aspects and local immunity. A. Rev. Microbiol. *35:* 595–638 (1981).

14 McNabb, P.C.; Tomasi, T.B.: Host defense mechanisms at mucosal surfaces. A. Rev. Microbiol. *35:* 477–496 (1981).

15 Nair, P.N.R.; Schroeder, H.E.: Retrograde access of antigens to the minor salivary gland in the monkey *Macaca fascicularis*. Archs oral Biol. *28:* 145–152 (1983).

16 Olsson, J.; Westergren, G.: Hydrophobic surface properties of oral streptococci. FEMS Microbiol. Lett. *15:* 319–323 (1982).

17 Pierce, N.F.; Sack, B.R.: Immune response of the intestinal mucosa to cholera toxoid. J. infect. Dis. *136:* suppl., pp. 113–117 (1977).

18 Schroeder, H.E.; Moreillon, M.-C.; Nair, P.N.R.: Architecture of minor salivary gland duct/lymphoid jollicle associations and the possible antigen – recognition sites in the monkey *Macaca fascicularis*. Archs oral Biol. *28:* 133–143 (1983).

19 Seward, M.: Local disturbances attributed to eruption of the human primary dentition. Br. dent. J. *130:* 72–77 (1971).

20   Walker, J.: Antibody responses of monkeys to oral and local immunization with *Streptococcus mutans*. Infect. Immunity *31:* 61–70 (1981).
21   Zickert, I.; Emilson, C.G.; Krasse, B.: Correlation of level and duration of *Streptococcus mutans* infection with incidence of dental caries. Infect. Immunity *39:* 982–985 (1983).
22   Orstavik, J.; Orstavik, D.: Influence of in vitro propagation on the adhesive qualities of *Streptococcus mutans* isolated from saliva. Acta odont. scand. *40:* 57–63 (1982).

B. Krasse, MD, Department of Oral Biology, University of British Columbia, Vancouver, B.C., V6T 1Y6 (Canada)

Cariology Today. Int. Congr., Zürich 1983, pp. 293–300 (Karger, Basel 1984)

Antimicrobials, Can They Be Effective

Walter J. Loesche

University of Michigan School of Dentistry, School of Medicine, Ann Arbor, Mich., USA

Introduction

For antimicrobials to be effective, therapeutic dosages must be delivered for a sufficient, but finite time period, to sites in which an infection is occurring. This simple therapeutic principle has rarely, until recently, been applied in dentistry to clinical trials of antimicrobial agents. This is because dentists have never had a treatment philosophy which had as its therapeutic goal the elimination or suppression of the microbes which specifically contributed to the decay process. This situation has changed with the demonstration that *Streptococcus mutans* and possibly lactobacilli and *Actinomyces viscosus* are important human odontopathogens [*Loesche,* 1982].

Nonspecific Plaque Hypothesis

Since 1890, when *Miller* introduced the chemoparasitic theory of dental decay, the caries process has been considered bacteriologically nonspecific. This opinion, referred to hereafter as the nonspecific plaque hypothesis (NSPH), views all bacterial species residing on the tooth surfaces as having the capacity to contribute to the acid attack on the enamel surfaces. As these bacteria are indigenous to the teeth and are found in all individuals, no need was seen for bacteriological diagnostic criteria to identify individuals at risk. Accordingly, no selection criteria for treatment were used, as the bacteria found in a patient with rampant caries were presumed to be similar to the bacteria found in a caries-inactive individual. The main difference between health and disease was the magnitude of the plaque accumulation.

Thus, in most clinical studies of antimicrobials performed under the NSPH, the subjects were not selected from a population that had active decay or periodontal disease, but from one which was most conveniently available. The therapeutic goal invariably was reduced or no plaque accumulation. Since plaque is continuously forming on the tooth surfaces, any successful agent would have to be used daily, and as all people form plaque, all people would have to be treated. Such an open-ended treatment schedule, in which all people should be more or less continuously treated, is unprecedented in antimicrobial therapy. No chemical antimicrobial agent with any degree of potency would be safe when administered in this fashion [*Loesche, 1976*].

Despite the problems inherent in the legacy of the NSPH, some promising drugs have been found, such as fluoride and chlorhexidine, which may make remarkable therapeutic agents. Thus, if these antimicrobial agents were used only in those patients with evidence of a dental infection, or known to be at risk to such an infection, i.e., patients with radiation xerostomia, then one might expect significant reductions in the caries score. Recent reports [*Zickert* et al., 1982; *Driezen and Brown, 1976*] indicate that these agents used in this focussed manner achieved impressive clinical reductions in dental decay.

The Specific Plaque Hypothesis

Keyes [1960] and *Fitzgerald and Keyes* [1960] demonstrated the microbial specificity of dental decay in animal models. These classic studies form the basis for the specific plaque hypothesis (SPH) [*Loesche, 1976*], which views certain plaques as being odontopathic, because they are colonized and/or dominated by one or more bacterial types which are responsible for a measurable amount of dental decay. These odontopathic species would include *S. mutans* and Lactobacillus species in coronal surface decay and *A. viscosus* and *S. mutans* in root surface decay [*Loesche, 1982*].

The SPH does not state that these bacterial species are responsible for all dental decay, but rather that they are responsible for a measurable amount of decay, with the expectation that this amount will be biologically significant. The SPH recognizes unique oral microbial ecosystems and the existence of a dynamic interplay of host and dietary variables which can cause changes in these ecosystems. Implicit in the SPH is the concept of a nondisease-associated plaque. For practical purposes this nondisease-associated plaque is simply plaque which is not dominated by known odontopathogens.

The goal of therapy is to suppress the cariogenic plaque(s) and to replace them with nondiseased plaques. This therapeutic goal may be realized, if antimicrobial modalities, such as mechanical debridement and chemical agents, can be applied with sufficient intensity, so as to achieve for short periods of time on the tooth surface some semblance of 'sterility'. If such 'sterilization' can be obtained, then the newly forming plaque will be derived from organisms in the bathing saliva and will contain high proportions of *Streptococcus sanguis* and *Streptococcus mitis* and low proportions of *S. mutans*. This is because the affinity of the saliva-coated tooth surface for *S. sanguis* and *S. mitis* is appreciably higher than its affinity for *S. mutans* [*van Houte and Green*, 1974; *Clark* et al., 1978]. In fact, if the salivary levels of *S. mutans* are below 10^3 colony-forming units (CFU) per milliliter, it is unlikely that even fissure surfaces will become colonized by *S. mutans* [*Svanberg and Loesche*, 1977].

Treatment According to the SPH

Diagnosis of an Odontopathic Infection

The essential criterion for treatment according to the SPH is a diagnosis of an odontopathic infection. In the past, this could only be made retrospectively by the numeration of the actual lesions. But now, given the documentation of the important role of *S. mutans* and Lactobacillus species in caries initiation and progression [*Loesche*, 1982], the diagnosis can and should be based upon both microbiological and clinical criteria.

Children with salivary *S. mutans* levels above 10^6/ml have been considered as having a high caries risk [*Bratthall*, 1980; *Zickert* et al., 1982]. Sterile occlusal fissures can be colonized by as few as 3,000 *S. mutans* per milliliter saliva [*Svanberg and Loesche*, 1977], whereas about 45,000 *S. mutans* per milliliter are needed to reliably colonize a smooth surface [*van Houte and Green*, 1974]. This would suggest that if the salivary levels of *S. mutans* were less than 10^4/ml, the patient's teeth are

Table I. Clinical trials of antimicrobial agents in which entry into study was based upon a diagnosis of high caries risk

Study	Diagnostic criteria	Treatment	Number of new lesions	Comment
Antibiotics				
Dreizen and Spies [1951]	high DFS	(1) no treatment (2) placebo (3) furadroxyl 7.5 mg/day	4.2/year 3.3/year 0.9/year	72% compared to placebo
DePaola et al. [1977]	plaque levels of *S. mutans*	(1) no treatment (2) 3% vancomycin gel daily at school	4.4/year 3.4/year	significant reduction
Loesche et al. [1977]	high DFS high *S. mutans*	(1) placebo (2) 5% kanamycin daily for 1 week	3.5/30 months 1.9/30 months	45% reduction
Fluoride				
Koch [1970]	high DFS	(1) OH (2) OH + 0.2% NaF dentifrice	9.5/year 3.7/year	60% reduction
Dreizen and Brown [1976]	radiation xerostomia	(1) OH + placebo gel (2) OH + 1% NaF gel daily (3) OH + 1% NaF gel + sucrose restriction	2.5/month 0.1/month 0.05/month	90% reduction compared to placebo
Loesche and Pink; cited in *Loesche* [1982]	high DFS high *S. mutans* in plaque	(1) placebo gel (2) 1.23% NaF gel daily for 1 week	5.9/30 months 4.0/30 months	32% reduction after 3 years

Combined modalities

Klock and Krasse [1978]	high salivary S. mutans and/or lactobacilli	(1) no treatment (2) OH + prof. cleaning with 5% MFP paste + dietary + sealants (a) above given once/month (b) above given twice/month	6.8/2 years 2.4/2 years 1.3/2 years	65–80% reduction in caries, but expensive
Zickert et al. [1982]	high salivary S. mutans and/or lactobacilli	(1) no treatment (2) 1% chlorhexidine for 2 weeks + sealant – retreatment with chlorhexidine when salivary S. mutans $> 2.5 \times 10^5$/ml	20.8/3 years 3.9/3 years	80% reduction in subjects with S. mutans $> 10^6$/ml

Preventive treatment

Kohler et al. [1982, 1983]	high salivary S. mutans in mothers of infants	(1) no treatment (2) OH + dietary + prof. cleaning with 0.2% NaF solution + daily use of 0.05% NaF rinse + caries excavation – treatment with 1% chlorhexidine for 2 weeks when salivary S. mutans $> 3 \times 10^5$/ml		63% of infants in no treatment group infected with S. mutans compared to 19% in treated group

OH = oral hygiene; MFP = mono-fluoro-phosphate.

not likely to become newly colonized by *S. mutans*. This value of 10^4/ ml could then be viewed as an idealized therapeutic end point of treatment. In practice, a more realistic goal has been to retreat patients, when the salivary *S. mutans* levels are greater than 2.5×10^5/ml [*Kohler* et al., 1982; *Zickert* et al., 1982].

Clinical Studies in High Caries Risk Patients

Topical fluorides reduce the incidence and severity of dental decay. It is apparent that some of these effects can be accounted for by an antimicrobial action of fluoride on the plaque flora. However, because most of these studies were not targeted upon high caries risk children in a population, they will not be considered in this brief review. Instead, only those clinical trails of antimicrobial agents in which patient entry into the study was based on either a clinical or a bacteriological diagnosis of high caries risk will be discussed.

Nine such studies are described in table I. All show impressive clinical reductions in caries ranging from 32 to 90% reduction, dependent upon the frequency of treatment. This beneficial effect can be obtained with antibiotics such as furadroxyl, vancomycin, or kanamycin, with several fluoride formulations, and with chlorhexidine.

The treatment efficacy of any one of these antimicrobials may be more a function of the initial level of *S. mutans* infection and the adequacy of treatment, rather than any unique antimicrobial action of the drug. This is best seen in the clinical trial of chlorhexidine and sealants used in 13- to 14-year-old teenagers [*Zickert* et al., 1982]. The treatment and no treatment groups were compared as a function of the initial salivary *S. mutans* levels. The treatment regimen caused a caries reduction of 2–4 surfaces in the groups that initially had less than 10^6 CFU/ml saliva, but a reduction of 17 surfaces in the group initially greater than 10^6 CFU/ml.

A caries reduction was obtained with treatment as minimal as 1 week unsupervised usage of 1.23% fluoride gel, immediately following the placement of dental restorations in young children who had rampant decay of the primary dentition [*Loesche,* 1982]. The unsupervised usage of these gels, for 1 week at 6- to 8-month intervals over a 3-year period resulted in about a 30% reduction in occlusal fissure caries in the newly erupting first molars. Part of this reduction was explained by assuming that the fluoride suppressed the *S. mutans* levels on the primary teeth to the extent that, when the molars erupted, they did not become initially infected with a cariogenic flora.

This scenario, predicted by the SPH, is analogous to the investigation being conducted in Sweden where mothers with high levels of salivary *S. mutans* are treated by combined mechanical and chemical modalities, so as to interrupt the passage of *S. mutans* to their infants [*Kohler* et al., 1982]. In those instances in which a reduction of *S. mutans* below the 3×10^5 CFU/ml saliva threshold was achieved in the mother, the establishment of *S. mutans* in her infant was prevented or delayed. 16 infants of successfully treated mothers have reached the age of 36 months. 3 of them are infected, versus 17 out of 27 in the control group [*Kohler* et al., 1983]. These findings show that the spread of *S. mutans* can be delayed or prevented by measures directed against the source of the infection. It now remains to be documented whether the children of the treated mothers have significantly less decay relative to the children of the untreated mothers.

These studies (table I) clearly demonstrate that antimicrobials can be effective in reducing dental decay when directed against a targeted organism such as *S. mutans*. It is likely that agents with some degree of substantivity on the tooth surface, such as fluoride or chlorhexidine, or are capable of penetrating the white spot lesion, such as fluoride [*Loesche,* 1982], will be the agents of choice.

References

Bratthall, D.: Selection for prevention of high caries risk groups. J. dent. Res. *59:* 2178–2182 (1980).

Clark, W.B.; Bammann, L.L.; Gibbons, R.J.: Comparative estimates of bacterial affinities and adsorption sites on hydroxyapatite surfaces. Infect. Immunity *19:* 846–852 (1978).

De Paola, P.F.; Jordan, H.V.; Soparkar, P.M.: Inhibition of dental caries in school children by topically applied vancomycin. Archs oral Biol. *23:* 187–192 (1977).

Dreizen, S.; Brown, L.R.: Xerostomia and dental caries; in Loesche, Stiles, O'Brien, Proc. Microbial Aspects of Dental Caries. Microbiology, suppl. 1, p. 263 (1976).

Dreizen, S.; Spies, T.D.: Effectiveness of a chewing gum containing nitrofuran in the prevention of dental caries. J. Am. dent. Ass. dento Cosmos *43:* 147–153 (1951).

Fitzgerald, R.J.; Keyes, P.H.: Demonstration of the etiologic role of streptococci in experimental caries in the hamster. J. Am. dent. Ass. dent. Cosmos *61:* 9–19 (1960).

Houte, J. van; Green, D.B.: Relationship between the concentration of bacteria in saliva and the colonization of teeth in humans. Infect. Immunity *9:* 624–630 (1974).

Keyes, P.H.: The infectious and transmissible nature of experimental dental caries. Archs oral Biol. *1:* 304–320 (1960).

Klock, B.; Krasse, B.: The effect of caries preventive measures in children with high numbers of *S. mutans* and lactobacilli. Scand. J. dent. Res. *86:* 221–230 (1978).

Koch, G.: Selection and caries prophylaxis of children with high caries activity. Odont. Revy *21:* 71–82 (1970).

Kohler, B.; Andreen, I.; Jonsson, B.; Haltquist, E.: Effect of caries preventive measures on *Streptococcus mutans* and lactobacilli in selected mothers. Scand. J. dent. Res. *90:* 102–108 (1982).

Kohler, B.; Bratthall, D.; Krasse, B.: Preventive measures in mothers influence the establishment of the bacterium *Streptococcus mutans* in their infants. Archs oral Biol. *28:* 225–231 (1983).

Loesche, W.J.: Chemotherapy of dental plaque infections. Oral Sci. Rev. *9:* 63–105 (1976).

Loesche, W.J.: Dental caries: a treatable infection (Thomas, Springfield 1982).

Loesche, W.J.; Bradbury, D.R.; Woolfolk, M.P.: Reduction of dental decay in rampant caries individuals following short-term kanamycin treatment. J. dent. Res. *56:* 254–265 (1977).

Miller, W.D.: The microorganisms of the human mouth (White Manufacturing Co., Philadelphia 1890).

Svanberg, M.L.; Loesche, W.J.: Salivary concentrations of *Streptococcus mutans* and *Streptococcus sanguis* and the colonization of artificial fissures in man. Archs oral Biol. *22:* 441–447 (1977).

Zickert, I.; Emilson, C.G.; Krasse, B.: Effect of caries prevention methods in children highly infected with *S. mutans*. Archs oral Biol. *27:* 861–868 (1982).

Walter J. Loesche, MD, University of Michigan School of Dentistry,
School of Medicine, Ann Arbor, MI (USA)

Cariology Today. Int. Congr., Zürich 1983, pp. 301–307 (Karger, Basel 1984)

Fissure Sealants – Then, Now and the Future

K. W. Stephen

Department of Oral Medicine and Pathology, University of Glasgow
Dental School, Glasgow, Scotland

In 1973, *Buonocore* [3] reported on the use of the UV-polymerized bis-GMA sealant, Nuva-seal (L. D. Caulk Co.), achieving 99% retention at 1 year and 87% at 2 years, only 1% of sealed surfaces becoming carious compared to 60% of controls. Other early studies also claimed high success rates but, of these, only *Ulvestad* [30] used erupting first molars of 5- to 7-year-olds, although 50% of these teeth have been shown to be carious within 1 year of eruption [14]. In addition, blind examination methods were not used by these academic/hospital-based staff.

In 1973, an attempt was made in Scotland to seal 573 such teeth under blind clinical field conditions by non-academic public dental service staff [23], using a new UV sealant TP2206 (since marketed as Alphaseal, Amalgamated Dental Ltd.), although most trials to date had used Nuva-seal. Unfortunately only 2.3% retention was found at 1 year. However, by 1975, others had reported poor Nuva-seal retention in 5- to 8-year-olds [6, 28, 31].

Early Laboratory Studies

In view of the poor TP2206 results, a series of investigations was initiated, these being directed both at the resins and their polymerizing sources. As a result, reasons for TP2206 (and Alphaseal) failure were demonstrated, both resins being incapable of setting at depth due to inclusion of a fluorescent dye and excessive catalyst [34]. Furthermore, while the UV output of the production Alphalite was superior to any Nuva-lite tested, the UV source used in the Scot's study was inferior and could have affected polymerization. Nonetheless, the Nuva-lite geometry was poor and the quartz tip had to be scanned for adequate UV distribution. The intensity of Nuva-lite bulbs varied and an exposure time of at least 45 s was required compared to the manufacturer's recommended 30 s [33]. The H_3PO_4 etchant concentration was not found to be critical [32], provided between 30 and 50% w/w was used with adequate post-etch washing [1], these laboratory measurements having been validated by enamel/sealant bond strength testing which proved superior to earlier predictions based purely on histological observation [19].

Thus, a further Nuva-seal study was undertaken where an unsupervised community therapist placed sealant in 241 first molars using a revised schedule. Here, 93.3% retention was obtained at 1 year [23], and a subsequent double-blind, contralateral trial showed 98.4% retention after a similar period, in 6- to 7-year-old children, compared to only 76.6% for Alphaseal [24].

Other Materials (Unfilled)

Of the unsealed self-curing (SC) resins, Delton (Johnson & Johnson Ltd.) has probably received most attention. However, results vary as UK data has shown it to be inferior to Nuva-seal. *Rock* et al. [16] achieved only 53% retention at 1 year although *Brooks* et al. [2] had 96.4% success with Delton in 5- to 8-year-olds, against only 86.3% for Nuva-seal. *McCune* et al. [10] reported 88% retention in similar teeth at 3 years and *Sheykholeslam and Houpt* [18], 85% at 2 years. It would seem that operator variability, perhaps coupled with geometry problems and inadequate exposure of the Nuva-lite, might explain these differences (see below).

In a further study with Delton and a new visible light (VL) polymerized non-filled sealant (ICI Ltd.), 2 academics had only 76% Delton retention at 1 year, with 75% for the ICI resin, in 8-year-olds [17]. A similar trial produced 84% Delton adherence compared to 74% for the ICI system [5].

The other non-filled SC resin in common use is the Concise White Sealant System (3M Co.) reported on by *Richardson* et al. [15] and *Simonsen* [20]. In the former paper, 86% success was claimed at 2 years in 7-year-olds while 96.1% was obtained in the latter study on 1019 teeth of 153 patients aged between 5 and 15 years. Also, at 1 year,

Simonsen [20] claimed 98.9% deciduous retention. Newer European products, e.g. Helioseal (Vivadent Schaan) (VL) and Contact-seal (Kerr-Sybron Corp.) (SC) have been introduced, but there is scant clinical data although their abrasion resistance is poor [29].

Filled Resins

The first commercially available filled resin was the SC Kerr Pit and Fissure Sealant (Kerr-Sybron Corp.), but only *Charbeneau and Dennison* [4] have reported a 79.2% retention rate at 1 year in 5- to 8-year-olds. When Nuva-cote (Caulk Co.) appeared, experiments showed its setting time, depth of polymerization, abrasion resistance and bond strength to be close to the heavily filled restorative, Nuva-fil (Caulk Co.), which was considered the best of a series studied [12]. The related experimental SC material, SCS (Caulk Co.), ran a close third while the unfilled resins Delton, Nuva-seal and Concise White Sealant were found to wear twice as rapidly. More recently, further filled resins have been marketed, e.g. Prismashield (Caulk Co.) (VL) and Estiseal (Kulzer GmbH) (SC and VL), laboratory testing indicating similar in vitro characteristics to Nuva-cote [*Strang* et al., unpubl.].

Clinical studies with these materials have been few although an initial investigation comparing Nuva-cote with Nuva-seal, gave 100% retention for Nuva-cote and 98.6% retention for Nuva-seal at 1 year [11]. Of course, this was not double-blind as appearances differed. Nonetheless the data confirmed thoughts that a well-polymerized filled material could contribute greatly to caries prevention.

When SCS became available, 438 sites were sealed with Nuva-cote and 439 with SCS in a double-blind trial [25]. At 1 year, there was 100% retention on Nuva-cote sites and only 1% loss from SCS teeth. It was also noted the cure rate could be accelerated by altering the catalyst concentration, a factor which could be beneficial for youngsters. To reduce further the overall application period, laboratory and clinical studies [26] using contralateral etch times of 60 or 20 s were undertaken in 6- to 8-year-olds. Here there was 95% retention on the 60 s sites compared to 100% retention on those etched for 20 s at 2 years. Thus substantial economic benefit could accrue as etching accounts for approximately 10% of the time required for sealant application. Unhappily, since this data was published, a decision has been taken not to market SCS. However, Nuva-cote is successful and, over a 4-year period, 1,539 deciduous molars have been sealed in 3- to 5-year-olds by a hygienist, with 81.5% retention and 99.2% caries inhibition [27].

The literature is deficient in Prismashield references but, in a further double-blind study with Nuva-cote, 100% retention has been obtained at 12 months with the latter, in erupting first molars, while 93.9% of Prismashield was intact [*Stephen* et al., unpubl.]. Again, losses were assessed to be due more to the bulk of the Prismalite guide rather than to deficiencies in the resin system. As yet, we are unaware of clinical data relating to Estiseal.

Polymerizing Systems

The fixed quartz guide Nuva-lite was devised to deliver UV emissions of 365 nm. However, it was soon realized this was of cumbersome design and early units had overheating problems. There were also geometrical and bulb difficulties which were capable of producing a UV output of $< 10 \text{ mW/cm}^2$, calculated as the absolute minimum to ensure adequate polymerization and subsequent retention, provided a 60 s exposure was allowed, although 30 mW/cm^2 was preferred [33].

The Alphalite, used conventional UV bulbs and its light-guide was a flexible fibre-optic, with a tip of 2.5 mm diameter compared to the 10 mm Nuva-lite. However, the guide was fragile and expensive to replace. Furthermore, while high output was obtained (100 mW/cm^2), due to its small diameter, it was still essential to scan the tip [33].

Since then a third generation of UV lights has emerged with timing units, UV monitoring facilities and flexible liquid-filled guidance systems of 6 mm tip diameter. The output from these, e.g. Lee-lite (Lee Pharmaceuticals GmbH), Bandelin (Bandelin Electronic KG), etc., has been assessed as $110–190 \text{ mW/cm}^2$ [13]. They are much superior to earlier designs.

As fears have been expressed regarding the use of UV emissions intra-orally, the most recent systems are dependent on visible light (440–448 nm), e.g. Prismalite, Espe Elipar (Espe GmbH) (UV and VL), Translux (Kulzer GmbH), Heliomat (Vivadent Schaan), etc. The bulbs are relatively inexpensive and polymerization and in-depth bonding has not suffered. However, the Prismalite is bulky and this could affect retention in awkward sites (see above). Generally, inadequate exposure may explain the differences obtained between SC, UV or VL resins as laboratory tests have consistently shown that, almost irrespective of light-source, 60 s polymerization is to be recommended [*Strang* et al., unpubl.]. Nonetheless, the geometry of some of the newer lights is more favourable.

Cost-Effectiveness

While few attempts have been made to assess cost-effectiveness, *Horowitz* [7] reported on a programme where approximately 100,000 teeth had been treated with only 5% loss at 6 months. The cost of placing each caries-inhibiting sealant was estimated as $ 12.25, this sum approaching that of a single restoration.

More recently, *Simonsen* [21] commented on Concise White Sealant 5-year data where 82% retention was recorded. Here, 94% of sealed surfaces were sound, and 59% of control sites were carious or restored. The cost for the sealed group was $ 10.23/child/annum while for controls, the sum was $ 21.15. *Leverett* et al. [9] also reported on 4-year data where 292 6- to 9-year-olds had contralateral quadrants Nuva-sealed or restored. The benefit-cost ratio for 'caries-inactive' subjects amounted to only 0.304 while for the 'caries-active' group it was 1.017. They concluded that for the caries-prone, sealing (even with Nuva-seal) was beneficial while if Nuva-cote had been employed, ratios would have been even more favourable.

However, the value of a successful sealant should not be costed in terms of clinical time and materials alone as the technique is atraumatic and presents the young subject with a painless procedure free from local anaesthesia and the use of terrifying high-speed equipment. Furthermore, no tooth damage occurs and, even if the sealant should fail, its replacement is rapidly achieved without further destruction.

For the future, we shall probably not witness a dramatic improvement in sealant properties as countless studies have shown that an adequately placed resin will totally inhibit caries and even inadvertent sealing of early or moderate caries can be beneficial [8]. Thus, by applying filled resins, retention of 5–10 years should be possible and it is only to be hoped that, internationally, the dental profession will correctly utilize the techniques and materials already proven by the work cited in this text.

References

1   Adipranato, S.; Beech, D.R.; Hardwick, J.L.: Effect of pretreatment of enamel on bonding to composite restorative materials. J. dent. Res. *54:* abstr. L354 (1975).
2   Brooks, J.D.; Mertz-Fairhurst, E.J.; Della-Giustina, V.E.; Williams, J.E.; Fairhurst, C.W.: A comparative study of two pit and fissure sealants: three-year results in Augusta, Ga. J. Am. dent. Ass. *99:* 42–46 (1979).
3   Buonocore, M.G.: Sealing of pits and fissures with an adhesive for caries prevention. J. Can. dent. Ass. *39:* 841–850 (1973).
4   Charbeneau, G.P.; Dennison, J.B.: Clinical success and potential failure after single application of a pit and fissure sealant: a four-year report. J. Am. dent. Ass. *98:* 559–564 (1979).
5   Conti, A.; Lotzkar, S.; Allan, X.; Marks, R.; Daley, R.: Evaluation of 'ICI' visible light cured dental fissure sealant. J. dent. Res. *62:* 222, abstr. 477 (1983).
6   Harris, N.O.; Moolenaar, L.; Hornberger, N.; Knight, G.H.; Frew, R.A.: Adhesive sealant clinical trial: effectiveness in a school population of the US Virgin Isles. J. prev. Dent. *3:* 27–37 (1976).
7   Horowitz, H.S.: Pit and fissure sealants in private practice and public health programmes: analysis of cost-effectiveness. Int. dent. J. *40:* 117–126 (1980).
8   Jensen, Ø.E.; Handelman, S.: Effect of an autopolymerising sealant on variability of microflora in occlusal dental caries. Scand. J. dent. Res. *88:* 382–388 (1980).
9   Levrett, D.H.; Handelman, S.L.; Brenner, C.; Iker, H.: Cost analysis of sealants: prevention and treatment of carious lesions. J. dent. Res. *61:* 225, abstr. 423 (1982).
10 McCune, R.J.; Bojanini, J.; Abodeely, R.A.: Effectiveness of a pit and fissure sealant in the prevention of caries: 3-year clinical results. J. Am. dent. Ass. *99:* 619–623 (1979).
11 Main, C.; Stephen, K.W.; Kirkwood, M.; Cummings, A.; Campbell, D.; Gillespie, F.C.; Thomson, J.L.; Young, K.C.: Comparisons between the UV resins, Nuva-seal and Nuva-cote by SEM studies, mechanical tests and clinical trial. Caries Res. *13:* 116 (1979).
12 Main, C.; Thompson, J.L.; Cummings, A.; Graham, E.C.; Kirkwood, M.; Stephen, K.W.; Gillespie, F.C.: Abrasion resistance of fissure sealants: in vitro and in vivo comparisons. J. oral Rehabil. (in press, 1983).
13 Main, C.; Cummings, A.; Moseley, H.; Stephen, K.W.; Gillespie, F.C.: An assessment of new dental ultra-violet sources and UV-polymerised fissure sealants. J. oral Rehabil. *10:* 215–227 (1983).
14 Miller, J.: Observations in clinical preventive dentistry. Br. dent. J. *94:* 7–9 (1953).
15 Richardson, A.S.; Waldman, R.; Gibson, G.B.: The effectiveness of a chemically polymerised sealant in preventing occlusal caries: two-year results. J. Can. dent. Ass. *44:* 269–272 (1978).
16 Rock, W.P.; Gordon, P.H.; Bradnock, G.: The effect of operator variability and patient age on the retention of fissure sealant resin. Br. dent. J. *145:* 72–75 (1978).
17 Rock, W.P.; Evans, R.I.W.: A comparative study between a chemically polymerised fissure sealant resin and a light cured resin. Br. dent. J. *152:* 232–234 (1982).
18 Sheykholeslam, Z.; Houpt, M.: Clinical effectiveness of an autopolymerised fissure sealant after 2 years. Community Dent. oral Epidemiol. *6:* 181–184 (1978).

19   Silverstone, L.M.: Fissure sealants: laboratory studies. Caries Res. 8: 2–26 (1974).
20   Simonsen, R.J.: The clinical effectiveness of a coloured sealant at 24 months. J. dent.
      Res. 58: 261, abstr. 675 (1979).
21   Simonsen, R.J.: Five-year results of sealant effects on caries prevalence and treat-
      ment cost. J. dent. Res. 61: 330, abstr. 1380 (1982).
22   Stephen, K.W.; Sutherland, D.A.; Trainer, J.: Fissure sealing by practitioners. Br.
      dent. J. 140: 45–51 (1976).
23   Stephen, K.W.; Kirkwood, M.; Young, K.C.; Gillespie, F.C.; MacFadyen, E.E.;
      Campbell, D.: Fissure sealing of first permanent molars. Br. dent. J. 144: 7–10
      (1978).
24   Stephen, K.W.; Kirkwood, M.; Young, K.C.; Gillespie, F.C.; Boyle, P.: Fissure
      sealing with Nuva-seal and Alphseal: two-year data. J. Dent. 9: 53–57 (1981).
25   Stephen, K.W.; Kirkwood, M.; Main, C.; Gillespie, F.C.; Campbell, D.: A clinical
      comparison of two filled fissure sealants after one year. Br. dent. J. 150: 282–284
      (1981).
26   Stephen, K.W.; Kirkwood, M.; Main, C.; Gillespie, F.C.; Campbell, D.: Retention
      of a filled fissure sealant using reduced etch time. Br. dent. J. 153: 232–233 (1982).
27   Stephen, K.W.; Boddy, F.A.; McCall, D.R.; Boyle, P.: Caries prevention in a
      hygienist-run practice – four-year data. XXX ORCA, abstr. 74 (1983).
28   Stiles, H.M.; Ward, G.T.; Woolridge, E.D.; Meyers, R.: Adhesive sealant clinical
      trial: comparative results of application by a dentist or dental auxiliaries. J. prev.
      Dent. 3: 8–11 (1976).
29   Strang, R.; Cummings, A.; Stephen, K.W.; McMenemy, P.; Wyper, D.J.: Laborat-
      ory evaluation of new fissure sealants – abrasion and enamel/sealant bond strengths.
      IADR (Brit. Div.), abstr. 90 (1983).
30   Ulvestad, H.: Fissurforsegling med lakkmaterialer: praktiske resultater. Norske
      Tandlægeforen. Tid. 83: 129–132 (1973).
31   Whitehurst, V.; Soni, N.N.: Adhesive sealant clinical trial: results eighteen months
      after one application. J. prev. Dent. 3: 20–22 (1976).
32   Young, K.C.; Hussey, M.; Gillespie, F.C.; Stephen, K.W.: In vitro studies of
      physical factors affecting adhesion of fissure sealant to enamel; in Silverstone,
      Dogon, Proc. Int. Symp. on The Acid Etch Technique, pp. 50–62 (North Central
      Publishing, Minnesota 1975).
33   Young, K.C.; Hussey, M.; Gillespie, F.C.; Stephen, K.W.: The performance of
      ultraviolet lights used to polymerise fissure sealants. J. oral Rehabil. 4: 181–191
      (1977).
34   Young, K.C.; Main, C.; Gillespie, F.C.; Stephen, K.W.: Ultraviolet absorption by
      two ultra-violet activated sealants. J. oral Rehabil. 5: 207–213 (1978).

Dr. K.W. Stephen, DDSc, Department of Oral Medicine and Pathology,
University of Glasgow Dental School, 378 Sauchiehall Street,
Glasgow G2 3JZ (Scotland)

Cariology Today. Int. Congr., Zürich 1983, pp. 308–316 (Karger, Basel 1984)

New Concepts in Therapeutic Cariology

F. Lutz

Department of Cariology, Periodontology, and Preventive Dentistry,
Dental Institute, University of Zurich, Switzerland

There is an abundance of incontrovertible data documenting a clinically significant and permanent decline in caries prevalence in many Western industrialized countries [1]. In addition, there is evidence that the occurrence of caries as well as the progression of periodontitis can be prevented in all age groups. Furthermore, a high level of oral hygiene of patients can be achieved and maintained by regularly repeated oral hygiene instruction and professional prophylaxis [2]. These facts inevitably have had, and continue to have, an impact on clinical dentistry. Among other effects, at an accelerating pace more and more dental patients of a new type are emerging: As to oral health they are well informed and highly motivated. Cost-effectiveness calculations have made them active participants in frequent recall programs. Consequently, little restorative work has to be done and potential carious lesions are diagnosed in an initial phase [1]. The patients' demands for esthetics and longevity of therapeutic measures, however, are high and difficult to meet actually begging for new concepts in therapeutic cariology.

The various modes of caries treatment (fig. 1) fall between two extremes: There is the preventive approach, *prophylaxis,* which is strictly nondestructive for dental hard tissue. Its effectiveness remains unchanged, if consistently maintained. In contrast, there is the purely

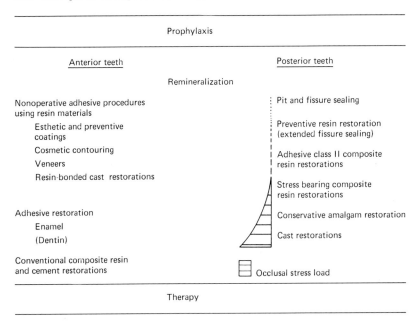

Fig. 1. Modes of caries treatments.

operative approach. Although the resulting restorations may be considered valid alternatives to progressing carious lesions, the placement of restorations as a *therapy* is basically irreversible and by nature destructive. Furthermore, the achieved, perhaps initially favorable results are short-lived because restorations have a limited longevity and are highly ineffective means for the prevention of the occurrence of new caries [2]. With regard to the above described type of dental patient, the caries treatments of choice should be as preventive and conservative as possible. In the following different treatments are evaluated paying particular attention to the above criteria.

Remineralization. Teeth are constantly subject to demineralization and remineralization. The higher the level of oral hygiene and the more intensive the recall program, the more likely remineralization will prevail. However, two requirements are still not yet satisfied: (1) a simple, active prophylactic treatment for initial proximal carious lesions favoring a fast, complete, and radiopaque remineralization, and (2) an effective local fluoride application for pits and fissures which would obviate fissure sealing [3–6].

Anterior Teeth

In anterior teeth, carious lesions are no longer a quantitative problem. However, the demands as to the quality of the respective treatments are difficult to meet; initial and long-term esthetics must be excellent; only virtually undetectable 'repairs' are considered acceptable. Progress was made by the adoption of the enamel acid etching technique, the marketing of translucent and colored sealers, and the advent of the microfiller technology.

Nonoperative Adhesive Procedures Using Resin Materials. Esthetic and prophylactic coatings, cosmetic contouring [7–9], veneers [10], and resin-bonded cast restorations [11] are mainly cosmetically orientated treatments and therefore primarily indicated in anterior teeth. Generally no cutting instruments are used for such adhesive procedures. Hence, they are ideally nondestructive and completely reversible. However, due to the mode of adhesion, these techniques are confined to the enamel shell. Furthermore, wear of resin materials limits their longevity. Nevertheless, these treatments are the procedures of choice in children and adolescent patients where pulp anatomy and gingival implications do not allow conventional fixed prosthodontic work. Whether resin-bonded cast restorations will also become a routine alternative in adults, particularly for economic reasons, remains to be seen [11].

Adhesive Restoration. According to present knowledge, the use of operative techniques is inevitable for the treatment of carious lesions with dentinal involvement. When using cutting instruments, however, a practitioner should always be aware of two basic principles: (1) 'primum nihil nocere', and (2) there is no restorative material that can compete with healthy dental hard tissue. Therefore, as little sound tooth substance as possible should be removed. This demand can be fulfilled due to the progress in oral hygiene and to the advent of adhesion to enamel: The four most destructive preparation rules given by G.V. Black, namely (1) establish outline form, (2) establish resistance form, (3) establish retentive form, and (4) extension for prevention, consequently can be relinquished. The solution is the adhesive preparation [8]. Only carious dentin and structureless enamel must be removed. The outline of the cavity is given by the carious lesion itself. Removal of sound dental hard tissue can be kept minimal except for the needs of access to the carious lesion and the preparation of a long bevel. It has recently been corroborated [12] that the adhesive restoration is superior to other types of operative resin restorations: it is the most conservative approach; there is no leakage; the percentage of 'excellent margin' is highest; and the impact of thermocycling is not significant. In combination with microfilled composite systems, particularly with incrementally applied light-cured versions, virtually undetectable restorations can be placed. It is estimated that more than half a million teeth have been treated with adhesive restoration and the 8-year clinical experience has been favorable.

The principles of adhesive restoration cannot, however, be employed wherever cavity margins are located in dentin. These segments of a carious lesion have to be restored conventionally. Macromechanical retentions and 90° butt joints have to be cut. This is a serious shortcoming of the current state of operative dentistry as the risk of root caries incidence will definitely increase in a population with an already increased life expectancy and with a greater number of retained teeth. Glass ionomer cements are not a valid alternative for two reasons: (1) the esthetic results are poor, and (2) their properties do not allow feathering [13]. Thus, despite their potential for adhesion to dentin, particularly eroded cervical areas need conventional restorations. Adhesive bonding to tooth structures, compatible with the currently used resin-based restorative materials, must consequently be regarded as a high priority item [14]. The clinical feasibility of multistep techniques using acidic mordant solutions and surface-active comonomers such as HNPM, NPGM, 4-MET, 4-META, and MPP is not proven yet [15, 16]. The bond strength achieved in vitro would be sufficient. However, the biocompatibility of the dentin cleanser as well as the chemical stability and durability of the bond under in vivo conditions are critical. With adhesive restorations in dentin even slight weakening of the bond would create an unacceptably high risk for caries, particularly under loosened feather edges and coatings.

Therefore, more long-term clinical data must become available before adhesive techniques can be routinely used on dentin.

Posterior Teeth

Pit and Fissure Sealing. Meticulous oral hygiene and optimal fluoride application can only delay fissure caries; its occurrence is unavoidable even in prophylaxis-oriented patients. There is an undisputed need for a treatment apt to prevent occlusal caries. Pit and fissure sealing, if used as a complementary individual prophylactic treatment, bridges the gap to the complete prevention of dental caries. Fissure sealing has initially been abused as a mass public health measure and promptly failed. That is why its clinical demise was prematurely proclaimed. Additional problems with fissure sealing stem from the fact that only prevention-oriented people can capitalize on it. These are participants in a recall program with a high level of oral hygiene and, as the success of fissure sealing is totally indication and technique dependant, practitioners with excellent knowledge in preventive dentistry and adhesive procedures. Generally, children with caries-free primary teeth are prime candidates for sealant applications: molars and premolars with sharp, deep fissures should be sealed individually immediately after tooth eruption [8, 9, 17, 18].

Preventive Resin Restoration (Extended Fissure Sealing). In the course of the continued search for most conservative restorative procedures, the preventive resin restoration has been developed. This technique enables restoration of occlusal carious lesions with only minimal removal of sound tooth structure while concurrently using the same material as a caries-preventive agent in adjacent pits and fissures. It is the treatment of choice for incipient or small carious lesions in occlusal surfaces of freshly erupted premolars and permanent molars. Thus, there is maximum preservation of sound dental hard tissue, a basic principle which is repealed in the usual 'extension for prevention' procedure. Superior esthetics is another fundamental advantage of the technique. Surprisingly, the long-term results are unequivocally excellent. This may be explained as follows: (1) preventive resin restorations are small and therefore well supported and protected by the surrounding natural tooth structure, (2) by definition, there is no occlusal stress load, and (3) the wear resistance of modern composite constructions in contact-free occlusal areas is comparable to that of amalgam, at least during the first 2–3 years [8, 9, 19–21].

Adhesive Class II Composite Resin Restorations. Initial proximal carious lesions can be restored using adhesive restoration. While the advantages are basically the same as with the preventive resin restoration, the procedure is technically more demanding. It is, however, justified in young patients with low caries activity exhibiting one or two initial proximal carious lesions which extend into dentin [8].

Stress-Bearing Composite Resin Restorations. For stress-bearing restorations the rationale for usage of composite resins may be twofold: (1) as esthetic restorative material, or (2) as a genuine resin-based amalgam substitute [14].

Resin-based stress-bearing esthetic restorations may be indicated as a compromise for cosmetic considerations usually in upper premolars. However, due to poor marginal adaptation, particularly along the gingivoproximal line-angle, such restorations bear a certain risk. Furthermore, the lack of adequate radiopacity may cause additional problems for quality control of the restorations. Above all, because of high wear, replacement is required every 2–3 years. Patients must be advised accordingly [14].

The advantages of composite resin materials are pleasing esthetics, low potential of toxicity, low thermal conductivity, and resource independence. However, although a considerable impetus has been given to this research, the following fundamental requirements for potential posterior composite resins remain to be met: (1) acceptable marginal adaptation, especially gingivoproximally, (2) sufficient radiopacity, (3) adequate wear resistance and form stability, (4) ease of manipulation, (5) finishability, and (6) color stability. Today, there is no genuine resin-based substitute for amalgam which can be used unrestrictedly as a restorative material for stress-bearing posterior restorations. In particular, amalgam-like wear resistance, excellent marginal adaptation and radiopacity greater than enamel are far from being realized simultaneously in one single composite construction [14, 20, 21].

Conservative Amalgam Restoration. Amalgam is the material of choice for stress-bearing posterior restorations because of favorable qualities, such as durability, wear resistance, ease of manipulation and the self-sealing properties due to corrosion. The conventional cavity preparations in teeth were designed to meet the needs of amalgam, with block-shaped cavities, edges with 90° butt joints, and retentions to lock each part of the restoration into the cavity. With modern amalgams, the principles of these preparation rules still hold true. However, a more conservative concept must be adopted [22]. The advantages of small amalgam restorations are overwhelming: (1) no weakening effect on the tooth, (2) less wear [21], (3) markedly increased longevity, and (4) superior esthetics. Key factors in this endeavor are oral hygiene and preparation technique. Proper usage of toothbrush, toothpaste and dental floss preclude the need for extension for prevention. Small and very small tungsten carbide burs in air motor handpieces and hand instruments are adequate for the preparation of occlusal outlines of only 1 mm in width and with an isthmus not wider than one fourth the intercuspal distance. The same instruments are suitable for the preparation of small self-retentive proximal boxes with the characteristic S-curve design and with only supragingival margins [23, 24]. Although widely used for cavity preparation, particularly in Europe, the combination 'air turbine–preparation diamond bur' is definitely too destructive and must not be used any longer for that purpose.

55 years of favorable clinical experience with the conservative amalgam restoration cannot be ignored [22]. The inclusion of this teaching in the curriculum of every dental school is overdue.

Conclusion

Unfortunately, in preventive and operative preventive dentistry the mode of treatment is often influenced by factors which are not patient related, such as skill and knowledge of the dentist, work load, motivation for quality, financial coverage of treatments, and availability of auxiliary personnel. However, according to the principles of ethics and the code of professional conduct, recently published by the American Dental Association [25], *dentists are morally bound to deliver quality care, competently and timely, within the bounds of the clinical circumstances presented by the patient.* Hence, our new prevention-minded type of patient has every right to expect the most prophylaxis-oriented and most conservative treatments possible. It is the dentist's obligation to provide them. In order to facilitate preventive and operative preventive dentistry, three measures have to be taken: (1) dental schools have to adapt their curriculums; prophylaxis-oriented concepts of treatment should be adopted and the respective techniques taught; (2) the profession and/or state-controlled institutions should train an adequate number of auxiliary personnel, and (3) changes in the current tariff system should be made allowing adequate coverage of prophylactic and prophylaxis-oriented treatments.

References

1   First International Conference on the Declining Prevalence of Dental Caries. J. dent. Res. 61: suppl., pp. 1304–1383 (1982).

2   Axelsson, P.; Lindhe, J.: Effect of controlled oral hygiene procedures on caries and periodontal disease in adults. J. clin. Periodontol. 5: 133–151 (1978).

3   Featherstone, J.D.B.; Rodgers, B.E.; Smith, M.W.: Physicochemical requirements for rapid remineralization of early carious lesions. Caries Res. 15: 221–235 (1981).

4   Nair, P.N.R.; Schroeder, H.E.: Schmelzkaries, ist sie heilbar? Schweiz. Mschr. Zahnheilk. 91: 633–647 (1981).

5   Belser, U.: Fluoraufnahme und Fluorretention des intakten oder angeätzten Oberflächenzahnschmelzes; Med. Thesis, University of Zurich (1974).

6   Tadoko, Y.; Iwaku, M.; Fusayama, T.: A laboratory report on vibration etching for fissure sealants. J. dent. Res. 61: 780–785 (1982).

7   Ibsen, R.L.; Neville, K.: Adhesive restorative dentistry; 1st ed. (Saunders, Philadelphia 1974).

8   Lutz, F.; Lüscher, B.; Ochsenbein, H.; Mühlemann, H.R.: Adhesive Zahnheilkunde; 1st ed. (Juris, Zurich 1976).

9   Simonsen, R.J.: Clinical applications of the acid etch technique; 1st ed. (Quintessence, Chicago 1978).

10 Faunce, F.R.: Bonded aesthetic dentistry – a laminate veneer handbook. 1st ed. (Plimark, Munich 1982).

11 Livaditis, G.J.; Thompson, V.P.: Etched castings: an improved retentive mechanism for resin-bonded retainers. J. prosth. Dent. 47: 52–58 (1982).

12 Lutz, F.; Lund, M.R.; Porte, A.; Swartz, M.L.: Cavity designs for compsite resin. Oper. Dent. (in press, 1983).

13 Phillips, R.W.: Science of dental materials; 8th ed., p. 486 (Saunders, Philadelphia 1982).

14 Phillips, R.W.; Lutz, F.: Status report on posterior composites. J. Am. dent. Ass. 107: 74–78 (1983).

15 Masuhara, E.: Die neuentwickelten haftfähigen Kunststoffe und ihre klinische Anwendung. Dt. zahnärztl. Z. 37: 155–159 (1982).

16 Bowen, R.L.; Cobb, E.N.; Rapson, J.E.: Adhesive bonding of various materials to hard tooth tissues: improvement in bond strength to dentin. J. Am. dent. Ass. *61:* 1070–1076 (1982).

17 Proc. Conf. Pit and Fissure Sealants: Why their Limited Usage? (American Dental Association, Council on Dental Materials, Instruments and Equipment, Chicago 1981).

18 Proc. Symp. Pit-and-Fissure Sealants: Is it Time for a New Initiative? (American Association for Dental Research and International Association for Dental Research). J. Publ. Hlth Dent. *42:* 295–336 (1982).

19 Simonsen, R.J.: Preventive resin restorations: three-year results. J. Am. dent. Ass. *100:* 535–539 (1980).

20 Lutz, F.: Beiträge zur Entwicklung von Seitenzahnkomposits; 1st ed. (KAR PAR PZM, Zurich, 1980).

21 Lutz, F.; Phillips, R.W.; Roulet, J.F.; Setcos, J.C.: In vivo and in vitro wear of potential posterior composites. J. dent. Res. (in press, 1983).

22 Prime, J.M.: A plea for conservatism in operative procedures. J. Am. dent. Ass. *15:* 1234–1246 (1928).

23 Rodda, J.C.: Modern class II amalgam cavity preparations. N.Z. dent. J. *68:* 132–138 (1972).

24 Almquist, T.C.; Cowan, R.D.; Lambert, R.L.: Conservative amalgam restorations. Oper. Dent. *29:* 524–528 (1973).

25 American Dental Association: Principles of ethics and code of professional conduct. J. Am. dent. Ass. *105:* 493–495 (1982).

F. Lutz, MD, Department of Cariology, Periodontology and Preventive Dentistry, Dental Institute, University of Zurich, CH-8028 Zurich (Switzerland)

Cariology Today. Int. Congr., Zürich 1983, pp. 317–326 (Karger, Basel 1984)

Is Health Promotion the Main Issue of Preventive Dentistry?

A. Thylstrup, V. Qvist[1]

Department of Cariology and Endodontics, Royal Dental College, Copenhagen, Denmark

Introduction

The greater part of common knowledge of dental caries and factors which influence the onset and progression of the disease, originates from clinical and epidemiological data. For example, common understanding of the effect of fluorides is predominantly based upon observations done in groups of individuals participating in clinical trials [*Heifetz*, 1978]. Unfortunately, epidemiologists have generally chosen to record dental caries in a way which favors standardization at the expense of accuracy. This means that attempts to transfer the complicated disease into operational categories have furthered a solidification of dental caries as being an either/or phenomenon in terms of sound versus decayed teeth.

Epidemiological data are consequently expressed in numbers of decayed, missing and treated (filled) teeth. Similarly, reductions in dental caries observed in clinical trials are expressed as reductions in treated or filled teeth, and the result related to the preventive procedure under investigation. It is therefore no wonder that caries prevention on a population basis has commonly been seen as an attractive and economical alternative to the much more expensive treatment of existing disease [*Burt*, 1978; *McHugh*, 1981]. For this reason a clear distinction has been generated in the literature between preventive dentistry and

[1] Sincere thanks are extended to our colleagues for their willingness to provide data on treatment behavior.

curative or restorative dentistry. As a result, preventive dentistry, presumably reinforced by its methodologies, has undergone the development of a speciality being mainly engaged with the task of keeping sound teeth sound in populations.

Treatment, on the other hand, is still pursued on an individual bio-surgical basis, yet regarded by specialists in preventive dentistry as inefficient as well as expensive [Burt, 1978; McHugh, 1981]. Even though we usually recognize the extremely complicated nature of dental caries, we may realize that, in the clinic as well as in common language, caries remain at the either/or level, treatment or no treatment. As we have seen, this tendency may have been reinforced by operational definitions of caries and seldom questioned simply because the either/or complex appears so familiar to the classical decision-making process performed by the individual dentist.

A discussion of the major issue of preventive dentistry, as raised by the organizers of this meeting, therefore requires a more elaborated definition of preventive dentistry and particularly what preventive dentistry represents to the individual dentist working within the contemporary structure of the dental health delivery service. Because goals for preventive dentistry, in principle, have been defined by the absence of treatment, it might be of importance to summarize the historical genesis of professional caries treatment. From primarily being devoted to relief of pain and illness, dental treatment during the first half of this century underwent rapid development, accellerated by improvements in methods in cutting of teeth and in restorative materials. Therefore, treatment of caries became synonymous with prevention of further progress of the disease [Hyatt, 1933; Dunning, 1981].

However, as is known, the concensus of recently conveyed reports on reduced dental caries has taught us that caries progression can be controlled in populations either resulting from the unspecific use of fluorides in terms of water fluoridation, fluoridated dentifrices, fortnightly rinsing programs, etc. [Birkeland et al., 1977; Glass, 1981; Brown, 1982; von der Fehr, 1982; Fejerskov et al., 1982; Koch, 1982; Thylstrup et al., 1982a] or by more specific procedures such as professional plaque control [Axelsson and Lindhe, 1977, 1978; Axelsson, 1981]. Therefore, it is considered relevant to examine the extent to which this decline in dental caries has had an impact on treatment practice. Or in other words, do dentists maintain a pattern of 'preventive treatment practice' that is in accordance with Hyatt's [1933] statement that 'the enamel defect of today is the carious cavity of tomor-row'? In an attempt to elucidate this hypothesis, data were collected by dentists participating in postgraduate courses in cariology. This com-munication only deals with principal aspects of the findings relevant to the discussion of today.

Material and Methods

The material was collected during the period 1981–1982. Prior to the courses two questionnaires were sent to the participating dentists. One questionnaire (approximal caries) dealt with actual tissue changes in approximal carious lesions as observed during operative treatment [*Thylstrup* et al., 1982b; *Bille* et al., 1983]. The other questionnaire (replacement of fillings) dealt with reasons for operative treatment with particular em-phasis on reasons for replacement [*Qvist* et al., 1983].

Approximal Caries
Each dentist was asked to record clinical and – when available – radiographic findings of the first five approximal surfaces which they restored in a given period. For each surface the following information was obtained. (1) Age of patient. (2) Type of tooth. (3) Treatment decisions as either based on radiographic findings, on clinical observations, or a combination of the two. (4) Clinical tissue changes. During the drilling process the treatment was stopped when the maximal extent of the lesion occurred in the gingival wall, cervical to the interproximal contact area. Observed clinical tissue changes were then classified according to a six-point scoring system [*Bille and Thylstrup*, 1982] illustrated in figure 2. Scores A and B indicate progressive changes in enamel; score C changes in dentine without cavity formation in enamel; scores D and E represent progressive cavitation in enamel, and score F that cavitation has reached dentine. (5) Radiographic findings were recorded by the dentists using the classification proposed by *Møller and Poulsen* [1973] (fig. 2).

A total of 263 dentists responded and information on 827 permanent approximal surfaces were obtained. Of these 660 radiographic findings were available.

Replacement of Fillings
The dentists were asked to record for each of the first 30 fillings placed in a given period information on whether a filling was made either due to primary caries or as a replacement of an old filling. In case of replacement the dentists were then asked to record information with respect to the type of old and new filling, filling material and approxim-ate age of the old filling in years. Finally, dentists were asked to classify their major reason for replacing a filling into one of the nine different categories indicated in table II. In addition information on patient age was recorded.

A total of 261 dentists responded, and information on 5,119 fillings placed in permanent teeth were obtained. In the following only information with respect to amalgam fillings will be given.

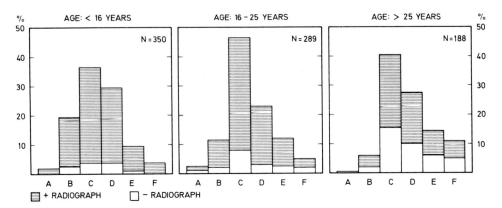

Fig. 1. Distribution of treated approximal caries in different age groups according to clinical tissue changes. The hatched part of the bars indicate the proportion where radiographs have been available. For explanation of abbreviations A–F, see text and figure 2.

Results

Approximal Caries

Of a total of 827 operative treatments recorded, 462 or 56% of the fillings were placed to arrest caries not yet having cavitated. About one third of these were classified as 'white spot' lesions involving only porous changes in the enamel. Figure 1 gives the percentage distribution of observed clinical tissue changes in relation to age. A marked tendency towards early diagnosis and prompt treatment of approximal lesions is observed among children less than 16 years of age. Consequently, only 13% of the restored lesions had obvious cavitation involving larger parts of the enamel and enamel and dentine (scores E + F). With increasing age of the patients, prompt treatment of enamel lesions becomes less pronounced, although still only 26% of the lesions on patients more than 25 years old showed obvious cavitation (score E + F). The hatched portion of the bars in figure 1 indicates the proportion where radiographs were available. The figure clearly shows that radiographs are more often available when children are treated than when treating adults.

Figure 2 illustrates the relationship between radiographic findings and the corresponding progression of lesions. Even though the classification of particularly the radiographic findings has to be considered

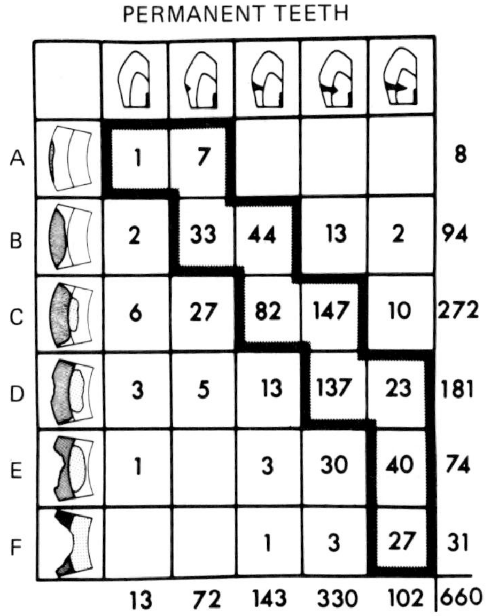

PERMANENT TEETH

A	1	7				8
B	2	33	44	13	2	94
C	6	27	82	147	10	272
D	3	5	13	137	23	181
E	1		3	30	40	74
F			1	3	27	31
	13	72	143	330	102	660

Fig. 2. Correlation between radiographic findings and clinical tissue changes in approximal carious lesions.

as somewhat arbitrary, it is interesting that a relatively fair agreement appears to exist between radiographic and clinical changes. Thus, small lesions correspond to small radiographic findings and larger tissue destructions to larger radiographic changes. In order to visualize this relationship a diagonal is framed in the figure. The framed area includes 82% of the observations.

Replacement of Fillings
Information on a total of 4,337 permanent teeth restored with amalgam were obtained. Of these 74% were performed to arrest primary caries or new caries in previously filled teeth (table I). Table II gives the percentage distribution of reasons for replacement of the remaining 1,112 failed fillings (26%) in relation to the age of the patients. About one third of the fillings in each age group is replaced due to secondary caries. Replacement due to marginal discrepancies accounts for another third in children less than 16 years of age, while this reason is less dominating for replacement of fillings in adults. In

Table I. Distribution of 4,337 amalgam restorations in permanent teeth according to the age of patients and the reason for treatment

Age of patient years	Reason for treatment with amalgams		
	primary caries	new caries in filled teeth	replacement of failed fillings
<16	2,446 (74%)	288 (9%)	571 (17%)
≥16	382 (37%)	109 (11%)	541 (52%)
Total	2,828 (65%)	397 (9%)	1,112 (26%)

Table II. Distribution (%) of replaced amalgam restorations according to the age of patients and the major reason for replacement

Reason for replacement of fillings	Age of patients, years	
	<16	≥16
Secondary caries	32	33
Discoloration	0	1
Marginal discoloration	2	0
Marginal discrepansies	29	15
Anatomic form	2	1
Fracture of filling	18	30
Fracture of tooth	3	10
Lost filling	8	7
Other reasons	7	4
Number of fillings	571	541

the same fashion more severe failures as fracture of filling and tooth account for only 21% of the replacement in children in contrast to 40% in the adult group.

Information on the age of the replaced fillings were given in 856 or 77% of the cases. It is then possible in figure 3 to draw curves illustrating the accumulated percentage distribution for time of replacement of amalgam fillings in permanent teeth for children and adults. The points at which the horizontal 50% line crosses the curves are thus representing the time on the abscissa where 50% of the fillings in the present material are replaced. On examining the curve for the adult

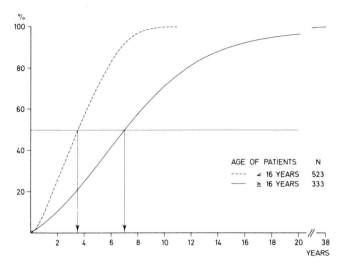

Fig. 3. Accumulated percentage distribution for time of replacement of amalgam fillings in permanent teeth.

patients, it is obvious that amalgam fillings may last or survive for extensive periods. It should be remembered on examining the curve illustrating the time of replacement in children that children leave the Public Child Dental Health Service at about the age of 16 years. Consequently, dentists have no opportunity to replace fillings more than 11 years old. It is obvious that these curves do not inform us about the 'theoretical durability' of fillings. On the other hand, the considerable amount of data showing no variation from course to course does provide us with important information with regard to the frequency with which fillings are being replaced. It should be noted, therefore, that the time of replacement of fillings in adults emerging from these data may closely approximate the 'actual durability' of fillings. With this in mind it is remarkable that only half of the fillings produced in adults survives for more than 7 years.

Discussion

Essentially, the data confirmed the hypothesis that a treatment philosophy based on early diagnosis and prompt treatment is still

prevailing, irrespective of the reduced progression of caries. To understand this phenomenon it is important to consider the essential role
which prevention of sequelae hitherto has played in the treatment of
caries. Thus, *Dunning* [1981] is presumably in agreement with the
majority of the dental profession when he states that 'in its broadest
sense, preventive dentistry is all of dentistry'. Accordingly, *Dunning* and
others operate with three levels of preventive dentistry with 'a basic
division between the prepathogenesis and pathogenesis stages of the
disease'. This division corresponds to primary and secondary prevention. Secondary preventive services are accordingly aimed at early
diagnosis and prompt treatment in order to prevent further progress
and extended loss of tooth structure [*Dunning, 1981*].

The data require, however, one further comment relevant to the
topic. In Denmark children up to 16 years of age receive free dental care
delivered by dentists and auxillaries employed by the municipalities.
Such a government-subsidized system is implicitly regarded as optimal
for the delivery of dental care to children. It is beyond any doubt that
the Public Child Dental Health Service has dealt successfully with the
backlog of dental caries with which it was faced when the service was
founded [*Hesselgren and Thylstrup, 1982*]. In an analysis of the Public
Child Dental Health Service founded in 1959, these authors showed
that the use of a wide spectrum of classical preventive measures in the
following decade successfully reduced the demand for fillings in children. However, in the next decade they observed an almost unchanged
level of produced fillings in spite of a considerably reduced progression
of caries in the population. The present data provide some explanation
of these findings as approximal lesions in children were treated with
fillings at a very early stage, and replacement of fillings due to, for
example, marginal defects were performed more frequently than among
adults.

The Danish Public Child Dental Health Service operates with a
broad spectrum of preventive measures, as do similarly organized
systems in other Scandinavian countries. The larger part of the preventive programs is carried out by dental auxillaries and directed to groups
of children. The individual dentist, on the other hand, is apparently still
operating within the frames of secondary and tertiary prevention and
accordingly gives treatment at early stages in order to prevent progress
of the disease. Consequently, the sharp distinction hitherto maintained
between preventive dentistry and restorative dentistry is not only in

contradiction to our actual knowledge of the disease, but also in conflict with the interest of the consumer.

These considerations have focussed on delivery of dental health as provided by the Public Child Dental Health Service, but they are applicable to the service delivered in private practice as well. It is of interest, however, for a further understanding of professional behavior that dentists working within the frames of a public system and thus independent of economy apparently adhere more to a traditional 'treatment for prevention' model than private practitioners do. Thus, the data suggest that the economical structure, within which dental care is delivered, plays a minor role relative to the traditional professional attitudes adopted during the educational process in its broadest sense. It is interesting, therefore, that many conflicting strategies for the improvement of delivery systems are being promoted while surprisingly little attention is being paid to the methodological focus of dentistry itself.

In summary, a serious conflict seems to exist between the highly problematic operational definition of dental health as being simply the absence of decay and current understanding of the carious process and possible ways of intervening without surgical treatment. Therefore, it is no wonder that at the same time we see some who 'treat' to 'prevent' while others 'prevent' to avoid 'treatment'. The major issue of contemporary preventive dentistry may therefore not be further oral health promotion, but a profound analysis and definition of oral health itself. We may then realize that an analysis of professional behavior and improvements in implementation of current knowledge and research becomes the major issue of preventive dentistry in the years to come.

References

Axelsson, P.: Concept and practice of plaque control. Pediat. Dent. 3: 101–113 (1981).
Axelsson, P.; Lindhe, J.: The effect of a plaque control program on gingivitis and dental caries in schoolchildren. J. dent. Res. 56: Special Issue C, pp. 142–148 (1977).
Axelsson, P.; Lindhe, J.: Effect of controlled oral hygiene procedures on caries and periodontal disease in adults. J. clin. Periodontol. 5: 133–151 (1978).
Bille, J.; Thylstrup, A.: Radiographic diagnosis and clinical tissue changes in relation to treatment of approximal carious lesions. Caries Res. 16: 1–6 (1982).
Bille, J.; Thylstrup, A.; Qvist, V.: Radiographic and actual tissue changes in approximal carious lesions at time for operative treatment. Abstract (ORCA, Dublin 1983).

Birkeland, J.M.; Broch, L.; Jorkjend, L.: Benefits and prognosis following 10 years of a fluoride rinsing program. Scand. J. dent. Res. *85:* 31–37 (1977).

Brown, R.H.: Evidence of decrease in the prevalence of dental caries in New Zealand. J. dent. Res. *61:* 1327–1330 (1982).

Burt, B.: The relative efficiency of methods of caries prevention in dental public health. Proceedings of a workshop (University of Michigan Press, Ann Arbor 1978).

Dunning, J.M.: Prevention of dental disease; in Jong, Dental public health and community dentistry, pp. 85–118 (Mosby, St. Louis 1981).

Fehr, F.R. von der: Evidence of decreasing caries prevalence in Norway. J. dent. Res. *61:* 1331–1335 (1982).

Fejerskov, O.; Antoft, P.; Gadegaard, E.: Decrease in caries experience in Danish children and young adults in the 1970s. J. dent. Res. *61:* 1305–1310 (1982).

Glass, R.L.: Secular changes in caries prevalence in two Massachusetts towns. Caries Res. *15:* 445–450 (1981).

Heifetz, S.B.: Cost-effectiveness of topically applied fluorides; in Burt, The relative efficiency of methods in caries prevention in dental public health. Proceedings of a workshop, pp. 69–104 (University of Michigan Press, Ann Arbor 1978).

Hesselgren, K.; Thylstrup, A.: Development in dental caries among children in 1961–79 in a Danish community with school dental service. Community dent. oral Epidemiol. *10:* 276–281 (1982).

Hyatt, T.P.: Prophylactic odontotomy (MacMillan, New York 1933).

Koch, G.: Evidence for declining caries prevalence in Sweden. J. dent. Res. *61:* 1340–1345 (1982).

McHugh, W.D.: Prevention in dental public health; in Slack, Dental public health; 2nd ed., pp. 11–50 (Wright, Bristol 1981).

Møller, I.J.; Poulsen, S.: A standardized system for diagnosing, recording and analyzing dental caries data. Scand. J. dent. Res. *81:* 1–11 (1973).

Qvist, V.; Thylstrup, A.; Mjör, I.A.: Reasons for operative treatment (in preparation, 1983).

Thylstrup, A.; Bille, J.; Bruun, C.: Caries prevalence in Danish children living in areas with low and optimal levels of natural water fluoridation. Caries Res. *16:* 413–420 (1982a).

Thylstrup, A.; Qvist, V.; Bille, J.: Kliniske og radiologiske forandringer i operativt behandlede approksimale cariesangreb. Tandlægebladet *86:* 617–625 (1982b).

A. Thylstrup, Prof., Royal Dental College, Jagtvej 160,
DK–2100 Copenhagen (Denmark)

Summaries of Panel Discussions

Note by the Editor

The last chapter of this volume contains the summaries of the discussions held during the 'Cariology 1983' conference and were written by the respective moderators of each session. The moderators were permitted unlimited freedom to accomplish this difficult task. The only conditions requested were a limitation in the space and the request not to produce a mere transcript of the discussion. Due to this degree of liberty, the differences between the approaches made were rather pronounced. The reader will notice that the lack of a uniform format adds to the flavour of this chapter. Those who are personally acquainted with the various authors will remark with amusement, how well the form and style of their contributions reflect the different characters of their personalities.

B. Guggenheim

Cariology Today. Int. Congr., Zürich 1983, pp. 328–331 (Karger, Basel 1984)

Epidemiology
Summary of Discussion

P.J. Holloway

Department of Child Dental Health, University Dental Hospital of Manchester, England

Dental epidemiologists seem confident that the prevalence of dental caries is decreasing in developed countries of Western European culture, particularly in children [*Glass,* 1982]. The trend is apparently so well-marked that it has become clear, despite a paucity of reliable, accurate data [*Downer,* 1984; *Carlos,* 1984]. This improvement is in direct contrast to changes occurring in developing countries, where seemingly caries prevalence is rapidly increasing. It has, in fact, been claimed that average caries levels in both cultures have now crossed, with those in developing countries being in general higher [*Barmes,* 1983]. This fact has alarming consequences for third world countries where the total health budget may be insufficient to support even the most basic type of dental service.

Although these assumptions seem indisputable, it should nevertheless be regretted that dental epidemiologists in the second half of the 20th century were not able to monitor these important changes more accurately, for their impact on dental services and dental education throughout the world will be fundamental. This failure is all the more surprising when it is appreciated that the science of dental epidemiology is now well developed through pioneers such as *Trendley Dean, Russell, Slack, Backer-Dirks* and the Zürich team under the guidance of Prof. *Mühlemann.*

It is to be hoped that in the future dental epidemiologists and public health workers will co-operate in monitoring changes in dental health in countries throughout the world, for changes will continue to occur both in adult and child populations, and services will need to be modified to accommodate to these, particularly in relation to the care of older people who will retain their teeth longer.

There is no reason at present to assume that the trends already noted will arrest. Although the rate of decrease in caries prevalence in developed countries may reduce, there is room for further improvement, and very recent figures would suggest that this is continuing to occur [OPCS, 1983]. In contrast, there is clearly scope for caries levels in developing countries to increase. The reasons for these changes are not fully understood, although where fluoridation has been initiated, the benefits are clear. Dental research workers and public health dentists may derive a certain self-satisfaction from reducing caries levels, but this must be tempered by the realisation that thorough studies into the phenomenon are lacking, and that they seem powerless to control the deteriorating situation in developing communities.

In general, the reasons might be quite different in the two cultures. Although perhaps not providing the full explanation, the use of fluoride must play a major role in the improvement in countries of Western European culture. Knowledge of the full effect of fluoride is only complete as far as fluoridation is concerned, for this is the only fluoride delivery system that has been monitored over the lifetime of individuals. It is possible that the results of 2- to 3-year controlled clinical trials underestimate the full effect of topical fluoride agents used routinely for a lifetime. However, although further benefits from fluoride can be anticipated in the future, these must eventually reach a maximum, for the benefits reduce progressively as each fluoride regimen is superimposed on the last [Marthaler, 1984].

Because the effect of fluoride has been measured scientifically, it should not, therefore, be assumed that this is the sole cause of the decline in caries. Other factors have been implicated, as diverse as changing patterns of sugar consumption [Jervis and Lennon, 1983], to loss of virulence of Streptococcus mutans [Bowen, 1984], but as none of these have been adequately investigated, much research remains to be done.

The cause of the deterioration in dental health in developing countries seems readily apparent [Sheiham, 1984]. Increasing industrialisation seems invariably linked to rising levels of sugar consumption and the inevitable breakdown of the dentition. This process merely mirrors similar changes in developed countries during the industrial revolution some 200 years ago. The consequences are well documented [Moore, 1983]. Although the cause of this change in dietary intake appears to be the result of changes in patterns of international trade, public health dentists seem reluctant to attempt to influence this process. Instead, they debate the difficulty of establishing fluoridation in primitive communities, the administrative problems of organising regular fluoride rinsing or tablet programmes, and the economic impossibility of marketing fluoride toothpaste or of providing an adequate dental workforce [*Gillespie,* 1984]. The answer (if there is one) will be found in an integrated, multi-factorial approach, combining proven methods of prevention, as and when these become practical, with fiscal and political decisions to limit the unnecessary consumption of sugar, to develop alternative uses of sugar in order to assist the economies of sugar-producing countries, and new technologies for the control of dental caries that can be applied to countries of very limited resources.

The improvement in the dental health of young people in Western democratic societies will confront research workers and public health dentists with new problems among high risk and older age groups, and it is important that answers are found [*Bowen,* 1984]. Yet these difficulties will pale to insignificance when compared to the public health problem now appearing in under-developed countries. Dental caries in the third world is rapidly assuming proportions that have been called 'frightening' [*Sheiham,* 1984] and urgent, fundamental measures are called for. An integrated approach to this problem is essential, and dental epidemiologists and public health workers must be in the forefront, measuring the problems, testing the preventive programmes and recording their impact on the communities at risk. Prevention as a public health activity must include political influence as well as technological transfer.

There is much to be done and little time to complete it. The international data base is still inadequate. Simple epidemiological methodology must be applied in more third world countries. Where caries levels are still low, active measures are required to retain these. Where caries prevalence is high, it must be reduced. Ingenuity is required to produce technologies appropriate to each situation, and alternative uses for sugar must be developed and sugar-based industries diversified.

Developed countries cannot afford to be complacent, for although clinical caries is beginning to come under control, nevertheless, early carious lesions are present that can develop if the challenge is increased or the protective factors removed. Cariogenic bacteria are present in the mouths of people in all communities, and root caries, abouth which little is known, is increasing as adults retain their teeth longer. Thus, fluoride delivery systems must be maintained and improved and people must be offered a wider choice of sugar-free products.

The dental profession itself must adapt to this changing picture. Levels of diagnosis may already have masked the reduction of caries in developed countries, while dental schools in developing countries are mistakenly training students to high technology repair rather than prevention. Dentists throughout the world must place the prevention of disease foremost in every activity they perform.

All these changes will require careful monitoring and guidance. It is essential that the sound, dental epidemiological principles developed in Zürich and other centres of excellence, under the scientific guidance of pioneers such as Prof. *Mühlemann,* are applied systematically on a world-wide basis for the good of humanity.

References

Barmes, D. E.: Indicators for oral health and their implications for developing countries. Int. dent. J., London *33:* 60–66 (1983).
Bowen, W. H.: Impact on research; in Guggenheim, Cariology today, pp. 49–55 (Karger, Basel 1984).
Carlos, J. P.: Epidemiological trends in caries: impact on adults and the aged; in Guggenheim, Cariology today, pp. 25–32 (Karger, Basel 1984).
Downer, M. C.: Changing patterns of disease in the Western World; in Guggenheim, Cariology today, pp. 1–11 (Karger, Basel 1984).
Gillespie, G. M.: Prevention of dental disease in developing countries; in Guggenheim, Cariology today, pp. 40–48 (Karger, Basel 1984).
Glass, R. L.: The first international conference on the declining prevalence of dental caries. J. dent. Res. *61:* special issue, pp. 1304–1383 (1982).
Jervis, P. N.; Lennon, M. A.: Sugar consumption in Britain. Proc. IADR (Br. Div.), Swansea, Abstr. 222 (1983).
Marthaler, T. M.: Explanations for changing patterns of disease in the Western World; in Guggenheim, Cariology today, pp. 13–23 (Karger, Basel 1984).
Moore, W. J.: Sugar and the antiquity of dental caries; in Holloway, The role of sugar in the aetiology of dental caries. J. Dent. *11:* 189–190 (1983).
Office of Population Censuses and Surveys: Children's dental health. Br. dent. J. *155:* 322–328 (1983).
Sheiham, A.: Dental caries in underdeveloped countries; in Guggenheim, Cariology today, pp. 33–39 (Karger, Basel 1984).

Prof. P. J. Holloway, Department of Child Dental Health, University Dental Hospital of Manchester, Higher Cambridge Street, Manchester M15 6FH (England)

Cariology Today. Int. Congr., Zürich 1983, pp. 332–339 (Karger, Basel 1984)

Saliva and Dental Caries
Summary of Discussion

Irwin D. Mandel

School of Dental and Oral Surgery, Columbia University, New York, N.Y., USA

Saliva is one of our natural resources. As with most such resources it is unappreciated until there is a shortage. It is not only the patients who are ungrateful, however; the profession treats saliva as an enemy – to be expunged, aspirated, or dammed. In actuality saliva is an ideal slow release device, fashioned by an ancient technology that is still in the public domain. It provides a spectrum of systems and activities that help maintain the integrity of the teeth and soft tissue surfaces. Salivary anticaries mechanisms include: (1) bacterial and food clearance; (2) direct bacteriostatic and bactericidal activity; (3) plaque pH regulation, and (4) modulation of enamel solubility. The various factors and systems act in a coordinated manner. Interference with delivery of saliva because of disease, surgery, or therapeutic interventions results in a rapid proliferation of the cariogenic flora and rampant caries in an unprotected mouth. Characterization of the salivary protective components and their interactions with each other, with plaque constituents, and with the tooth surface is a dynamic area of research, described at the conference by active researchers who are recognized authorities in their respective fields.

In the first paper of the session, Dr. *Leo Sreebny* discussed salivary flow rate and caries. He reviewed the reasons that have made it difficult for investigators to determine accurately the correlation between flow of saliva and caries in situations other than severe impairment of gland function and suggested that new approaches be developed. In his view, consideration should be given not only to influx of saliva, but pooling, distribution, availability, and efflux of saliva as well. This dissection of the fluid flow process in the oral cavity has led Dr. *Sreebny* to a set of studies on salivary clearance of dietary carbohydrates which he described in some detail. Hopefully, in time, similar considerations will be given to bacterial clearance, an area in which the immunochemical and biochemical mechanisms have usurped the mechanical.

Dr. *Colin Dawes* reviewed the relation to caries of the inorganic constituents in saliva and stressed the importance of the buffering role of bicarbonate and the concentration of calcium and phosphate ions, and he related state of saturation of saliva to flow rate and to the interaction with the fluid phase of plaque. He pointed out that except for chloride most of the plaque fluid components were manyfold higher than their counterparts in saliva. Recent studies on the characterization of plaque fluid and its relation to salivary composition were described. Dr. *Dawes* also discussed his mathematical model of salivary clearance of sugar and identified (as did Dr. *Sreebny*) the importance of swallowing frequency and residual volume, as well as salivary influx, on the clearing process.

Dr. *Per Brandtzaeg* provided a comprehensive review of the human studies on secretory IgA levels and caries, the pathways for generation of antibodies against cariogenic organisms, and the possible mechanisms by which the IgA antibodies can affect plaque formation and caries initiation. The specifics of sIgA protection, however, still remain unclear. Despite its low concentration in the salivary secretions per se, IgG, as well as sIgA, can have an impact in the oral cavity because of its high concentration in gingival crevicular fluid. Even in the absence of overt inflammation this fluid can become incorporated into supragingival pellicle and plaque as well as whole saliva. Research in a number of laboratories attests to the efficacy of both the sIgA and the humoral IgG systems in providing protection against caries in rodents and primates via vaccination. A positive feeling about the potential clinical value has to be tempered, however, by concerns over safety in the long term.

Dr. *Roland Arnold* examined the recent information on the operation of the nonimmunological antibacterial factors in saliva and described the actions and interactions of the systems involving lysozyme, lactoperoxidase, and lactoferrin. Interaction of a series of chaotropic ions in saliva (bicarbonate, thiocyanate, chloride, fluoride) with lysozyme can amplify its affect and result in disruption of cell membranes and eventual lysis of a number of oral organisms, including *Streptococcus mutans*. Lactoperoxidase operates in the mouth largely by converting thiocyanate to hypothiocyanite, using hydrogen peroxide liberated by oral bacteria for the process. The hypothiocyanite results in a reduction of bacterial acid production as an immediate consequence of interference with glycolysis and/or the phosphotransferase system.

Perhaps the most exciting of the recent developments has been Dr. *Arnold's* research on the bacteriostatic (via 'nutritional immunity', competing for iron) and bactericidal properties of lactoferrin (in the presence of iron) and its interaction with the sIgA system. The new findings strongly suggest that lactoferrin can be synergistic or antagonistic, depending on the specific antigens involved and the numbers of organisms present in the milieu. The data indicate that the lactoferrin sIgA interaction favors the maintenance of a commensal flora and the control of potentially pathogenic organisms. In the case of *S. mutans* the implication is that with low numbers of the organism the reaction between lactoferrin and sIgA is antagonistic, with high numbers it is synergistic. Further developments in the new approach to population control are awaited eagerly.

Dr. *Donald Hay* described the range of proteins in parotid and submandibular saliva, many of which have only been characterized in recent years. He considered them primarily from a functional point of view but stressed the need for additional information of structure at the molecular level in order to understand more fully the relationships between structure and function. In addition to the antibacterial activities already described by Drs. *Brandtzaeg* and *Arnold,* saliva also contains a group of macromolecules (mucins) which can prevent adherence of bacteria to tooth and tissue site by masking bacterial adhesions or successfully competing with them. They can also effectively clump or aggregate bacteria, reducing their ability to adhere. Mucins have other protective properties, helping to guard soft tissues against abrasion, infection, and ulceration.

A set of proteins in saliva seem uniquely suited for maintenance of hard tissue integrity. They help provide a driving force for remineralization of early subsurface lesions while preventing spontaneous precipitation from the supersaturated saliva. Saliva also contains a set of components (and systems) that help regulate the pH of plaque. These not only include the well-known bicarbonate buffer system, urea and ammonia, but also arginine- and lysine-containing peptides. These latter molecules can serve as substrate for plaque bacteria with the resultant formation of ammonia and the polyamines cadaverine and putrescine. Base formation in plaque is an area worthy of increased attention.

Dr. *Kirsten Eggen* provided further information on the composition of acquired enamel pellicle in vivo, describing recent studies with Dr. *Rölla*. In contrast to in vitro studies with hydroxyapatite, in which proline-rich proteins are the major proteins adsorbed, pellicle scraped from teeth 2 h after cleaning contained a different major anionic component. This protein, very high in serine, glycine, and glutamic acid, was very similar to a phosphoprotein from submandibular saliva described by *Boat* et al. in 1974. The protein cross-reacts with a recently described family of phosphoproteins which contains cysteine [*Shomers* et al., 1982]. The in vivo pellicle preparation also contained immunoglobulins, lysozyme, amylase, albumin, and glucosyltransferase. Further exploration of the specific nature of the pellicle, individual variation, and quantitation are areas of ongoing research. The biological properties of pellicle are potentially a mix of good news and bad news with a diffusion barrier to acid penetration in the former category and adherence of cariogenic microorganisms in the latter. It is ever thus.

The discussion on the relation of salivary flow rate and inorganic constituents to caries dealt mainly with sugar clearance and remineralizing potential. It was suggested that functional measurements of clearance would have to consider such factors as: (1) the volume of saliva in the mouth before and after swallowing; (2) the impact of the ingested food on the stimulation of salivary flow rate; (3) the effects of tongue and cheek movement on food clearance, and (4) loss of sucrose and glucose because of bacterial metabolism. The use of a nondisappearing marker such as chromic oxide was recommended as a means of charting and quantitating clearance. A new generation of 'flow rate' studies is anticipated, studies that measure physiological activity.

Dr. *Leach* presented data on the effect of sugar substitutes, apparently operating via salivary stimulation and remineralization, on impeding caries progression in rodent model systems. The model involved induction of caries by a high sucrose diet, amelioration of the attack by starch replacement of the sucrose, and then cessation and even reversal by sucrose substitutes. He suggested that after early demineralization, remineralization may result in increased protection above the normal level because the remineralized enamel was less soluble than the original.

Reservation was expressed on the clinical impact of salivary stimulation by high sugar concentration in the oral cavity. Although it could dampen the potential cariogenicity of sugars in solution, sugars retained on teeth would be likely to encourage *S. mutans* colonization, proliferation, and plaque buildup. Given the multifactorial nature of caries, looking at the salivary effects alone is inappropriate.

It was suggested that an important effect of reduced flow rate in xerostomia was the failure to supply an adequate amount of total calcium and phosphorus for remineralizing needs. There was disagreement by those who considered the critical factor to be the concentration of calcium and phosphorus in the plaque fluid, rather than the total store. It was suggested that, for protection of normal enamel surfaces, the plaque fluid concentration would be the determining factor, but if there was a prior demineralization, an available store of calcium and phosphorus was essential. Availability of an appropriate level of fluoride was also important. Fluoride concentration in the oral cavity was not only dependent on its introduction and/or secretion but on its mucosal absorption as well. Fluoride disappeared very quickly from under the tongue for instance. Clearance and remineralization had to consider the mouth as a functioning unit, not merely as a mathematical hole.

The saliva-plaque fluid interaction is attracting more attention by investigators and there was some discussion of the high concentration of inorganic constituents in plaque fluid, relative to saliva. Consideration was given to the possibility of a diffusion inhibitor, adsorption to organic components, and release of intracellular components from bacteria, mainly potassium, magnesium, and phosphorus. The ability of the plaque to maintain its high osmolarity is clearly a subject for further research.

Discussion of the role of antibodies in saliva focused on the relative value of the local secretory IgA versus the systemic IgG routes for vaccination against caries and the possible side effects of both procedures. Dr. *Brandtzaeg* expanded on his reservations about safety of the parenteral use of an *S. mutans* antigen (with adjuvant) because of the possibility of an autoimmune response (to kidney and heart) and the exacerbation of gingival disease resulting from immune complexes-affecting complement. Although he had less concern over the IgA approach, he continues to point out our lack of information on the long-term nature of the IgA response and the failure to examine the possible contribution of IgG antibody in the IgA vaccination studies.

Dr. *Bowen* offered the view that a secretory IgA route should work in primates and an IgA response has not been clearly demonstrated in monkeys because, when they come in from the wild, they have antibodies in saliva to food components that cross-react with *S. mutans* antigens. He suggested that modest increases in sIgA antibodies to specific antigens may confer considerable protection despite the inability to quantitate this phenomenon. In human experiments at NIDR, feeding *S. mutans* resulted in only a small increase in IgA antibodies but produced a dramatic effect on colonization of these organisms. Once the specific antigen is identified and becomes available for measurement in an ELISA or similar procedure, antibody measurement would be more meaningful. Dr. *Bowen* also reported on a current study on vaccination in primates in which *S. mutans* was introduced in the drinking water or by gastric intubation to generate an sIgA response. At the end of 2 years there is a marked reduction in tooth infection and in caries.

Dr. *Bowen* does not share Dr. *Brandtzaeg's* concerns over safety. He pointed out that in primate experiments employing intravenous or subcutaneous inoculation of *S. mutans* over a 10-year period he has not seen an exacerbation of gingival inflammation. He also noted that *Russell* et al. [1980], in England, have isolated an *S. mutans* antigen which does not cross-react with heart muscle and are about to start a full-scale clinical trial in children using parenteral administration.

Other discussers questioned whether sufficient IgG antibodies could enter the oral cavity in the absence of gingival inflammation to provide adequate protection against cariogenic organisms and, once in the oral cavity, whether it would remain functional in the proteolytic environment of the plaque. Indeed, if it resisted proteolysis, was there adequate complement and polymorphonuclear leukocytic activity to affect the target organisms? These questions remain to be answered, but there was some agreement that only small amounts of antibody directed to a specific antigen could have a profound effect. It was noted that *Challacombe* and colleagues in England had recently reported (in an abstract) that there was an inverse relationship between caries activity and IgG antibody titer to *S. mutans* in gingival crevicular fluid.

In the discussion of the lactoferrin-sIgA interactions described by Dr. *Arnold,* it was noted that most of the work to date has been done

on samples from colostrum. In saliva, both lactoferrin and sIgA levels
are lower and interacting ions may be present. The findings with
colostrum, however, should be applicable to the oral cavity. The combination of an immunological and a nonimmunological system
provides a flexibility and a regulatory impact on the oral flora not
available with either system acting alone.

In response to a question on the importance of sequencing the
various salivary proteins that have been isolated in pure form in recent
years, Dr. *Hay* described experiments on the structure-function relationship of the acidic proline-rich proteins. He showed that the negatively charged first 30 residues contained the crystal growth inhibitor
activity which helps prevent random mineralization in the oral cavity.
It was pointed out that other factors also affect calculus formation, e.g.
plaque pH, presence of bacterial inhibitors, nucleating molecules such
as calcium phospholipid phosphate, etc. Calculus formation (as well as
demineralization-remineralization of the enamel) involves a number of
pathways.

The discussion on pellicle formation pointed up some of the differences between in vitro and in vivo findings. In vitro, anionic proline-
rich proteins are selectively adsorbed; not in vivo. It may depend,
however, on the method of removing the pellicle in vivo since *Bennick*
et al. have reported that proline-rich proteins bind so tenaciously to
enamel that they are not removed by curetting but will come off
when the outermost layer of enamel is dissolved by acid [*Bennick*
et al., 1983].

Dr. *Rölla* presented additional data on the presence of bacterial
glucosyltransferase in 2-hour pellicle in vivo. It is his view that this
could provide a mechanism for sucrose-enhanced colonization and
proliferation of *S. mutans*. Other mechanisms of bacterial attachment
were discussed as well. Dr. *Eggen* did not think that the anionic
phosphoprotein that was the major component in their pellicle samples
provided specific receptors for *S. mutans* or *S. sanguis*. She speculated
that some of the minor proteins, which showed considerable individual
variation in concentration, were more likely candidates. The possibility
was also discussed of hydrophobic interactions between bacteria and
lipids in pellicle (glycolipids, phospholipids, and lipid covalently bound
to mucin). A provocative speculation was also offered that polysaccharides on the tooth surface, precipitated as the pH falls, could physically entrap bacteria. In summation, colonization could be enhanced

by electrostatic interaction, specific affinities, hydrophobic interaction, and physical entrapment.

References

Bennick, A.; Chau, G.; Goodlin, R.; Abrams, S.; Tustian, D.; Madapallimattam, G.: The role of human salivary acidic proline-rich proteins in the formation of acquired dental pellicle in vivo and their fate after adsorption to the human enamel surface. Archs oral Biol. *28:* 19–28 (1983).
Boat, T.F.; Wiesman, U.N.; Pallavicini, J.C.: Purification and properties of a calcium-precipitable protein in submaxillary saliva of normal and cystic fibrosis subjects. Pediat. Res. *8:* 531–539 (1974).
Russell, M.W.; Zanders, E.D.; Bergmeier, L.A.; Lehner, T.: Affinity purification and characterization of protease-susceptible antigen I of *Streptococcus mutans.* Infect. Immun. *29:* 999–1006 (1980).
Shomers, J.P.; Toboc, L.A.; Lenive, M.J.; Mandel, I.D.; Ellison, S.A.: Characterization of cystein-containing phosphoproteins from human submandibular sublingual saliva. J. dent. Res. *61:* 764–767 (1982).

I.D. Mandel, DDS, School of Dental and Oral Surgery, Columbia University, 630 West 168th Street, New York, NY 10032 (USA)

Cariology Today. Int. Congr., Zürich 1983, pp. 340–352 (Karger, Basel 1984)

Diet and Dental Caries
Symposium Overview

E. Newbrun[1]

Department of Stomatology, University of California, San Francisco, Calif., USA

Introduction

At this conference honouring Prof. *Hans Mühlemann,* it is appropriate that one session was devoted to the role of diet in dental caries and that such topics as the influence of trace metals, plaque pH biotelemetry, sugar substitutes, and the rodent model to test cariogenicity of foods were discussed. Investigators at the Experimental Caries Research Laboratory in Zürich under the leadership of Prof. *Mühlemann* have been in the vanguard of dental research on all these topics. Indeed, much of the pioneer work on telemetric methods to monitor plaque pH changes in vivo originated in Zürich. Similarly, the standardization of the rat caries model with respect to microflora, caries scoring, and programmed feeding to control the frequency of eating were pioneered at the Dental Institute of the University of Zürich. These landmark contributions to the progesss of caries research are directly due to the imagination, creativity, and scientific acumen of Prof. *Mühlemann.*

It is not the purpose of this overview to abstract the excellent presentations of this symposium, nor to transcribe verbatim the ensuing, often lively, discussion. Rather, I have attempted to summarize the important points brought out during the discussions and highlight the main areas of agreement and disagreement among the panelists and the audience. I have also taken the liberty of raising some questions concerning the role of diet in root caries, a topic that has largely been ignored.

---

[1] I am indebted to Ms. *E. Leash* for her editorial assistance.

Compatibility of Nutritional and Dental Dietary Goals

The issue of whether a diet that is noncariogenic or of low cariogenicity (ideal dental diet) is compatible with overall nutritional goals has been reviewed [2,52]. Sometimes, we in the dental profession find ourselves on the horns of a dilemma when we recommend peanuts or potato chips as safe or acceptable snacks. These items are usually salted and contain considerable fat. However, the intake of both salt and saturated fats should be reduced [62]. Incidentally, recent findings indicate that hypertension may not be sodium dependent but sodium chloride-dependent [33]. Total daily per caput salt (sodium chloride) intake averages between 12 to 14 g, of which about $1/3$ occurs naturally in food, $1/3$ is added during processing, and $1/3$ is added at the table. This per caput intake should be lowered to about 8 g/day. The food industry has parallel responsibilities to help reduce salt and sugar intake, both of which are major food additives. Nevertheless, in some countries salt is used as a vehicle for nutritional supplementation of diets with iodine and also fluoride. Salted peanuts are dentally safe snacks because they are nonacidogenic and can also abort the pH drop that occurs after eating sugary snacks [13]. The salt acts as a sialagogue, although chewing of the peanuts per se may suffice to stimulate salivary flow.

Role of the Food Industry and the Dental Profession

Food manufacturers have an important role to play in developing dentally safe, noncariogenic snacks [41]. Although some researchers think we do not yet know what to tell industry, we actually have more than enough findings from biochemical and microbiological experiments in animals and from clinical and epidemiological studies on humans to support the case for reducing sugar (particularly sucrose and/or monosaccharides) in foods [17,44,53,55]. The dental profession also has a responsibility to work with industry in providing objective tests to evaluate the dental safety of foods. Some of those tests are discussed later. Although it may be extremely difficult to change an *individual* patient's dietary and snacking habits, considerable alterations in a *society's* pattern of food intake has occurred during wartime rationing [59,61]. Furthermore, even in peacetime, marked changes in the intake of sugars have resulted from altered manufacturing practices. In the USA within the past decade, high fructose corn syrups (HFCS) have jumped from less than 1 to 15% of the caloric sweetener market [62]. As is often the case, money is the best motivator. When the price of sucrose rose sharply in the mid-1970s, food manufacturers, especially the producers of soft drinks, had a palpable incentive to decrease the sucrose content of their product. But from a dental viewpoint, HFCS are anything but safe. The important lesson from this is that those who state that we 'can't change people's diets' are wrong; diets have changed radically and will continue to change.

The dental profession also has a responsibility to influence governmental authorities and food regulatory agencies to recognize that some foods are noncariogenic (dentally safe) and that labelling of foods with respect to cariogenic potential is desirable and in the best interests of the consumer [43]. Manufacturers face tremendous problems because there are no uniform standards of dental acceptance of food products, and labelling regulations vary in different countries [23]. As a first step in resolving some of these difficulties, we should insist on dental representation along with medical, nutritional, and toxicological expertise on all such regulatory committees. Methods of testing cariogenicity of foods should be universally acceptable, which implies a need for compromise among those of us involved in caries research. We cannot allow ourselves the luxury of saying that since we do not have a perfect test of food cariogenicity, nothing can be done about regulations or labelling. It is improbable that any single test, whether in vivo or in vitro, can adequately measure all the factors involved in the carious process [42]. However, a combination of tests may be useful in predicting the cariogenic potential of a food or beverage [3,36].

Animal Model

The advantages of using animals to assay cariogenicity of foods are obvious with respect to low cost, speed with which lesions are formed, and avoidance of moral or legal problems that arise with human subjects. The rodent model for cariogenicity testing has undergone considerable modification in order to control as many variables as possible (animal strain, age, infection, caries scoring system, randomization of animals on diet, programmed feeding) [34,38,60]. Unfor-

Table I. Mean enamel buccal caries scores ($\pm$ SD) in rats one same diet[1] showing variation between experiments

Experiment No.	Diet No.	
	456 and SSL	305
I	10.4 $\pm$ 1.2	16.4 $\pm$ 0.9
II	6.6 $\pm$ 1.2	11.2 $\pm$ 1.4
III	4.0 $\pm$ 0.8	12.4 $\pm$ 1.8
IV	1.5 $\pm$ 1.1	21.4 $\pm$ 0.8
V	8.0 $\pm$ 1.5	19.2 $\pm$ 1.3
VI	14.2 $\pm$ 1.5	12.3 $\pm$ 1.1
Mean	8.9 $\pm$ 3.6	15.5 $\pm$ 4.2

[1] Diet No. 456 and SSL in programmed feeder or diet 305 ad libitum [40].

tunately, the method described by *Navia* [39] in which the test food is offered alternately with gel diet No. 456 does not maintain a high degree of reproducibility. In spite of attention to details and standardization of all procedures and manipulations, there is a disturbing variation from experiment to experiment, especially for buccal smooth surface scores (table I) [40]. In 6 separate experiments the groups were fed either the 'control' diet SSL alternately with diet No. 456 by controlled frequency feeding [16], or diet No. 305 ad libitum. The differences in results between experiments were greater in some cases than between diets in the same experiment. The sucrose content (5% dry wt.) of diet No. 456 contributes to the caries process so that baseline data are 'noisy' and may be the reason that 'minor differences' in the cariogenicity of snack foods could not be distinguished by this method.

Plaque pH Measurement and Acidogenicity of Foods

Considerable discussion centered on the technique of intraoral plaque pH telemetry as well as on how to interpret such data. In all of the studies, whether conducted by the group in Minnesota [49] or in Zürich [22], no attempt was made to control the diet during the 3–7 days that the plaque is being formed on the glass electrodes. Accordingly, the composition of the microflora in those preformed plaques is a result of influences other than that of the food being tested. Both the amount of plaque formed [4] and the proportions of *Streptococcus mutans* are influenced by the preceeding dietary sucrose intake [21,56,58]. Although we understand a great deal about the effect of sugars on colonization of plaque by *S. mutans* and lactobacilli, we know little else concerning the role of diet on plaque bacterial ecology.

Most of the subjects in plaque pH telemetry studies have been adults with a history of caries, but not necessarily with active lesions. The morphology of plaque covering glass electrodes has been described [22]. No quantitative data have been published concerning the taxonomy of the flora on these electrodes, other than a comparison of total colony-forming units and proportion of streptococci recovered from glass and enamel surfaces [25]. *Streptococcus sanguis* was the predominant group of streptococci isolated from plaque on the electrodes by the Minnesota group. Very few if any *S. mutans* were found, although 1 subject had a high lactobacillus count, which did not appear to alter the pH response. In studies using pure cultures, lower pH values were found in the agar beneath colonies of *S. mutans* than beneath colonies of *S. sanguis* or *Streptococcus mitis* [45]. One reason advanced for permitting test subjects an unrestricted diet during the formation of plaque on the electrodes was that food to be tested would act on a 'normal' plaque. Dr. *Schachtele* explained that a 'standardized' plaque simply meant that a similar pH response occurred irrespective of preceding diet. He had no information as to the thickness of the plaques formed on the electrodes, either interproximally or buccally. Obviously a range of thickness might be formed in different subjects, and diffusion in and out of the plaque would be affected.

Biofilm (acquired pellicle) formed on glass differs in composition from that formed on enamel [54] and could affect bacterial colonization on these surfaces. The pH response seen with glass electrodes might be a 'hyperresponse', since glass is inert whereas enamel consists of hydroxyapatite which could dissolve and thereby buffer the acid formed. Such an idea was rejected by Dr. *Schachtele,* who stated that there was no difference in the pH response of plaque on buccal tooth surfaces whether measured by indwelling glass electrodes, antimony or glass touch electrodes in vivo, or by plaque sampling and measuring pH response in vitro [48]. However, plaque pH recorded by built-in electrodes at interproximal sites gave lower minimal values and slower return to resting pH than buccal sites on the same tooth [24].

Plaque pH telemetry can be used to classify food items into non-acidogenic, hypoacidogenic, and acidogenic products. The former, as the name implies, do not lower plaque pH at all. Hypoacidogenic products (e.g. ribose, xylose, sorbose, melibiose, polydextrose, coupling sugar) are fermented slowly and do not depress plaque pH below 5.7 either during ingestion or up to 30 min thereafter. Acidogenic foods cannot satisfactorily be classified on the basis of minimum pH reached, as many of them drop close to 4.0. *Schachtele and Jensen* [49] have attempted to group foods into least and most acidogenic categories by calculating units of pH less than 5.7 multiplied by time (min). Because of the logarithmic relationship between pH and hydrogen ion concentration (cH), it would be more appropriate that the data should be converted to cH values and calculated as 'proton-hours' or 'cH area' [12,47]. Unfortunately, for statistical testing cH data show markedly non-Gaussian distribution [11]. Even when cH area is used, any ranking of foods within the acidogenic group is still just that, an *acidogenicity* scale. It cannot be directly equated with *cariogenicity* [22]. This limitation should not in any way detract from the value of plaque pH telemetry as a means of identifying dentally safe products.

Trace Elements

Human epidemiological surveys of caries prevalence in relation to the presence or absence of a particular trace element have not always been confirmed when tested by adding that particular element to, or excluding it from, the diet of experimental animals. This could be due to erroneous interpretation of the original data. For example, in a community with a soft-water supply, the low pH acting on copper pipes can raise the copper content of the water. An apparent relationship between high copper ingestion and high caries prevalence is not warranted, however, as the soft water may be deficient in another unidentified element which is the real cause of the high caries prevalence. If one finds an association in a human epidemiological study between a trace element and caries, it should be tested in the animal model. If the association holds up, it is still necessary to go back to human studies either in a controlled clinical trial of the trace element or in a test of the hypothesis in a different population, preferably in another part of the world.

The rodent model itself presents problems, for example, when used to test the effect of a trace metal dietary supplement. If the pups are fed the element post-weaning, both first and second molars have already calcified. Prior to birth and weaning the mother cannot always transfer the element through the placenta or the milk.

Trace elements other than fluoride may influence caries by being systemically absorbed from the diet and incorporated into enamel. However, trace elements (e.g. strontium) may also have a topical posteruptive effect and be incorporated during maturation of the enamel or remineralization [8]. Furthermore, some trace elements (e.g. zinc, copper) interfere with plaque bacterial metabolism and could affect caries in this way. Finally, the ionic state of the element is important. Stannous ions reduce caries, whereas stannic ions do not.

Diet and Root Caries

The preceding discussion and most of the available dental literature has dealt with the role of dietary factors in the development of coronal caries. Although root caries has afflicted man since ancient times, our understanding of its etiology is limited, particularly concerning the role of diet. Root caries has been noted on the teeth of ancient skulls of North American Indians [35], Fiji Islanders [5], Hawaiians [28], pre-Columbian Peruvians [57], and early Anglo-Saxons [6,18,37]. Generally these same teeth had few, if any, coronal caries. The usual explanation offered for this difference in caries prevalence between ancient man and modern man living in an industrial society is that primitive diets contained far less sucrose. Certainly sucrose was not cultivated in Hawaii 200–500 years ago, nor in the pre-Columbian Americas. Starches such as taro root and corn were a staple of these primitive diets. However, any conclusion as to the importance of starch versus sucrose in root caries based on these limited findings would be purely speculative.

The prevalence of root caries has also been found to exceed the prevalence of coronal caries in certain present-day populations. By the time they reach 30–39 years of age, natives of Lufa, Papua, New Guinea have more root caries than coronal caries [50]. The principal food of this population is sweet potatoes, supplemented with a variety of vegetables, fruits, nuts, and occasionally with meat [51]. A higher rate of root caries has also been found among narcotics addicts and has been attributed to the general avitaminosis, excessive consumption of refined carbohydrates, and poor oral hygiene of this population [19]. However, the diet history of these addicts was not analyzed quantitatively nor were objective measurements of vitamin levels obtained. Decreased salivary flow due to habitual use of narcotics could also account for the increase in root caries.

The Vipeholm dental caries study is one of the few in which dietary factors were relatively well controlled. In those groups receiving sugar supplements between meals (22 caramels or 24 toffees daily) the frequency of root caries was high; in the toffee group, root caries accounted for 25% of all lesions. However, these goups were also slightly older than the other test groups [17].

More recently, *Hix and O'Leary* [20] reported that in patients with periodontal disease, both treated and untreated, those that had the most root caries gave a diet history indicating significantly more exposures to fermentable carbohydrates per week. Unfortunately, no attempt was made to quantify the amount or types of sugars ingested; only the frequency of ingestion of 'readily fermentable carbohydrate' was scored.

King [32] reported that golden hamsters developed root caries whether fed a predominantly cereal diet (whole meal flour, whole meal bread, or white maize) or a high (65%) sucrose diet. Caries, if present, was due to the indigenous flora, but less than 7% of the molar teeth were affected. None of the animals developed primary coronal caries. Conventional hamsters infected with filamentous bacteria (subsequently identified as *Actinomyces viscosus* T6) developed root caries on a fine-powdered, high-sugar diet 2000 (sucrose 56%, skim milk powder 28%, whole meal flour 6%, yeast 4%) originally formulated by *Keyes* [30]. When the diet was changed to a commercial laboratory chow, the plaque mineralized and root caries did not progress [31]. Root caries was induced in rats monoinfected with a *Streptococcus salivarius*-'like' strain SS2 or 1A when fed diet 2000, whereas diet 585, a coarse-particle diet (sucrose 25%, whole milk powder 30%, yellow hominy grits 42%) induced only fissure caries [14,29]. However, in earlier studies with a more virulent organism, *S. mutans* GS5, root caries as well as coronal caries was obtained with monoinfected rats on diet 585 [15]. In most subsequent studies, both with conventional rodents [10,46] or monoinfected rats [7,26,27], diet 2000 has been used to obtain root caries. *De Palma* et al. [9] compared the ability of different foods (toffee, butter

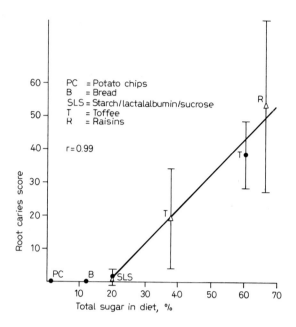

Fig. 1. Root caries scores in the rice rat fed different diets with various sugar content. Regression line plotted for data from starch/lactalbumin/sucrose, toffee (2 kinds), and raisins [9].

crackers, bread, raisins, potato chips) to induce root caries in the rice rat. They found a direct relationship between root caries scores and the total sugar content of the test food item. Calculation of the correlation coefficient (r = 0.99) shows it to be highly significant (see fig. 1).

Clearly, there is a paucity of well-controlled animal studies or quantitative data in humans on the importance of dietary factors in root caries. Based on epidemiological findings in ancient civilizations and primitive societies, *Banting and Courtright* [1] concluded that root caries can occur in populations whose diets have little sucrose. However, most animal and some human data suggest that root caries will increase, as will coronal caries, with increased amount and frequency of sugar intake. This hypothesis needs to be confirmed using both modern techniques of computerized diet history analysis and experimental variation of animal diets.

Conclusion

The goal of a nutritionally adequate diet is compatible with one of low cariogenic potential. The food industry should be encouraged to manufacture foods, especially snacks, that contain nonacidogenic or hypoacidogenic sugar substitutes. Such products should be labeled accordingly as 'dentally safe'. The dental profession should advise patients to consume these foods in preference to sugary snacks. Foods can be evaluated for cariogenicity by well-controlled animal tests, but cariogenicity in humans also depends on individual consumption patterns. Plaque pH response in vivo after ingestion of individual foods can be used for identifying foods that are safe for teeth (nonacidogenic), but ranking of acidogenic foods by this method would be premature. Other factors besides acid production are involved in the carious process. Trace elements other than fluoride affect dental caries and may act systemically and/or topically by incorporation into enamel or by antimicrobial action. Whereas there is compelling evidence for the role of sucrose and other fermentable sugars in coronal caries, we know less concerning dietary factors in the etiology of root caries.

References

1   Banting, D.W.; Courtright, P.N.: The distribution and natural history of carious lesions on the roots of teeth. J. Can. dent. Ass. *41:* 45–59 (1975).
2   Bender, A.E.: Nutrition and diet in a changing society; in Guggenheim, Cariology today. Int. Congr., Zürich 1983, pp. 119–124 (Karger, Basel 1984).
3   Bibby, B.G.; Goldberg, H.J.V.; Chen, E.: Evaluation of caries-producing potentialities of various foods stuffs. J. Am. dent. Ass. *42:* 491–509 (1951).
4   Carlsson, J.; Egelberg, J.: Effect of diet on early plaque formation in man. Odont. Revy *16:* 112–125 (1965).
5   Chappel, H.G.: Jaws and teeth of ancient Hawaiians. Mem. Bernice P. Bishop Mus. *9:* 251–268 (1927).
6   Corbett, M.E.; Moore, W.J.: Distribution of caries in ancient British populations. J. dent. Res. *50:* 663 (1971).
7   Crawford, A.C.R.; Socransky, S.S.; Smith, E.; Phillips, R.: Pathogenicity testing of oral isolates in gnotobiotic rats. J. dent. Res. *56:* Abstr. 275, p. B120 (1977).
8   Curzon, M.E.J.: Influence on caries of trace metals other than fluoride; in Guggenheim, Cariology today. Int. Congr., Zürich 1983, pp. 125–135 (Karger, Basel 1984).
9   De Palma, J.; Rosen, S.; Harper, D.S.: Specific foods as etiological factors in bone loss and root caries. J. dent. Res. *62:* Abstr. 1136, 295 (1983).

10   Doff, R.S.; Rosen, S.; App, G.: Root surface caries in the molar teeth of rice rats. II. Quantitation of lesions induced by high sucrose diet. J. dent. Res. *56:* 1111–1114 (1977).

11   Edgar, W.M.: The role of saliva in the control of pH changes in human dental plaque. Caries Res. *10:* 241–254 (1976).

12   Edgar, W.M.: Duration of response and stimulus sequence in the interpretation of plaque pH data. J. dent. Res. *61:* 1126 1129 (1982).

13   Geddes, D.A.M.; Edgar, W.M.; Jenkins, G.N.; Rugg-Gunn, A.J.: Apples, salted peanuts and plaque pH. Br. dent. J. *142:* 317–319 (1977).

14   Gibbons, R.J.; Banghart, S.: Induction of dental caries in gnotobiotic rats with a levan-forming streptococcus and a streptococcus isolated from subacute bacterial endocarditis. Archs oral Biol. *13:* 297–308 (1968).

15   Gibbons, R.J.; Berman, K.S.; Knoettner, P.; Kapsimalis, B.: Dental caries and periodontal bone loss in gnotobiotic rats infected with capsule-forming streptococci of human origin. Archs oral Biol. *11:* 549–650 (1966).

16   Guggenheim, B.; Schmid, R.; Mühlemann, H.R.: Programmed feeding; in Tanzer, Animal models in cariology, sp. suppl.: Microbiology Abstracts, pp. 391–401 (Information Retrieval Inc., Arlington 1981).

17   Gustafsson, V.E.; Quensel, C.E.; Lanke, L.S.; Lundqvist, C.; Grahnen, H.; Bonow, B.E.; Krasse, B.: The Vipeholm dental caries study. The effect of different levels of carbohydrate intake on caries activity in 436 individuals observed for 5 years. Acta odont. scand. *11:* 232–364 (1954).

18   Hardwick, J.L.: The incidence and distribution of caries throughout the ages in relation to Englishmen's diet. Br. dent. J. *108:* 9–17 (1960).

19   Hecht, S.S.; Friedman, J.: The high incidence of cervical dental caries among drug addicts. Oral Surg. *2:* 1428–1442 (1949).

20   Hix, J.O.; O'Leary, T.J.: The relationship between cemental caries, oral hygiene status and fermentable carbohydrate intake. J. Periodont. *47:* 398–404 (1976).

21   Hoover, C.; Newbrun, E.; Mettraux, G.; Graf, H.: Microflora and chemical composition of plaque from patients with hereditary fructose intolerance. Infect. Immunity *28:* 853–859 (1980).

22   Imfeld, T.N.: Identification of low caries risk dietary components. Monogr. oral Sci., vol. 2, pp. 1–28 (Karger, Basel 1983).

23   Imfeld, T.: Non-acidogenic and non-cariogenic sugar substitutes and sweeteners; in Guggenheim, Cariology today. Int. Congr., Zürich 1983, pp. 147–153 (Karger, Basel 1984).

24   Jensen, M.E.; Schachtele, C.F.; Polansky, P.J.: Indwelling pH electrodes: analysis of human dental plaque response at different sites; in Hefferren, Ayer, Koehler, Foods, nutrition and dental health, vol. 3, pp. 103–114. (Pathotox, Park Forest South 1981).

25   Jensen, M.E.; Polansky, P.J.; Schachtele, C.F.: Plaque sampling and telemetry for monitoring acid production on human buccal tooth surfaces. Archs oral Biol. *27:* 21–31 (1982).

26   Jordan, H.V.; Hammond, B.F.: Filamentous bacteria isolated from human root surface caries. Archs oral Biol. *17:* 1333–1342 (1972).

27 Jordan, H.V.; Keyes, P.H.; Bellack, S.: Periodontal lesions in hamsters and gnoto-
    biotic rats infected with *Actinomyces* of human origin. J. periodont. Res. *7:* 21–28
    (1972).
28 Keene, H.J.: Dental caries in ancient and modern Hawaii. J. Hawaii dent. Ass. *7:*
    9–14 (1974).
29 Kelstrup, J.; Gibbons, R.J.: Induction of dental caries and alveolar bone loss by
    a human isolate resembling *Streptococcus salivarius*. Caries Res. *4:* 360–377 (1970).
30 Keyes, P.H.: Dental caries in a Syrian hamster. VIII. The induction of rampant
    caries activity in albino and golden hamsters. J. dent. Res. *38:* 525–533 (1959).
31 Keyes, P.H.; Jordan, H.V.: Periodontal lesions in the Syrian Hamster. III. Findings
    related to an infectious and transmissible component. Archs oral Biol. *9:* 377–400
    (1964).
32 King, J.D.: Dental cavities in the golden hamster. Br. med. J. *i:* 876–877 (1950).
33 Kurtz, T.W.; Curtis-Morris, R.: Dietary chloride as a determinant of 'sodium-
    dependent' hypertension. Science *222:* 1139–1141 (1983).
34 Larson, R.H.; Amsbaugh, S.M.; Navia, J.N.; Rosen, S.; Schuster, G.S.; Shaw,
    J.H.: Collaborative evaluation of a rat caries model in six laboratories. J. dent. Res.
    56: 1007–1012 (1977).
35 Leigh, R.W.: Dental pathology of Indian tribes of varied environmental and food
    conditions. Am. J. phys. Anthrop. *8:* 179–199 (1925).
36 Matsukubo, T.; Newbrun, E.; Maki, Y.; Miyake, S.; Takaesu, Y.: Evaluation of
    cariogenicity of foods based on a combination of four variables; in Hefferren,
    McEnery, Foods, nutrition and dental health, vol. 5 (American Dental Association,
    Chicago, in press 1984).
37 Miles, A.E.W.: The dentition of the Anglo-Saxons. Proc. R. Soc. Med. *62:*
    1311–1315 (1969).
38 Navia, J.M.: Animal models in dental research (University of Alabama Press,
    University 1977).
39 Navia, J.M.: The value of animal models to predict the caries-promoting properties
    of human diet or dietary components; in Guggenheim, Cariology today. Int.
    Congr., Zürich 1983, pp. 154–165 (Karger, Basel 1984).
40 Navia, J.M.; Lopez, H.: Rat caries assay of reference foods and sugar-containing
    snacks. J. dent. Res. *62:* 893–898 (1983).
41 Newbrun, E.: The role of food manufacturers in the dietary control of caries. J. Am.
    Soc. Prev. Dent. *4:* 43–44 (1974).
42 Newbrun, E.: Criteria indicative of cariogenicity or non-cariogenicity of foods and
    beverages; in Guggenheim, Proc. ERGOB Conf. Health Sugar Substitutes, pp.
    253–258 (Karger, Basel 1978).
43 Newbrun, E.: Criteria of cariogenicity for labeling foods. J. Am. dent. Ass. *105:*
    627–630 (1982).
44 Newbrun, E.: Sucrose in the dynamics of the caries process. Int. dent. J., London
    32: 13–23 (1982).
45 Onose, H.; Sandham, H.J.: pH changes during culture of human dental plaque
    streptococci on mitis-salivarius agar. Archs oral Biol. *21:* 291–296 (1976).
46 Rotilie, J.A.; McDaniel, T.; Rosen, S.: Root surface caries in the molar teeth of rice
    rat. III. Inhibition of root surface caries by fluoride. J. dent. Res. *56:* 1498 (1977).

47   Rugg-Gunn, A.J.; Edgar, W.M.; Geddes, D.A.M.; Jenkins, G.N.: The effect of different meal patterns upon plaque pH in human subjects. Br. dent. J. *139:* 351–366 (1975).
48   Schachtele, C.F.; Jensen, M.E.; Human plaque pH studies: estimating acidogenic potential of foods. Cereal Foods Wld. *26:* 14–18 (1981).
49   Schachtele, C.F.; Jensen, M.E.: Can foods be ranked according to their cariogenic potential? in Guggenheim, Cariology today. Int. Congr., Zürich 1983, pp. 136–146 (Karger, Basel 1984).
50   Schamschula, R.G.; Barmes, D.E.; Keyes, P.H.; Gulbinat, W.: Prevalence and interrelationships of root surface caries in Lufa, Papua New Guinea. Community Dent. oral Epidemiol. *2:* 295–304 (1974).
51   Schamschula, R.G.; Keyes, P.H.; Hornabrook, R.W.: Root surface caries in Lufa, New Guinea. I. Clinical observations. J. Am. dent. Ass. *85:* 603–608 (1972).
52   Shaw, J.H.; Witschi, J.C.: Is the ideal diet for preventing dental caries physiologically adequate? in Guggenheim, Cariology today. Int. Congr., Zürich 1983, pp. 166–172 (Karger, Basel 1984).
53   Sheiham, A.: Sugars and dental decay. Lancet *i:* 282–284 (1983).
54   Sonju, T.; Glantz, P.-O.: Chemical composition of salivary integuments formed in vivo on solids with some established surface characteristics. Archs oral Biol. *20:* 687–691 (1975).
55   Sreebny, L.M.: Sugar availability, sugar consumption and dental caries. Community Dent. oral Epidemiol. *10:* 1–7 (1982).
56   Staat, R.H.; Gawronski, T.H.; Cressey, D.E.; Harris, R.S.; Folke, L.E.A.: Effects of dietary sucrose levels on the quantity and microbial composition of human dental plaque. J. dent. Res. *54:* 872–880 (1975).
57   Stewart, T.D.: Dental caries in Peruvian skulls. Am. J. phys. Anthrop. *15:* 315–326 (1931).
58   Stoppelaar, J.D. de; Houte, J. van; Backer Dirks, O.: The effect of carbohydrate restriction on the presence of *Streptococcus mutans, Streptococcus sanguis,* and iodophilic polysaccharide-producing bacteria in human dental plaque. Caries Res. *4:* 114–123 (1970).
59   Takeuchi, M.: Epidemiological study on dental caries in Japanese children before, during and after W.W. II. Int. dent. J., Lond *11:* 443–457 (1961).
60   Tanzer, J.M.: Animal models in cariology, sp. suppl.: Microbiology Abstracts (Information Retrieval Inc., Arlington 1981).
61   Toverud, G.: Child dental health. Br. dent. J. *160:* 299–304 (1964).
62   US Department of Agriculture, Economics and Statistics Service: Sugar and sweetener report, vol. *6:* pp. 1–49 (1981).
63   US Senate Select Committee on Nutrition and Human Needs: Dietary goals for the United States, p. 12 (US Government Printing Office, Washington 1977).

Prof. E. Newbrun, Department of Stomatology, HSW-604, University of California, San Francisco, CA 94143 (USA)

Cariology Today. Int. Congr., Zürich 1983, pp. 353–361 (Karger, Basel 1984)

Dental Plaque
Highlights of the Discussion

R.J. Gibbons

Forsyth Dental Center, Boston, Mass., USA

The topic of dental plaque is central to any discussion of cariology because it is these bacterial accumulations on the teeth which actually cause dental decay. While the cariogenic activities of plaque bacteria can be significantly influenced by the diet or by the flow and composition of saliva, it is the bacteria that are cariogenic and not other factors per se. The session on plaque considered the types of bacteria which seem to be important in the caries process, and it reviewed some of the parameters which affect their colonization, metabolism, and cariogenicity. The following summary highlights some points of interest which arose during the discussions involving panel members and the audience.

Relationship of Streptococcus mutans *to Dental Caries*

Considerable evidence suggests that organisms of the *S. mutans* group are among the most important etiologic agents of dental caries in humans. They are highly acidogenic and aciduric bacteria and their cariogenic potential is well-established in animal models. Also, *S. mutans* preferentially colonizes the teeth, and is found in especially high proportions in pits, fissures, contact points, and other retentive areas. Thus, its pattern of colonization parallels the recognized susceptibility of these sites to dental decay. In addition, several investigators have demonstrated that the presence and proportions of *S. mutans* on specific tooth surfaces often correlate with caries development. However, as pointed out by Dr. *G. Bowden,* the association of *S. mutans* with human dental decay is not a simple one-on-one relationship. Many tooth surfaces harbor *S. mutans* and yet do not decay and, conversely, surfaces monitored over time occasionally develop decay in the absence of detectable *S. mutans*.

Several reasons were suggested which could account for these observations. Because the prevalence of dental decay has been declining dramatically in the USA and Europe during the past decade, possibly due to the widespread use of fluoride, the potential of *S. mutans* for initiating decay is being combated. Thus, one may expect to find *S. mutans* on sound enamel surfaces with increasing frequency. It was also pointed out that *S. mutans* colonizes in a remarkably localized way, and this makes it difficult to associate the presence of *S. mutans* with decay developing on a specific tooth site. Dr. *Bowden* drew an analogy with the distribution of the orange-tipped butterfly in England. He observed that one can find large numbers of such butterflies near the Essex Bridge, but none can be found down the road. Likewise, *S. mutans* can often be found in high proportions in plaque removed from one small area of a tooth, and yet it can be undetectable just a few millimeters away. This suggests that caution must also be used in interpreting observations regarding the development of incipient carious lesions in the apparent absence of *S. mutans*.

Others commented that strains of *S. mutans* derived from humans vary considerably in their virulence, at least as assessed in animal models. *S. mutans* strains have also been observed to become altered in virulence while colonizing experimental animals. When a highly virulent strain is introduced into the mouths of gnotobiotic rats, isolates of altered virulence can readily be obtained within a few weeks. It is thought that the host responds immunologically to the dominating types of *S. mutans* cells present, and then these initially virulent types become suppressed and other antigenic subtypes are selected. Such antigenic and physiologic variation has been observed with other bacteria, especially those associated with chronic infections. Certain bio- or genetic types of *S. mutans* have also been suggested to be more pathogenic than others. However, data to substantiate this possibility are not available, and it would be quite difficult to obtain because of the variation that exists between strains of the same type.

Is S. mutans *Normal or a Pathogen?*

Considerable discussion centered on whether *S. mutans* should be considered an autochthonous member of the oral flora or a pathogen. Most agree that *S. mutans* can be isolated from the teeth of a very high percentage of older children and adults, and therefore, it is clear that it is common. Its prevalence has led to one view that *S. mutans* is 'normal', and the development of dental caries is the result of an ecological imbalance, or a shift in the proportions of the normal oral flora induced by factors such as the frequent ingestion of sucrose-containing foods. The opposing view is that *S. mutans* is no more 'normal' than is dental decay; both are 'common', but neither should be considered 'normal'. For example, approximately 40% of humans may harbor group A streptococci and 60% *Candida albicans*. These organisms are therefore also relatively 'common', but they are not considered to be normal or autochthonous. In addition, *S. mutans* has invasive properties, and it has been associated with subacute bacterial endocarditis.

These two views represent in part semantic differences, and in part different philosophies. However, it may be easier to motivate the public to adopt caries-preventative procedures if the infectious nature of the disease is emphasized. Dr. *D. Bratthall* attempted to mediate the discussions. In considering whether *S. mutans* was 'normal' or an 'invader', he stated that he believed it was now a 'normal invader'. However, if the percentage of humans who become infected by *S. mutans* could be reduced by interfering with its transmission, or by chemotherapeutic, immunologic, or other means, then *S. mutans* would be less prevalent and therefore no longer as 'normal' as it now appears.

What is Unique about S. mutans *in Regard to Cariogenicity?*

It is generally recognized that many plaque bacteria in addition to *S. mutans* produce acids from the fermentation of dietary carbohydrates, and the question arises as to what is unique about *S. mutans* to account for its postulated role in caries etiology. Several comments were made in this regard. Although there are bacteria other than *S. mutans* which produce caries in experimental animals, some, such as *Streptococcus salivarius* and *Streptococcus faecalis,* are not found in high numbers on human teeth. In addition, strains of *S. mutans* are frequently much more virulent than other bacteria in experimental animals. Dr. *W. Bowen* commented that lactobacilli usually require 100 days to produce the same degree of cavitation in animals that *S. mutans* can induce within 30 days. In addition, monkeys have a flora similiar, though not identical to that of humans, which includes lactobacilli, yet they develop only minimal dental caries when free of *S. mutans,* even when fed diets known to be highly caries-conducive. Dr. *W. Loesche* also pointed out that *S. mutans* is much more acidogenic and aciduric than most other plaque bacteria, and these properties may be reflected in the overall metabolism of plaque. For example, plaques harboring high proportions of *S. mutans* from carious sites metabolize sucrose up to 6 times faster than plaques from sound surfaces which have low proportions of *S. mutans*. Another unusual feature of *S. mutans* pointed out by Dr. *Loesche* is its ability to tolerate very high concentrations of sucrose. This is used to advantage in the formulation of selective media. Thus, mitis salivarius bacitracin (MSB) medium contains 20% sucrose, and other selective media for *S. mutans* contain as much as 50% sucrose as a selective agent. While all of these features likely contribute to the cariogenic potential of organisms of the *S. mutans* group, it should be pointed out that other yet unknown factors may also be important.

Interfering with the Transmission of S. mutans

Many infectious diseases have been controlled by interfering with the transmission of the infecting organism. Efforts to use such an approach for controlling *S. mutans* and dental caries have recently been reported by *Kohler, Bratthall, and Krasse* [Archs. oral Biol. *28:* 225, 1983]. They identified mothers with high salivary *S. mutans* levels ($> 10^6$/mlP) and treated them with chlorhexidine and fluoride until the numbers of the organism were decreased by an order of magnitude. They noted that significantly fewer infants of treated mothers became infected with *S. mutans* than did infants of untreated mothers. Dr. *Krasse* further commented that this study is continuing and the effect observed is still apparent 3 years later. Also, much less caries developed in the children who were free of *S. mutans*. Thus, children infected with *S. mutans* at 1 year of age averaged 10 decayed or filled tooth surfaces when 4 years of age. However, children who remained free of *S. mutans* had only 0.3 such surfaces. Dr. *D. Bratthall* elaborated that it has not been possible to eliminate *S. mutans* from the mouth once it has colonized. The best professional toothcleaning does not get rid of it, and intensive application of antibacterial agents such as chlorhexidine or iodine produces only a temporary suppression. Therefore, interfering with transmission may prove to be a very important approach. Administration of vaccines to infants may be another way of interfering with *S. mutans* transmission, though there have been few studies in this area.

What if S. mutans *Could Be Eliminated?*

The question arose as to what would happen if *S. mutans* could be eliminated? There were two somewhat divergent views. One was that *S. mutans* fills a 'functional niche' within the overall ecology of the dental plaque, and if it were eliminated, the void would be filled by some other organism. It was theorized that the organism coming in would likely have metabolic and physiological features similar to those of *S. mutans*. It was also suggested that lactobacilli might take over and assume more importance. Proponents of the opposing view argued that monkeys and humans exist without detectable *S. mutans*, and they have no apparent problems; they exhibit minimal or no dental decay, and no new cariogenic organisms have appeared. Furthermore, lactobacilli colonize fissures and other retentive sites, but they are not usually found on sound enamel surfaces or associated with white spots lesions. Also, they often disappear from the mouth when carious lesions are restored. Therefore, their colonization appears to be favored by the prior existence of a carious lesion, and their potential for initiating lesions seems to be low. Though it is conceivable that some degree of decalcification could be initiated by bacteria other than *S. mutans* which might foster colonization of lactobacilli, this does not appear to have occurred to a significant extent in either *S. mutans*-free monkeys or humans, or for that matter, on areas of teeth which do not have detectable levels of *S. mutans* in otherwise infected individuals.

Diffusion Properties of Plaques

Histological and electron microscopic observations have left little doubt that dental plaques in situ have a definite structure, and that the bacteria present frequently exist as microcolonies. However, investigations of the diffusion properties of plaque have used pooled samples scraped from several tooth surfaces. This causes some concern, particularly to microbiologists, because there is reason to suspect that initial areas of demineralization develop under certain microcolonies, i.e., those of *S. mutans,* and the diffusion properties of microcolonies of one organism may be quite different from those of another. While attempts have been made to study the diffusion of isotopes in intact plaques, it has not always been possible to differentiate mobile from bound molecules of the diffusing substance, and therefore these studies have been difficult to interpret. A further complication is that the tortuosity of diffusion pathways varies greatly in plaques and is influenced by the density of bacterial cells present.

Dr. *J. Featherstone* pointed out that an array of complex diffusion reactions take place which are relevant to the caries process. Dietary carbohydrates must diffuse into the plaque and be taken up by bacterial cells. The carbohydrates are then converted to acids which must pass out of the bacteria into the plaque matrix and then diffuse either through the pellicle to the enamel or else out to saliva. Since plaque is saturated with calcium and phosphate ions, these ions will not diffuse out of enamel unless the pH of plaque drops and thereby lowers the saturation levels. Then acid must diffuse through the pellicle to enamel, and calcium and phosphate ions must diffuse out of the enamel through the pellicle and into the plaque. All of these diffusion processes occur rapidly, probably within minutes or even seconds. They all should be considered in regard to caries development and the reversal of incipient lesions.

It has been observed that mutants of *S. mutans* which no longer produce highly insoluble alpha 1 : 3-linked glucans are no longer cariogenic, and it has been suggested that these polymers may alter the diffusion of acids in plaques. In addition, lipoteichoic acids, which are strongly negatively charged, may become entrapped in glucans and thus impart ion-exchange properties to the plaque matrix. However, studies to date have found that glucans from *S. sanguis,* which may not contain large amounts of alpha 1 : 3 linkages, do not restrict diffusion of acids or sugars in in vitro models. Dr. *D. Geddes* commented out that while glucan does not appear to greatly affect diffusion in plaque, one should not confuse 'diffusion' with 'penetration', i.e., the time it takes for a molecule to penetrate through the plaque. The thickness of the plaque is significantly increased by glucan synthesis, and an increase in thickness of 12% would increase the penetration time of a molecule through the plaque by 25%.

In spite of the technical problems in studying the diffusion properties of plaques, the recent studies in this area seriously challenge the notion that plaque serves as an important diffusion-limiting barrier. Rather, the studies to date suggest that fluoride ions and acetic and lactic acids are able to diffuse through plaque within seconds to either saliva, or to the tooth surface.

This raises the question that if lactic acid can diffuse out of plaque so quickly, how does caries ever develop? Dr. *D. Hay* pointed out that the size of the 'sink' into which diffusion is occurring must be considered. In the case of plaque this 'sink' is a thin film of saliva over its surface. Dr. *C. Dawes* elaborated that if 0.7 ml of saliva is assumed to be present at any given time, and the oral cavity is estimated to have a surface area of 200 cm², then the thickness of the salivary film would be 0.1 mm or less. Acids in plaque probably quickly establish an equilibrium with the small quantity of saliva present, and the rate of removal of acid then becomes dependent on the rate by which saliva moves across the plaque. This can explain the apparent dilemma arising from the in vitro studies which suggest that acids can diffuse out of plaques quickly, and yet carious lesions develop underneath plaques due to their high acid concentrations. Dr. *W. Bowen* also commented that it is not necessary to postulate the need for a plaque diffusion barrier for the development of caries in fissures or at contact points where most lesions form. By virtue of their morphology, these sites may be 'diffusion-limiting systems'.

Aspects of Plaque Metabolism

Ingestion of a wide variety of foods results in low pH values in dental plaques in situ. This is thought to reflect the widespread occurrence of readily fermentable sugars in foods, and it indicates that bacteria need be exposed to relatively low concentrations of sugar to produce sufficient acid to lower the plaque pH. The metabolism of carbohydrate storage compounds is also thought to contribute to the acid content of plaque. Though rinsing plaques with water appears to rapidly remove acid, its concentration quickly builds up due to the metabolism of carbohydrate storage materials.

Most individuals agree that metabolic studies involving samples of pooled dental plaque removed from the mouth should be interpreted with caution. Plaques taken from the mouth lose their structural integrity and, therefore, their uniqueness. In addition, the metabolic potential of the bacteria may become altered. Dr. *J. Carlsson* pointed out that the pyruvate-formate-lyase pathway of streptococci, which is responsible for the production of formic and acetic acids from pyruvate under conditions of low sugar concentration, is very sensitive to oxygen. Streptococci exposed to air for as little as 2 min show little or no pyruvate-formate-lyase activity.

In the presence of high concentrations of sugar, streptococci form large quantities of lactate acid in addition to acetic and formic acids and ethanol. This is because lactic dehydrogenase becomes activated by the elevated levels of fructose diphosphate which accumulate in the cell, and pyruvic acid is converted to lactic acid. This is the so-called 'lactate gate', and it is thought to help drain the pool of metabolic intermediates. Dr. *Carlsson* has suggested that the lactate gate and the elaboration of glucosyltransferases represent important mechanisms which enable streptococci to cope with the feast or famine conditions of the mouth and avoid 'substrate accelerated death' or 'sugar killing' due to the accumulation of intracellular metabolites. However, mutants of *S. mutans* which are defective in the production of either glucosyltransferase or of lactic dehydrogenase are able to colonize conventional animals fed high sugar-containing diets. Thus, they appear to compete effectively with other bacteria, and in some cases, even with wild type *S. mutans* strains. Therefore, neither glucosyltransferase nor the lactate gate appear to be essential per se for protecting against sugar killing.

The metabolism of nitrogenous compounds is an important feature of plaque which has received relatively little attention. Oral bacteria probably have continuous access to high concentrations of proteinaceous material present in saliva and crevicular fluid. The content of free amino acids in saliva is low – generally too low to support growth of most bacteria, but the concentration of free amino acids in plaque fluid is approximately 30 mM and is 10–15 times higher than that in saliva. This is thought to reflect proteolytic activities of plaque bacteria acting upon salivary components.

The metabolism of amino acids usually results in the formation of fatty acids and ammonia. Thus, the pH of plaques does not drop during the course of amino acid metabolism and, in fact, may rise. However, amino acid metabolism by pure cultures is often repressed by the presence of glucose. Therefore, it may not be feasible to attempt to supplement carbohydrate-containing foods with fermentable amino acids to attempt to maintain the pH homeostasis of plaque.

R.J. Gibbons, MD, Forsyth Dental Center, Boston, MA 02115 (USA)

Cariology Today. Int. Congr., Zürich 1983, pp. 362–374 (Karger, Basel 1984)

Fluoride and Enamel

Summary of Session and Panel Discussion

O. Fejerskov

Department of Dental Pathology and Operative Dentistry, The Royal Dental College, Aarhus, Denmark

Summary of Chairman's Introduction

Fluoride is still the predominant component in the prevention and treatment of dental caries, but after more than 50 years of intensive research with innumerable publications we do not really know how fluoride excerts its cariostatic effect(s). Nevertheless the last decade has provided us with a spectrum of scientific data based on physicochemical experiments, laboratory studies, animal experiments, microbiological studies and experimental human studies, which has enabled us to reinterpret clinical observations. In 1983, therefore, we should be able to use fluoride in cariology based on solid scientific knowledge rather than on slogans such as: 'if little is good more is better.' However, extremely costly clinical trials are constantly being conducted and tremendous effort is invested in testing the effect of a variety of fluoride regimes in which the concentration of fluoride is empirically chosen, time sequence of application varies, various vehicles are used, and pH and other variables are furthermore played around with.

It is evident that most epidemiologists and manufacturers operate on the basis of the concept that fluoride prevents dental caries by being incorporated into the enamel apatite. This has been the predominant concept – in other words, fluoride prevents caries by increasing the resistance of the tooth. We are all familiar with postulates such as 'fluoride-deficient teeth', 'optimally mineralized teeth', etc. This has been a tempting and pleasantly simple explanation, and the well-known data showing a relationship between a slight increase in water fluoride concentrations and a decrease in caries prevalence originating from the time period where we had no topical fluorides like dentifrices are well established. However, these classical data only tell us that fluoride interferes with the carious processes, but not how. Nevertheless, it was obvious to link these caries data to the observation that the fluoride concentration in the surface enamel layers was increased in teeth developed in areas with slightly elevated fluoride in the water supplies. At the same time we knew from crystallographic studies on bone apatite that fluoride gives rise to more perfect crystals, and also that the substitution of the hydroxyl ion with fluoride reduces the dissolution rate of the apatite. It was therefore concluded that increased systemic intake of fluoride during tooth formation gives rise to an increased fluoride concentration in surface enamel, which explains an increased resistance of the enamel to caries attack. This concept was very easy for the dental profession to understand and for us as clinicians to pass on to the public. It would really be prevention of a disease.

When the systemic use of fluorides for various reasons could not be established in many parts of the world, the attempts at developing various topical fluoride products and regimes were therefore in principle all based on the above-mentioned concept of trying to incorporate fluoride into the enamel apatite to protect the tooth against acid attack. However, basic research during the last decade has raised serious doubt as to the validity of caries prevention being a simple function of enamel fluoride concentration. As an example I would like to draw your attention to a few considerations:

(1) Although there is an apparent relationship between enamel fluoride concentration and in vitro solubility reduction in laboratory experiments, there is no evidence that this has any clinical significance.

(2) The amount of fluoride incorporated into surface enamel in individuals born and reared in areas with 1.0–1.5 ppm of fluoride in their drinking water as compared to that of individuals from low-fluoride areas is of a magnitude which by no way can explain the difference in caries reduction as a simple result of decreased solubility.

(3) Using in vivo biopsy methods no relationship has been established between enamel fluoride content and caries prevalence and incidence of the individual. One problem here is of course that we can only measure fluoride in vivo on free smooth surfaces.

(4) There is no relationship between the capacity of topical treatments to incorporate fluoride into sound enamel and their caries-reducing effect.

We have therefore to discuss today what we really know about the interaction between fluoride and enamel. Before doing so, it is of importance to draw your attention to the fact that during this conference we have been discussing dental caries without specifying when we were talking about the disease as it may be recorded in epidemiological surveys, and when we were considering it at light or even electron microscopical levels. When we in the clinic and also in most histological studies are talking about incipient white spot lesions, we are in reality dealing with the results of innumerable intermittent pH drops, the result of which is a distinct loss of mineral with pronounced porosity of the enamel deep to a relatively unaffected surface layer as observed in the light microscope. At the ultrastructural level and from a molecular point of view dramatic changes with exchange of ions take place at the enamel surface and within the enamel long before we ever record this in the clinic.

Summary of Papers

John Weatherell: There seems to be no such a thing as absolute resistance to caries attack. The review was very difficult to write, because I did not believe very much of the data. I apologize for saying that to the many colleagues who have spent a lifetime in doing research in this field. Based on the literature and our own experiments we conclude that fluoride is acting in the liquid phase and not simply by stopping dissolution because it is incorporated into the enamel. We think that fluoride in the environment moves into the enamel and acts in a way on the initial translucent zone so that the surface zone in the caries lesions is a remineralized translucent zone from which carbonate and magnesium has been lost. In this context it is important to realize that the enamel surface is in contact with a solution which is supersaturated with whatever mineral is there. So what fluoride does – we think – is that it facilitates the process of remineralization at the liquid/enamel interface. Therefore the fluoride incorporated into the enamel may be of limited interest, although it may dissolve into solution and thereby act in the way just described as caries develops.

Jim ten Cate: Firstly, the effect of fluoride on demineralization as observed in our experiments indicates that fluoride acts by being present in the liquid phase during the process of demineralization. In a three-dimensional diagram we consider the calcium loss as a function of the acidity of the buffer and the fluoride content in the buffer. The concentrations and pH values we are dealing with in our in vitro model are within physiological levels in the oral cavity. The results of these experiments show that if fluoride is present even at low concentrations during acid attack, it significantly decreases the loss of calcium from the solid. We calculated the solubility product for the various fluoride salts which may form a various pH. The critical stage is whether fluorapatite may form or not under the varying conditions. However, it is remarkable that the condition where we have the liquid supersaturated or unsaturated with respect to fluorapatite does not make that much of a difference, whereas if we look at calcium fluoride, there seems to be a particular relationship between conditions under which the liquid is supersaturated with calcium fluoride and those where loss of calcium is prohibited. So, may be the presence of calcium fluoride is more important at the time of acid attack than is fluorapatite.

Secondly, fluoride affects the type of lesion formed. The principal difference between a lesion formed without the presence of fluoride and that formed when fluoride is present, so that the liquid is supersaturated with respect to fluorapatite, is that in the latter case the lesion develops as a subsurface type of lesion opposite to an erosion. With 0.5 ppm fluoride in the liquid the surface layer becomes more pronounced and a double layering pattern in mineral distribution within the lesion is in itself of interest. The lesion is less deep, i.e. there is a smaller loss of mineral. With 1 ppm of fluoride, this is even more pronounced and at 2 ppm under these conditions, lesion formation is totally prohibited.

Thirdly, we know that calcium and phosphate will deposit in a lesion if the artificial saliva is supersaturated with respect to calcium and phosphate salts. In principle, if fluoride is present at 1 ppm, the deposition of calcium is enhanced with a fluoride-to-calcium ratio which indicates that a highly fluoridated apatite is formed. The thermal dynamic driving force if fluoride is present is greater and therefore remineralization occurs. The degree of supersaturation determines whether the mineral is deposited throughout the lesion or mainly restricted to the surface. The mechanisms by which this happens are much more complex, but the principles of remineralization are as indicated here.

Joop Arends: Firstly, I will question whether we can distinguish between sound and initial carious enamel. At pH 7 fluoride in low concentration (< 10 ppm) diffuses into the spaces of the enamel at a speed of approximately 50 μm/day and absorbes or reacts with the apatite. The enamel is quite porous and the diffusion constantly continues. Secondly, pH is never stable and the minerals are constantly lost and redeposited. We do not know at present why fluoride does not go through the enamel more quickly nor why the gradients are built up so slowly. Thirdly, not all fluoride present within the enamel is reactive. The evidence we have at present shows that fluoride which diffuses in the liquid phase between the crystals or may even be adsorbed to the surface of the crystals is active in affecting demineralization. This is of great importance as the data indicate that if fluoride is present at concentrations of 1 ppm in the intercrystalline liquid phase, the protection is much higher than if it is present in more than 1,000 ppm in the solid phase. The significance of this is of tremendous importance as it shows, as the chairman already indicated, that more fluoride is not necessarily better. Once the fluoride is present in the liquid phase it prevents dissolution, however, as time goes on, it will deposit in the crystallites and will no longer be effective in reducing caries dissolution. So from a clinical point of view, this means that to maintain caries protection we will have continuously to have fluoride available, but at low level. Above approximately 50 ppm of fluoride calcium fluoride is deposited not as a mineral as such, but in tiny globules in the magnitude of 10–50 Å at the surface and possibly also within the porous enamel. The small size of a calcium fluoride globule is of importance as we all know that the smaller the size the higher is the reactivity and solubility of the salt. The calcium fluoride dissolves in the course of time, and diffuses both into the enamel and out into saliva.

Leon Silverstone: In our model system in vitro we have been able to reproduce all the zones which are known to be present in caries lesions in vivo. The lesion is in fact dynamic. Thus it is possible by changing the conditions to change the size and configuration of the lesion significantly. The crystal size in the body of the lesion is much smaller than in sound normal enamel whereas the crystals of a previous body of the lesion after remineralization exhibit crystal sizes 4–5 times larger than that of normal enamel. In our system we can increase remineralization by 100% by adding 1 ppm of fluoride to the calcifying fluid. Under these conditions the various precursor phases tend to precipitate at the surface thereby limiting the degree of remineralization. If the supersaturation in the liquid is diminished so that it is just supersaturated with respect to the apatite, but not the precursor phases, a reduction both in depth of the lesion and in porosity of approximately 70% is found. Increasing the fluoride to 10 or 100 ppm in this system did not increase the rate of remineralization. Even in vitro, the demineralization can reach the dentine without the lesion being able to being detected under classical clinical trials. Under in vitro conditions with a very sensitive radiographic technique, the histological examination shows that we may have rather extensive lesions in the enamel which we cannot detect radiographically. This means that patients who we clinically say are caries-free may have 10 or 15 lesions in the mouth. Therefore the term 'caries-free' is a bad term. We should rather say that the patient is free from clinical caries.

We can thus in our system take a lesion which is histologically large, but clinically small, and reduce that histologically to a much smaller lesion. But what is of significance is that we make the lesion more difficult to progress. In fact the rate of progression of the remineralized lesion is only one tenth of that of the unremineralized control. This surely must be of clinical significance.

John Featherstone: If we have not had plaque, you would not have the caries lesion. The mineral of the enamel comprises densely packed crystals each of which actually extends from the very enamel surface to the dentino-enamel junction. In between the crystals we have corresponding to the margins of the prisms larger diffusion pathways. In sound enamel, if that ever exists, we have 10% by volume of water. We have about 15% by volume of spaces through which acid can diffuse in and minerals out of the enamel, which is a porous and highly active substance. If lipid is covering the enamel crystallites, ions will have difficulties in passing though it. Continuous exposure of enamel to an acid acetate buffer, pH 5, gives rise to a distinct demineralization, but if fluoride is present in the liquid, almost no loss of mineral takes place. Carbonated hydroxyapatite is very different from pure hydroxyapatite. If you put fluoride into the carbonated hydroxyapatite, it has almost no effect on the dissolution of the crystals in the acetate buffer. This is a key point. However, if you add fluoride to the buffer and measure the dissolution rate, there is a dramatic effect. With 1 ppm of fluoride in the buffer the dissolution rate is cut by approximately 35%. To sum up, fluoride inhibits crystal dissolution if present in the liquid. Concerning remineralization fluoride enhances uptake of calcium and phosphate.

Jan Ekstrand: Most of the systemic fluoride regimes are based on empiricism. We do not know anything about the actual plasma concentration of fluoride which gives rise to a maximum uptake of fluoride into enamel or which gives a maximum protection against caries, or what causes enamel fluorosis. Several factors influence the concentration of fluoride in plasma, i.e. time of blood sampling, absorption, age, site of sampling, etc. When we are dealing with fluoride being used systemically, we are therefore dealing with a very complicated system. There is ample evidence that the active fluoride in the oral environment is that present in saliva, crevicular fluid and the plaque fluid. The concentrations in the first two are directly related to that of plasma and are important factors for the concentration in plaque fluid. Elevated salivary concentrations of fluoride give rise to a significant caries reduction and I think in man that we should tend to increase the salivary fluoride concentration. The concentration of fluoride in artificially fluoridated waters should be very carefully monitored. In contrast to *Dean's* populations, people today have access to a variety of fluoride sources such as dentifrices, rinsing programs, varnishes, gels, etc. There is no particular treshold apparently below which we can be sure that dental fluorosis does not occur. The concentrations in gels have been determined purely from empirical considerations and when applying prefabricated trays, it is apparent that the fluoride concentration in plasma following these regimes by far exceeds what should be considered as acceptable. As there is no evidence that fluoride gels should be superior to any other fluoride regime from a cariostatic point of view, it seems surprising that this system has developed. In conclusion, it is obvious that much more pharmacologic data are needed before we can determine the most proper use of fluoride systemically to achieve a maximum caries reduction.

Discussion

Fejerskov: Does enamel resistance as such exist? And if so, how should we define it? If it does exist can we then significantly interfere with it?

Weatherell: When talking about the initial caries attack, I am thinking of the event taking place at the very enamel surface with loss of magnesium and carbonate and in this context, I do not think that enamel resistance as such plays any significant role.

Arends: I do not think that there is any significant difference in enamel resistance between the surface and the inner part of the enamel except if we are talking about the outer 100 Å of enamel surface.

Silverstone: I think enamel resistance or caries resistance is a misleading term. 5–10 years ago we published some work where we showed that it was more difficult to produce a lesion on remineralized, sound enamel than on adjacent control-enamel. It is not a resistant tooth, but we slow down the rate of attack. In the laboratory we can reach a stage of remineralization where progression is slowed down to such an extent that we can no longer create a lesion under these conditions. A resistant tooth does not exist. The many hundred teeth I have examined all exhibited histologically caries lesions, but frequently without any macroscopical evidence of a white spot lesion.

Featherstone: We have recently taken teeth from high and low caries people and from high and low caries towns, and developed artificial caries lesions in them. We found absolutely no difference in their intrinsic reactions. So the basic intrinsic composition of the enamel did nothing to the resistance, at least in our artificial caries model. The differences in speed of lesion development were absolutely dramatic only when fluoride concentration in the liquid varies.

Silverstone and Featherstone: There is no relationship whatsoever between the fluoride content and the resistance to artificial caries lesions.

Rölla: Let us take a retention site covered with plaque and add sucrose to the individual 5 times a day and at the same time add fluoride to the cycling process. Would that not after 10 years give rise to a more resistant area as compared to that let us say 1 month after eruption? And how high would the content of fluoride in that area be?

ten Cate: If you take teeth with natural white spot lesions and expose them to artificial caries in the laboratory, apparently the already carious area becomes less attacked than the remaining tooth. Concerning incorporation of fluoride into the enamel we have carried out some experimental recycling studies in the laboratory which show that by adding even lower amounts of fluoride to the liquid during the experiment you can incorporate far more fluoride into the enamel than by applying frequent gel treatments to the teeth.

Weatherell: Areas covered by plaque exhibit enhanced fluoride uptake. However, any area of the tooth which may be porous will take up fluoride, so whether it is because of its porosity of the pH cycling, I do not know. The fluoride levels vary so much that I do not think it is possible to correlate the fluoride content to the actual resistance of any area to caries attack.

Arends: We think that the shape of the fluoride gradient in a given part of the enamel may determine the direction and rate of progression.

Silverstone: There is simply much fluoride in enamel where a given area is porous. If you in the laboratory make an artificial lesion and look at the fluoride profile in the enamel as compared to normal enamel, the surface fluoride corresponding to the caries lesion has almost disappeared into the body of the lesion, whereas if you take a natural caries lesion, you find a relatively well-mineralized surface zone with a high fluoride content. Misleadingly people have thought that this is the reason for the maintenance of the surface. But that is not so, it is just because the enamel is highly porous and the fluoride comes in. However, the fluoride in the lesion is of importance when demineralization occurs as it becomes released and thus interferes with demineralization.

Mobley: We have at Procter & Gamble recently carried out a clinical trial comparing two different fluoride regimes with a placebo group and collected the deciduous teeth in the various groups for fluoride analysis. In sound enamel we did not find any significant difference in fluoride content between the three study groups. Of more interest, however, was our findings of fluoride content in white spot lesions in the teeth collected. In the sodium fluoride group which showed a 41% caries reduction, there was a significantly higher fluoride content in white spot lesions as compared to the placebo group. However, this only shows that in this group the fluoride ion activity has been higher at the time of caries development. Of even greater importance was the observation of a correlation coefficient of 0.21 between the fluoride content of white spot lesions and the caries increment of the individual. This shows that there is a higher fluoride activity in those individuals showing the greatest caries reduction, but it also seems to show that the site where the fluoride has its primary activity is in the form of slowing down caries progression or enhancing remineralization.

ten Cate: This is a nice approach. Too many people have tried to correlate caries incidence with fluoride content of drinking water, tablets and fluoride in the enamel. We should rather compare caries experience and exposure to fluoride, which is a totally different thing. Frequency of fluoride intake or fluoride in white spot lesions is more relevant.

König: Have we paid too little attention to the organic part of the enamel when discussing its susceptibility to caries attack?

Featherstone: The pellicle is a very strong inhibitor of surface enamel dissolution. The crystals are surrounded by proteins and lipid, so whatever acid or molecule or ion has to pass through it to get to the crystal surface. My uneducated guess would be that both lipid and protein with its phosphate groups stick to the crystals, and the acids one way or another have to compete with it. Lipid constitutes 1% by weight. There is a twofold increase in lesion progress rate if most of the lipid is extracted before exposing teeth to artificial caries lesion development.

Weatherell: We believe that the more protein the less caries-susceptible is the enamel. On the other hand, others have not been able to demonstrate any correlation between protein content and caries susceptibility.

Fejerskov: In highly porous fluorotic enamel the depth of artificial caries lesions is much less than in well-mineralized enamel.

Silverstone: Saliva is a highly powerful remineralizing solution, but saliva and the protein components of saliva restrict penetration of the mineral into the lesion.

Geddes: Caries occurs under plaque, I do not think the panelists can brush the clinical situation away. Does plaque act as a barrier to fluoride or is it a slow release system?

Weatherell: We really do not know where the fluoride in plaque comes from. Part of the fluoride may come from the enamel. I personally feel very hesitating when considering plaque as a slow fluoride release system.

Birkeland: We have ample evidence that fluoride should be constantly present in the oral fluid to exhibit its cariostatic effect. If a fluoride regime is stopped, 3 or 4 years later the caries increment in the previous experimental group versus the previous control appears very similar. What is the panel's comments on this?

Silverstone: Paradoxically we have to have an initial caries lesion to get remineralization, i.e. to get the crystals to grow, we have to have pores in the enamel to get areas with greater crystal size.

Arends: I think there is a discrepancy. In in vivo remineralization we seldom observe crystal growth. There may be a slight increase in crystal size about 10%, but the increase in mineral is a result of a reprecipitation of minerals in the lesion. The amount of fluoride within the lesion is not really of great importance. It is a question of availability of the fluoride. The fluoride content within the crystals can be very high and still caries progression very rapid. Unless fluoride is available at the interface between crystals and the liquid phase, it may have limited effect.

Marthaler: I very much sympathize with all what has been said. In particular, statistical analysis of clinical data indicates that erupting teeth exhibit a greater caries reduction in clinical trials than teeth already erupted at the start of the experiment. As an epidemiologist and biostatistician, I must say that we should handle these data with some precaution. Teeth erupting during study have a shorter exposure time to fluoride. Therefore, if as we now think fluoride interferes with the progression of lesions, in the fluoride group these teeth may not be present in the oral environment for a sufficient time to develop a lesion. In the fluoride group there may not be sufficient time to develop lesions whereas in the control group some lesions will develop. This can be very well demonstrated from early studies with water fluoridation. Some studies have shown a caries reduction of 80–90% in 6-year-old children after the introduction of fluoride. This is certainly an artifact. This figure is obtained on the basis of fissure caries in first molars.

Fejerskov: We have to distinguish between the effect of topical fluoride on clinically sound enamel and on enamel which already is undergoing significant caries dissolution. One painting with 2% NaF in vivo on clinically sound buccal surfaces gives rise to calcium fluoride formation to an extent whereby the fluoride ion level in saliva in that mouth is maintained high up to 8–12 h after. We have previously shown that this is of a magnitude high enough to enhance remineralization significantly in vivo. This indicates that the calcium fluoride reservoir even on relatively sound surfaces may have clinical significance by maintaining a slight increase in salivary fluoride. But what level is desirable? This is the next point I would like to have the panelists' comments on.

Arends: This question is highly important. There is apparently a difference between the level necessary to prevent demineralization and that being important for remineralization. The data we have available from in vivo studies at present indicate that remineralization is optimized by fluoride levels in the order of a half to a tenth of 1 ppm locally in the oral cavity. Note that we never know what the concentration is inside the actual lesion. The maximum concentration to protect against caries dissolution may be one or two orders of magnitude higher, so there is a discrepancy there which may keep us busy for another decade.

ten Cate: Based on our recycling experiments, it appears that concentrations about 0.1–0.4 ppm are important to achieve remineralization. From a clinical point of view we shall realize, however, that when we are talking about de- and remineralization, we are not just talking about making big lesions and repairing them. De- and remineralization is going on constantly at the very surface. So what is important is to have fluoride available at the site where you have the greatest pH drop, because here you get the greatest porosities and therefore the greatest chance for having calcium fluoride deposited and the results of the largest crystal growth. In these cases the concentration is probably not that important because the porosity is so great that it would pick up fluoride anyhow.

Ekstrand: What should be the therapeutic level in the oral cavity? Here comes the question of the role of the plaque, and whether we should use a slow release device. Recently we have shown by using fluoridated chewing gum and measuring pH in the plaque that a level of 0.06–0.08 ppm is sufficient to have a significant effect. This concentration apparently has nothing to do directly with the effect on remineralization, so we have to have much more in vivo studies to know more about various mechanisms.

Weatherell: We have recently made some oral clearance studies which show great variation depending on where saliva is sampled in relation to where fluoride is applied. After a fluoride rinse with a 1,000-ppm solution you would have in the upper buccal sulcus a significant increase even 20 min after application whereas sublingually it has disappeared. I think research is urgently needed concerning what I would call rheology of the mouth.

Bowen: I share the concern concerning the repeated use of clinical trials on gels, rinsing programs and other sorts of ad hoc topical programs. Could we have some comments on ions which might have an adverse effect on remineralization as compared to the beneficial effect of fluoride.

ten Cate: What we should look at is really plaque fluid which is completely different in ion strength and calcium and phosphate content from saliva. And in this context the pH is very important.

Featherstone: Ionic activity is what it is all about. The diffusion from saliva into plaque will be totally dependent on the volume of each and the concentration within each component. The diffusion into plaque from saliva is much quicker than into enamel.

Arends: An increase in factor 2–3 above normal level is a significant one. The flow within the mouth is also very important, and we have evidence that the diffusion of fluoride even within millimeters within the mouth is almost not existing.

ten Cate: Concerning adverse effects on remineralization, there is not much to say except that an increase in other ions would diminish the possibility for remineralization. Carbonate would influence crystal size and crystal diameters, but I think the main effect would be from inhibitors present in saliva.

Silverstone: When the tooth erupts into the mouth, it is very important to have fluoride available. We earlier used the word posteruptive maturation which really is early remineralization of initial porous areas. Concerning inhibitory effect, I can only speak about in vitro systems and carbonate and copper certainly inhibit remineralization.

Midda: Many clinicians think that the dentifrices explain the major reduction in caries around the world. A lot of it is being swallowed and therefore not incorporated into the enamel, but at the same time the salivary concentration will be elevated. Will the panel like to comment on whether swallowed dentifrices could account for a pool of fluoride explaining the decrease in caries? I consider it as a slow release device when being swallowed and therefore it may act this way.

Ekstrand: The elevation in saliva as a result of elevated plasma levels is almost insignificant as compared to the 100- to 1,000-fold increase in saliva immediately following a topical treatment.

Eggen: Based on the studies we have done and others, I think we should keep in mind that pellicle formed when fluoride is present may have a different composition from that of pellicle without fluoride present.

Fejerskov: Let me take that question one step further. If the pellicle is changed in composition, will that affect initial microbial colonization? Either the composition of the microbiota or the speed by which colonization takes place?

Kilian: Based on our studies in vivo we did not find any effect of fluoride on bacterial colonization irrespective of whether it was present in high amounts of fluor hydroxyapatite or calcium fluoride or in the form of free fluoride ion based on frequent rinsing during the experimental period.

Gibbons: Some years ago we made experimental studies on compressed discs of fluorapatite versus hydroxyapatite and studied the colonization on these. We studied the ratio absorption of *Streptococcus sanguis* and *Streptococcus salivarius* to them and we could detect no difference.

Rölla: In relation to your very strong arguments this morning, it is apparently a waste of time to try to apply fluoride preeruptively. Before we leave this room, could you please try to develop a clear answer to whether this is true or not.

Ekstrand: The concentration of fluoride in tablets was adjusted to mimic the amount ingested if children live in 1-ppm areas. However, if you look at the plasma curves of fluoride of individuals living in a fluoridated area, it is constantly slightly elevated above normal whereas if you compare it with plasma curves following ingestion of a fluoride tablet, there is a rapid increase and then a relatively rapid elimination. Pharmacologically there is no comparison between the systemic effect of fluoride in the water supply and that of a tablet.

Silverstone: The scientific evidence for need of prenatal fluoride supplementation is totally lacking. Concerning preeruptive effect, it is purely hypothetical and at this present time, I really do not know whether I will recommend systemic use of fluoride. As we have stressed today, the important thing is to have topical fluorides available at the time of eruption of the teeth. The actual concentration we should aim at, we do not know at present.

Featherstone: I would like to refer to two pieces of work. The first is that of *Ken and Stephen*, who for many years have been working with the effect of fluoride tablets. To the best of my knowledge they concluded that the cariostatic effect was almost exclusively a result of the topical effect of the fluoride. Secondly, 2 years ago, *Fejerskov* et al. provided a very good summary of the art concerning the current status of use of fluoride and they concluded and convinced a lot of people that the major cariostatic effect of fluoride is a result of the topical effect. I certainly believe that the systemic effect is very, very minimal.

Fejerskov: Let me emphasize that we are not opposing water fluoridation. Water fluoridation is an excellent way of obtaining caries reduction. The explanation for the caries reduction appears to be, however, that we elevate the fluoride ion activity in the oral environment sufficiently to interfere with ongoing de- and remineralization processes.

Arends: I will be very brief. I think the major effect is a topical effect. I think the preeruptive, systemic effect is minimal.

ten Cate: I have little to add. The difficulty in comparing data 20–50 years ago with those of today is that we now have so much fluoride available from a variety of extra sources that it may totally mask the situation today. It will still be of interest to know whether fluoride given systemically and incorporated into the enamel may have a beneficial effect on people later exhibiting rampant caries, but the major cariostatic effect of fluoride is certainly that of a topical one.

Weatherell: Fluoride appears to interfere with what we call stage 3 in enamel development corresponding to a certain stage of enamel maturation. If we intend to get fluoride adsorbed to the enamel at that stage and thereby enrich the enamel with fluoride, we have to accept that we at the same time interfere with enamel formation and develop dental fluorosis. So if we have to use fluoride preeruptively, it has to be used just prior to eruption. But the effect achieved can just as well be obtained by giving fluoride at the time of eruption. So my weight is also on the use of fluorides immediately preeruptively and mainly posteruptively.

Fejerskov: It would have been beneficial right now to have another 3 h discussion on the actual clinical implications of what we think and believe today. In my introduction I purposely used the word prevention, but based on the discussion we have had today realizing that caries is a dynamic process, it may be more reasonable to consider fluoride as a therapeutic agent with which we treat ongoing caries processes subclinically and clinically.

Silverstone: The audience today possibly comprises the most outstanding researchers in the field of cariology in the western world today. I do not think we should leave this meeting without stressing to our colleagues in fields like operative dentistry that you do not grasp a bur and drill a hole today as soon as you see a caries lesion. Therefore I think it is of paramount importance to get the message through to our students of today that any procedure should be based on thorough scientific background.

O. Fejerskov, MD, Department of Dental Pathology and Operative Dentistry, The Royal Dental College, Vennelyst Boulevard, DK-8000 Aarhus C (Denmark)

Cariology Today. Int. Congr., Zürich 1983, pp. 375–379 (Karger, Basel 1984)

Prevention and Therapy – Where from Here?
Summary of Session and Discussion

Harald Löe

National Institute of Dental Research, National Institutes of Health, Bethesda, Md., USA

This last session dealt with caries prevention and caries therapy. An update on both these topics seemed timely in view of the reports from several countries that caries in children and youth is on the decline. This historical decrease in caries prevalence represents a landmark accomplishment and is apt to impact dramatically on the dental health of populations. Also, it is anticipated that this change in morbidity and mortality of teeth must influence profoundly dental education and dental practice.

The observation was made, however, that although some countries are experiencing a reduction in caries in the young, there are no data to show that this reduction will be sustained during adult life. Secondary caries in the adult continues to be a problem and the prevalence of root surface caries among elderly patients is probably high and little understood. Thus, there are still problems to be researched and there is still knowledge to be transferred to clinical use.

One important area where both research and technology transfer are needed is the behavior science as this relates to the prevention of oral and dental diseases.

Dr. *Klaus König* spoke of behavioral modifications in the context of acceptance and nonacceptance of individual preventive measures and emphasized that on an individual basis prevention must be accepted, adopted, and performed by the patient every day throughout life. People are changing their behavior toward their general health. The motivation would be much greater if one could combine the oral and general health message.

The suggestion was made that it would be desirable to devote the main efforts to target risk groups and to provide adequate financial incentives. It was felt that organizationally school-based programs would continue to be an important component of the system of dental disease prevention, especially in identifying high risk patients. It was suggested that it would be more productive to have the dentist leave his/her office and work with the children in the classroom in order to instill an appropriate level of appreciation for the concept and prac-ticalities of caries prevention.

In terms of caries prevention, the following strategies were suggest-ed: target group I: whole populations, through which one would gain more good for more people; target group II: high risk individuals, where one identified individuals and intervened; target group III: secon-dary prevention.

How Does One Identify Risk Groups or Individuals at High Risk?

There are certain stages in the natural history of any disease which may serve to identify susceptible persons. It is well known that caries is most active during childhood and adolescence, after which the disease rate is reduced, and there is smaller risk. Also, at the individual level there are a number of ways by which persons at high risk can be identified: (1) *Clinical examination* would indicate to some extent the historical and current levels of caries activity. (2) *Bacterial tests* are now available.

There is evidence from clinical studies that combined clinical and bacterial data provide the best basis for making predictions about future caries experience. A simplified test for *Streptococcus mutans* counts is being developed (*Bratthall*). It was mentioned that one tech-nician could process bacterial tests for 300 patients in 2 days at very low cost. It was agreed that persons with 1 million *S. mutans*/ml saliva are at high risk.

Is Vaccination against Caries a Dead Issue?

Scientific studies in animals have shown that immunization may result in production of antibodies and increased protection against streptococcal infection and caries. So, why don't we have a vaccine already?

Dr. *Bo Krasse* listed the following three problems relative to vaccine developing:

(1) *S. mutans* is an important but not the only source of antigen. Consequently, a *S. mutans* vaccine would provide only partial protection.

(2) *S. mutans* is acquired during childhood and remains as an indigenous microorganism for life. The implication is that the immune system must be constantly responsive, and it is possible that this leads to the development of a tolerance or immune exclusion.

(3) Colonization of tooth surfaces does not bring the microorganisms into contact with the immune system and, therefore, there is no stimulation of the immunoglobulins at an early stage of the disease.

Despite these limitations, the fact remains that immunization against caries is feasible. The following reasons were articulated for continued support of anticaries vaccine development:

(1) Risk groups with high *S. mutans* counts would benefit from such a preventive measure.

(2) Caries in Third World countries is on the increase. Since dentist/population ratios are unfavorable and other preventive technologies essentially unavailable, vaccination against caries could be added conveniently to already existing immunization programs.

(3) The search for an anticaries vaccine will continue to increase our basic understanding of oral immunology and in particular the secretory immune system.

Dr. *Krasse* concluded that vaccination against dental caries is not a dead issue.

The discussion generally supported this conclusion. The point was made that a similar debate occurred relative to justification of the development of vaccines against pneumonia. Even with the existence of effective antibiotic therapies against pneumonia, it was felt that vaccines were needed, especially for high risk patients.

Can Antimicrobials Be Effective in the Prevention and Treatment of Caries?

Dr. *Walter Loesche*, in his remarks, stressed the necessity of establishing a firm diagnosis of a cariogenic infection before attacking the plaque with antimicrobials and the need to monitor the efficacy of the treatment based on the absence, presence, and quantity of the specific bacterial species. Fluorides and chlorhexidine were mentioned as suitable antimicrobials. Treatment might extend for 1 week. Retreatment is often necessary, and emphasis should be placed on combining antimicrobial therapy with dietary and mechanical treatment modalities. Prophylactically, antimicrobials may be used to intervene in the transmission of cariogenic microorganisms from parents to infants and/or from primary teeth to the permanent dentition.

The question was raised as to the evidence for the efficacy of antimicrobial agents in the prevention of caries in humans, as most population studies also have involved instruction in oral hygiene and restriction in carbohydrate consumption. It was mentioned that in one study the protocol called for an initial reduction in *S. mutans* counts through sucrose restriction. Two-thirds of the participants complied, one-third did not. The latter group were then treated with fluoride gel. If the bacterial counts were still high, the individuals were treated successfully with chlorhexidine.

What about Sealants?

In his presentation, Dr. *Kenneth Stephen* made mention of the fact that the early studies on sealants drew criticism because the sealants were placed in children who might not have needed them. Today, there is consensus that primary and permanent molars can be successfully sealed and that the sealant should be applied at the time of eruption of these teeth. The materials and technologies used in sealing pits and fissures have improved greatly over the years. It was concluded that, from a clinical point of view, there is no doubt that successful sealing of fissures inhibits occlusal caries and that unsealed molars were more than 20 times at risk of developing caries.

The discussion brought out the question as to whether or not every child would be a candidate for sealant procedures and, if not, how should one decide who should receive such treatment. It was concluded that there was little hope of avoiding massive application of sealants without establishing a firm clinical and bacterial diagnosis.

New Concepts in Treating Caries

Dr. *Felix Lutz* suggested that the concept that all dental care is preventive dentistry is unacceptable. Only primary prevention is prevention in the true sense of the term. In the past, dental curricula, lack of auxiliary personnel, and the fee system have continued to promote repair of damage and have retarded the introduction of primary prevention as a significant component of private practice. Good oral hygiene and dietary counseling are basic prerequisites for good operative dentistry. If prevention fails and 'white spot' caries lesions develop, attempts should be made to promote remineralization. The treatment of choice for small cavities in posterior occlusal surfaces is the placement of resin fillings, preserving a maximum of tooth substance. Composites are still not available as a substitute for amalgam in case of larger cavities. However, in the preparation of the cavities, every effort should be made to conserve dental tissues. For anterior teeth the adhesive restoration is superior, since it requires minimal removal of tissue.

The discussion mentioned that for approximately 100 years *G. V. Black's* principles for cavity preparation have been standard approach to operative dentistry. The time has come to revise these principles and to agree on new concepts for cavity preparation.

Dr. *Anders Thylstrup* mentioned that early diagnosis used to be important, since, if not treated, the lesion would progress rather rapidly to a large lesion. Today, the rationale has changed. Thanks to multiple exposures to fluoride and to plaque control, the progression of caries from subclinical levels is slow and in most instances the lesion can be remineralized. Nevertheless, a survey of how the dentists deal with incipient caries lesions showed that less than 20% of fillings were made in teeth exhibiting true cavitation and that approximately 80% of the fillings were placed in white spots or incipient lesions, essentially confirming that early diagnosis followed by prompt placement of a filling is the prevailing approach. It was Dr. *Thylstrup's* opinion that there is an enormous gap between the current scientific knowledge and the actual application in clinical practice in this area and that an improvement in the communication between researchers and practitioners would be in order.

H. Löe, MD, National Institute of Dental Research, Bethesda, MD 20205 (USA)

Author Index

Subject Index